Vascular Anaesthesia: a practical handbook

Vascular Anaesthesia: a practical handbook

Lawrence Caldicott MB BS FRCA

Andrew Lumb MB BS FRCA

Deirdre McCoy FFARCSI

*St James's University Hospital, Leeds Teaching Hospitals NHS Trust
Beckett Street, Leeds, UK*

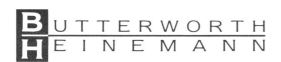

BUTTERWORTH
HEINEMANN

OXFORD   AUCKLAND   BOSTON   JOHANNESBURG   MELBOURNE   NEW DELHI

Butterworth-Heinemann
Linacre House, Jordan Hill, Oxford OX2 8DP
225 Wildwood Avenue, Woburn, MA 01801-2041
A division of Reed Educational and Professional Publishing Ltd

 A member of the Reed Elsevier plc group

First published 1999

British Library Cataloguing in Publication Data
A catalogue record for this book is available from the British Library

Library of Congress Cataloguing in Publication Data
A catalogue record for this book is available from the Library of Congress

ISBN 0 7506 3468 5

Composition by Genesis Typesetting, Rochester, Kent
Printed and bound in Great Britain by MPG Books Ltd, Bodmin, Cornwall

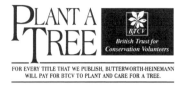

Contents

Foreword

This handbook was written with the objective of improving anaesthetic care provided for patients undergoing major vascular surgery. This patient population tends to be elderly, with a high incidence of co-existing cardiac, respiratory, renal and endocrine disorders. Patients with cardiac disease undergoing vascular surgical procedures have benefited from many innovations developed from cardiac surgery including invasive haemodynamic monitoring, transoesophageal echocardiography and continuous ambulatory ECG detection of myocardial ischaemia. Cardiac and thoracic anaesthesia are well recognized subspecialties. Vascular anaesthesia, in contrast, has been slow to develop its own identity, but clearly its time has arrived.

The content of this book ranges from the pre-operative management of vascular surgical patients and patients with cardiac disease undergoing major vascular surgery; choice of anaesthetic technique; patient monitoring and cardiovascular support; the specifics of the various surgical procedures and the post-operative care in intensive care/high dependency units.

Despite the fact that practically all anaesthetists provide anaesthesia for vascular surgery, there has been, until recent times, a distinct lack of informaton published about this particular topic. Perioperative mortality is a direct result of the intraoperative and postoperative care rendered by the anaesthetist. This practical handbook was written by three clinicians working in the field of vascular anaesthesia and reflects the scientific foundation of this specialty and, while providing a rational basis for clinical practice, avoids advocating one institution's unique preferences. The handbook complements established texts such as Joel Kaplan's *Vascular Anesthesia* and Michael F. Roizen's *Anaesthesia for Vascular Surgery*. Institutions have put in place fellowship programmes and specialty module rotations in vascular anaesthesia. The advent of the Vascular Anaesthesia Society of Great Britain and Ireland and the Journal of Cardiothoracic and Vascular Anesthesia are all manifestations of an increasing interest in and awareness of the complexities of management of patients undergoing major vascular surgery.

I wish Drs Caldicott, Lumb and McCoy success with their venture and I am sure that individual anaesthetists and departments will find the handbook a useful resource.

Anthony J. Cunningham MD, FRCPC
Dublin

Preface

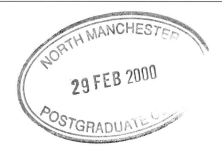

The prevalence of vascular disease in the population is high, and likely to increase alongside life expectancy. With almost a third of adults in the UK continuing to smoke for much of their life, vascular disease looks set to remain a major health problem well into the next millenium.

Recent advances in the management of vascular patients have led to the establishment of specialist centres, with the arrival of surgeons who are involved only in vascular surgery. However, the high prevalence of vascular disease, and the often acute onset of symptoms, means that almost all hospitals will need to continue providing surgery for these patients. Advances in surgical treatment of vascular disease have been greatly assisted by developments in anaesthesia, including the use of epidural anaesthesia and improved perioperative care to facilitate prolonged and complex surgery. Interest in anaesthesia for vascular surgery as a sub-specialty has followed the surgical trend for specialization, as evidenced by the existence of a Society for Cardiovascular Anesthesia in the USA and the recent establishment of the Vascular Anaesthesia Society of Great Britain and Ireland.

That vascular anaesthesia presents a challenge is undisputed. A vascular patient who *does not* smoke or have ischaemic heart disease is unusual, and will normally be treated with great suspicion by the vascular anaesthetist. Perioperative mortality and serious morbidity for elective major arterial surgery is around 5%, a figure which exceeds most other surgical specialties, including cardiac surgery. In addition, as already stated, many procedures are performed in non-specialist hospitals often by non-specialist, or even trainee, anaesthetists.

We feel there is a need for an up-to-date and concise book outlining some of the recent developments in vascular anaesthesia. We hope that this book will provide all anaesthetists with some assistance when asked to provide anaesthesia for vascular surgery. For the trainee and non-specialist, chapters on specific vascular procedures will give an outline of the surgical requirements and contemporary anaesthetic techniques, whilst for the specialist, recent advances in vascular surgery are detailed and references provided.

Andrew Lumb
Lawrence Caldicott
Deirdre McCoy

1

Cardiovascular physiology and pathophysiology

Cardiac output

Myocardial contraction

Anatomy

Myocardial cells are branched and nucleated, containing numerous mito-chondria and a sarcoplasmic reticulum in intimate association with the contractile units, the sarcomeres (Figure 1.1).

Sarcomeres are banded structures containing the proteins actin and myosin. These are closely arranged and, during contraction, 'slide' over each other to shorten the cell and produce myocardial contraction (Figure 1.2).

Physiology

Myosin is a long, 'thick' protein, with multiple lateral protrusions arranged in a helical pattern along its length. Actin is a 'thin' protein, which has active sites along its length that are inhibited from interacting with the heads of the

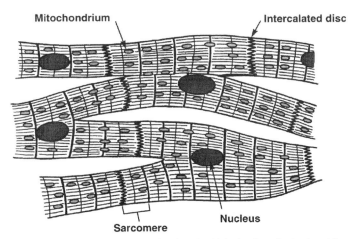

Figure 1.1 A group of myocardial cells showing the high density of mitochondria and the contractile units, the sarcomeres.

Relaxed

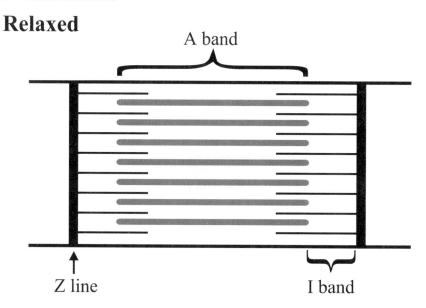

Contracted

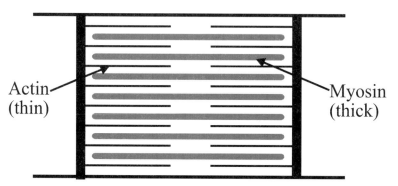

Figure 1.2 Diagram of a relaxed and contracted sarcomere showing how the contraction is due to the 'sliding' of actin and myosin proteins over each other, resulting in the shortening of the sarcomere.

myosin protrusions by the tropomyosin/troponin complex. During depolarization of the myocardial cell, an initial fast influx of sodium ions is followed by an influx of calcium ions during the plateau phase of the action potential. This triggers the release of more calcium ions from the sarcoplasmic reticulum, and the concentration of calcium inside the cell rises to 100 times its previous value. Calcium interacts with the tropomyosin/troponin complex, allowing exposure of the previously hidden active sites on the actin molecule. The heads of the protrusions on the myosin molecule now interact with the active sites on the actin and bend to move the myosin relative to the actin, resulting in shortening of the sarcomere and myocardial contraction as shown in Figure 1.3. Myocardial cells exhibit a 'stretch-dependent calcium sensitivity', meaning that they become more sensitive to calcium ions at increasing initial fibre lengths, resulting in increased subsequent contraction. The exact mechanism has not been elucidated, but could be due to the exposure of more active sites on the actin molecule with increased fibre length. This is of crucial importance in the intact heart, and is the basis of Starling's law of the heart.

Relaxation of the myocardium requires energy (up to 15% of the total energy expended during one cardiac cycle), to force the calcium ions back into the sarcoplasmic reticulum, allowing the tropomyosin/troponin complex to cover up the active sites on the actin and permitting relaxation.

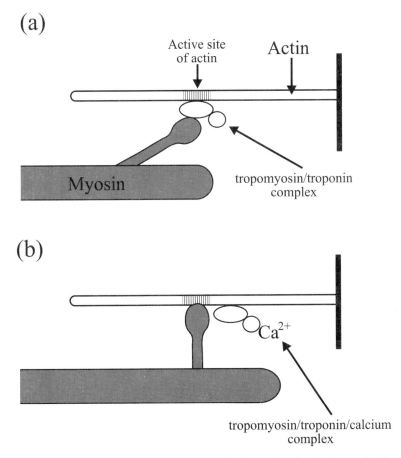

Figure 1.3 A diagram showing actin and myosin proteins (a) in the relaxed phase, and (b) in the contracted phase. Note how the presence of calcium allows the tropomyosin/troponin complex to move and expose the active site on the actin molecule. This allows the side arm of the myosin molecule to interact with the active site on the actin, and produces shortening of the sarcomere.

Stroke volume

Stroke work

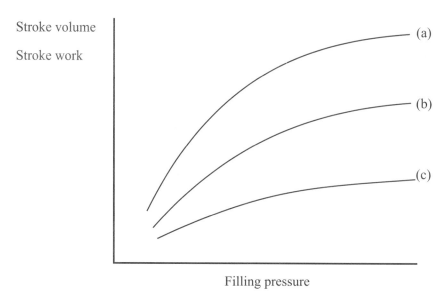

Filling pressure

Figure 1.4 Ventricular performance curves showing changes in ventricular work/stroke volume for curves representing fibres at differing states of contractility: (a) normal myocardial fibre; (b) fibre at a reduced level of contractility; (c) fibre at a grossly reduced level of contractility consistent with the curve produced by a failing heart.

Starling's Law. In 1894 and 1918, Frank, and later Starling, conducted experiments on isolated fibres of rabbits' hearts to elucidate the performance of the myocardium. Their results are summarized in Starling's law;

> The subsequent force of contraction of a myocardial muscle cell is dependent on the initial stretch of that fibre.

Ventricular performance curves can be constructed to show these results. If filling pressure or end diastolic volume (which are indirect measures of myocardial stretching) are plotted against cardiac output, stroke volume or ventricular work, a ventricular performance curve can be constructed as shown in Figure 1.4.

Cardiac output

Cardiac output is defined as the amount of blood the heart pumps in 1 minute, and is therefore the product of the stroke volume and the heart rate. The normal value in adults varies from about 4 to 6 l/min when the body is at rest. To allow for different body shapes and sizes, it is usually standardized to body surface area in the cardiac index. This is defined as cardiac output per square meter of body surface area. Surface area can be obtained from nomograms or, usually, is calculated in the monitoring equipment being used to measure cardiac output. A value of about 1.8 m^2 is average, giving a normal cardiac index of 3.0 l/m^2.

Cardiac output is constantly changing with the body's state of arousal and activity, and is limited by the disease processes of the heart–as is often the case in the vascular patient.

Stroke volume

Stroke volume is determined by three main factors. The preload on the heart and the contractility of the myocardium will determine the energy of contraction of the myocardial cells. This is opposed by the afterload on the heart, which is the energy required to raise the pressure inside the ventricle above that of the aorta and eject blood from the heart.

Preload determines the initial stretch of the myocardial cell prior to contraction. The greater this initial stretch, the greater the subsequent force of contraction of that myocardial cell–Starling's law of the heart. The exact mechanism of this change is still not fully understood, but is probably due to increased sensitivity to calcium ions as the myocardial cell is stretched[1]. In clinical practice it is not possible to measure 'stretch' of the left ventricular myocardium end diastole, but what can be measured are the central venous pressure (CVP) and the pulmonary capillary wedge pressure (PCWP). The relationship between these pressure measurements and ventricular stretch is outlined in Figure 1.5. Clinically, the preload can be assumed roughly to be proportional to the CVP for the right ventricle and the PCWP for the left ventricle. In most clinical situations, trends in CVP and PAWP can be used as a guide to changes in the filling pressures of the relevant ventricle.

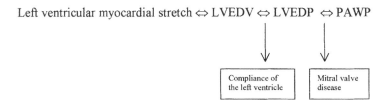

Left ventricular myocardial stretch ⇔ LVEDV ⇔ LVEDP ⇔ PAWP

| Compliance of the left ventricle | Mitral valve disease |

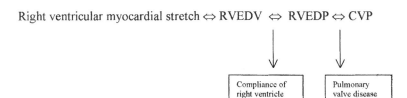

Right ventricular myocardial stretch ⇔ RVEDV ⇔ RVEDP ⇔ CVP

| Compliance of right ventricle | Pulmonary valve disease |

Figure 1.5 The relationship between myocardial stretch, central venous pressure (CVP) and pulmonary artery wedge pressure (PAWP). These pressures are only an estimate of ventricular stretch, and the accuracy depends on the compliance of the appropriate ventricle and any associated atrioventricular valvular disease. LVEDV, left ventricular end-diastolic volume; LVEDP, left ventricular end-diastolic pressure, RVEDV, right ventricular end-diastolic volume; RVEDP, right ventricular end-diastolic pressure.

Contractility. The state of contractility (or inotropic state) of the myocardial cell determines the energy of contraction of that cell at a given amount of stretch. Fibres at a higher state of contractility will contract more from the same 'starting point' than fibres at a lower state of contractility. Contractility is raised with positive inotropic agents, either endogenously from the adrenal medulla and sympathetic nerves or exogenously. Depression of contractility occurs with negative inotropes, which may include drugs such as beta blockers or calcium channel blockers, or can occur with developing hypoxia and acidosis.

Afterload. In 1806, Laplace described the relationship in a spherical body between the wall tension, the wall thickness, the radius of curvature and the resultant pressure inside the sphere. Although not a sphere, this relationship can be applied to the human ventricle.

$$\text{Laplace's Law: } P = \frac{2Tw}{r}$$

where P is the pressure inside a sphere; T is wall tension; w is wall thickness; and r is the radius.

T can be thought of as the afterload. This is the tension that must be created by the myocardial cells to generate the intraventricular pressure, P, which must be slightly greater than arterial pressure to allow blood to be ejected from the heart. Rearranging the equation, we get:

$$T(\text{afterload}) = \frac{Pr}{2w}$$

The afterload can be seen to depend directly on arterial pressure and radius of curvature of the ventricle. If the radius were to double, the wall tension (T) would also have to double to produce the same intraventricular pressure (P). This is why dilated hearts are at a huge mechanical disadvantage. Increases in wall thickness of the ventricle will help to reduce afterload.

Heart rate

Increases in heart rate result in reduced systolic and diastolic times. At heart rates of about 180 beats per minute in the healthy heart, the reduction in diastolic time is such that adequate filling of the ventricle can no longer occur and cardiac output will fall. Similarly, at very low rates cardiac output will fall, as stroke volume can only increase so much. The exact contribution of stroke volume and heart rate to cardiac output varies with the clinical situation. In exercise, both heart rate and stroke volume increase to produce large increase in cardiac output. In patients with coronary artery disease, this increase in heart rate is much reduced and results in lower cardiac outputs being achieved despite a similar increase in stroke volume when compared to normal hearts. In hypovolaemia, the tachycardia is a compensatory mechanism to try to support cardiac output in the face of a falling preload and reduced stroke volume. The overall cardiac output will remain the same or fall.

The cardiac cycle

Rhythmic contraction and relaxation of the heart can be broken down into four distinct phases to aid understanding, and these are shown in Figure 1.6.

1 *Ventricular filling* (diastole): Initially there is rapid filling, because the elastic elements of the heart are recoiling after contraction and blood is almost sucked in. In the last third of diastole, the atria contract and force another 20% of blood into the ventricle. This contribution is lost in atrial fibrillation. The normal end diastolic volume of the left ventricle is approximately 120 ml.
2 *Isovolaemic contraction*: During this phase the ventricles contract and there is a rapid increase in intraventricular pressure, which results in closure of the atrioventricular valves. When the pressure in the ventricle exceeds the pressure in the systemic and pulmonary circulation, then the aortic and pulmonary valves respectively will open.
3 *Ejection phase*: Initial ejection is rapid, and the peak pressure in the ventricle becomes the peak pressure in the systemic circulation. The aorta can not accommodate all the blood, and initially it expands as it is filled.

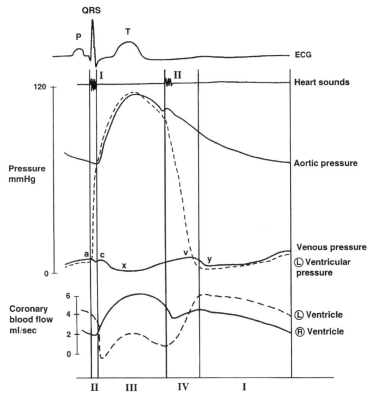

Figure 1.6 The four phases of the cardiac cycle related to the electrocardiogram (ECG). See text for details. Note that most left ventricular blood flow occurs in diastole.

Ejection then slows down, and ventricular pressure actually falls slightly below systemic pressure during the latter stages of ejection, causing a slowing down of the blood flow from the ventricle. Eventually ejection stops and there is a small recoil of blood back into the ventricle, which catches the aortic valve leaflets and closes them. This produces the dicrotic notch visible in the arterial waveform. The average stroke volume is about 80 ml, giving a normal left ventricular ejection fraction of about 67%.

4 *Isovolaemic relaxation.* There is a rapid fall in the pressure inside the ventricle with relaxation of the myocardium. When intraventricular pressure is below atrial pressure, the atrioventricular valves will relax and blood will start to fill the ventricular cavity.

Central venous trace

Central veins are in communication with the right atrium, and exhibit pressure changes that reflect right atrial pressure. Figure 1.6 shows this to be a triphasic wave, with three peaks and two descents. The 'a' wave coincides with atrial contraction. In nodal rhythm or complete heart block, contraction

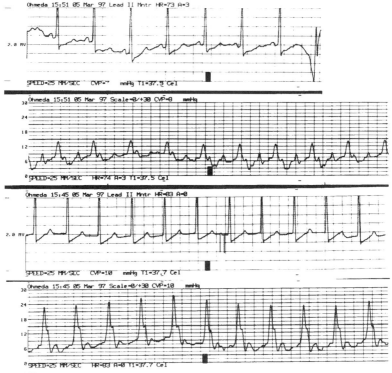

Figure 1.7 A patient under anaesthesia with intermittent episodes of nodal rhythm. A normal central venous pressure trace can be seen when the patient is in sinus rhythm, but once nodal rhythm occurs the P wave disappears into the QRS complex and the atria and ventricles contract at the same time. The produces large 'cannon' waves in the CVP trace, which are visible in the lower figure.

of the atrium against a closed a-v valve will produce giant 'a' waves, as can be seen in Figure 1.7. The 'c' wave is caused partly by the bulging of the tricuspid valve into the atrium, and partly by transmitted pulsations from the carotid artery. The 'v' wave is due to atrial pressure rising during atrial filling. Giant 'v' waves can be due to tricuspid regurgitation. The 'x' descent is due to atrial relaxation, and the 'y' descent to rapid atrial emptying at the start of ventricular filling.

Ejection fraction

The ejection fraction is the fraction of the end diastolic volume that is ejected with each contraction, and equals stroke volume/end diastolic volume (%). It is afterload- and preload-dependent, but is extensively used as a measure of ventricular performance[2]. These changes in ejection fraction with loading conditions are not, however, linear, and ejection fraction is maintained in the normal range until the loading conditions are severely abnormal. The same is true with contractility, and ventricular function has to be greatly reduced before resting ejection fraction will fall. Studies have shown that a low ejection fraction after a myocardial infarction is a poor prognostic indicator, but other studies looking into the ability of the ejection fraction to predict postoperative cardiac events have failed to show consistent results (see p. 100). However, measurement of ejection fraction is easy to perform and will detect poorly functioning myocardium, and is frequently used in the preoperative assessment of patients. The ejection fraction is usually 0.67 (or 67%), and this figure represents the maximal mechanical efficiency of the normal left ventricle ejecting into a normal arterial tree[2].

Blood pressure

The flow of blood around the body is proportional to the pressure difference between the two points considered, and inversely proportional to the resistance of the blood vessels carrying the blood.

Flow = Pressure gradient/Resistance

This is analogous to Ohm's law of electricity, E = IR, and can be rewritten;

Blood pressure = Cardiac Output × Peripheral Resistance

Using the knowledge of the factors responsible for maintenance of cardiac output, an overview of the whole cardiovascular system can now be produced in one diagram (Figure 1.8).

Overall control of the cardiovascular system is coordinated by the brain via the sympathetic and parasympathetic nervous systems, in response to afferent impulses from peripheral receptors.

Peripheral pressure receptors

Arterial baroreceptors. These are non-encapsulated nerve endings present in the adventitial layer of the aortic arch and the carotid sinus at the lower end

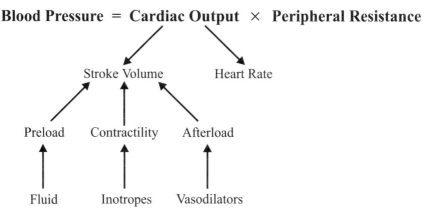

Figure 1.8 An overview of the cardiovascular system, showing the relationship between blood pressure, cardiac output and peripheral resistance. Stroke volume is determined by preload, contractility and afterload, and these in turn can be altered by giving fluid, starting inotropes, or adding in vasodilators.

of the internal carotid artery. Fibres from the aorta join the vagus (Xth cranial) nerve, while fibres from the carotid sinus join the glossopharyngeal (IXth cranial) nerve. The central axons of both terminate in the nucleus tractus solitarius. The receptors respond to stretch of the arterial wall, which is interpreted as a rise in blood pressure. They will also react to a fall in blood pressure by not firing. Baroreceptors vary in their threshold for response and the range over which they will respond. Stimulation of arterial baroreceptors results in a reflex vasodilatation and bradycardia mediated via efferents in the vagus nerve, which results in a lowering of the blood pressure.

Veno-atrial stretch receptors. These nerve endings are present at the junction of the atria and large veins of the chest. Their myelinated nerve fibres travel in the vagus nerve. They are stimulated by increasing cardiac filling, and can be thought of as 'central volume receptors'. Stimulation results in a reflex tachycardia from sympathetic stimulation of the sino-atrial node, and a diuresis from the action of atrial natriuretic hormone, which is released.

Chemosensitive fibres. These unmyelinated vagal and cardiac sympathetic afferents respond to bradykinin, prostaglandin lactic acid and potassium ions. Cardiac sympathetic chemosensitive afferents are thought to transmit the pain of angina.

Arterial chemoreceptors. These are present in the aortic and carotid bodies, which are small nodules lying beside the aorta and the carotid sinus. They are highly vascularized (probably the most vascularized tissue in the body on a blood flow to weight basis), and respond to hypoxia, hypercapnia and acidosis. Their cardiovascular effects are therefore minimal under normal circumstances, but in conditions of extreme hypotension and/or haemorrhage they are stimulated and elicit a sympathetically mediated vasoconstriction that helps to support the blood pressure.

Skeletal muscle receptors. Receptors present in skeletal muscle are stimulated by potassium and hydrogen ions released from exercising muscle.

This stimulation results in a reflex tachycardia and an increase in myocardial contractility and vasoconstriction in non-active muscle. This helps to raise blood pressure and increase perfusion of the exercising muscle.

Central integration and control

This is complex and still not fully understood. However, in the control of the cardiovascular system, the medulla, cerebellum and hypothalamus are all involved in the integration of afferent impulses and the generation of an efferent response. The nucleus tractus solitarius of the medulla is the site of reception of almost all the afferent fibres. There are pathways from here to the cerebellum, hypothalamus and the nucleus ambiguus in the medulla, which is the site of efferent vagal neurones that supply the heart. The rostral ventrolateral neurones of the medulla exert a sustained excitatory effect on the sympathetic neurones in the spinal cord, and this acts to maintain blood pressure.

Areas in the cerebellum are involved in maintaining the tachycardia, muscle vasodilatation, renal vasoconstriction and pressor responses to exercise.

In the hypothalamus, the perifornical region (probably activated by the amygdala of the limbic system) is responsible for the 'fight or flight' response seen to extremes of danger. This results in the tachycardia, hypertension, splanchnic vasoconstriction and skeletal muscle vasodilatation that occurs. The above information has been incorporated into Figure 1.9.

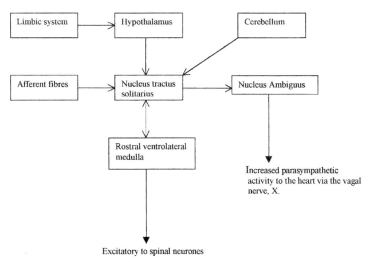

Figure 1.9 Central control of the cardiovascular system. The concept of a single 'vasomotor' centre is probably too simplistic, and final cardiovascular control is a complex interplay between afferent impulses and the hypothalamus, cerebellum, limbic system and nucleus tractus solitarius. The final sympathetic pathway is initiated from the rostral ventrolateral medulla, but the exact connections are unknown. The nucleus ambiguus is the site of initiation of increased parasympathetic tone to the heart, mediated via the vagal nerve.

Sympathetic nervous system

The sympathetic nervous system is part of the efferent limb of the central control of the cardiovascular system, and is summarized in Figure 1.10. It is composed of vasoconstrictor and vasodilator nerve fibres, and arises in the brainstem. The fibres travel in the bulbospinal tract to synapse with preganglionic neurones in the intermediolateral columns of the spinal cord grey matter at levels T1–L3. The fibres of the preganglionic neurones pass via the ventral nerve roots to synapse with the postganglionic neurones in the sympathetic chain, which lies anterior to the spine. The sympathetic chain extends above and below the levels T1–L3 because some preganglionic fibres travel up or down a few levels before synapsing. Some other preganglionic fibres pass through the sympathetic chain to synapse at more distant ganglia, such as the coeliac or hypogastric ganglia or the adrenal medulla. Non-myelinated postganglionic fibres travel with peripheral nerves or run with the larger blood vessels down to the level of the larger arterioles. Veins are usually much less richly innervated. The main preganglionic neurotransmitter is acetylcholine, and the postganglionic neurotransmitter is noradrenaline, which acts on alpha$_1$ receptors on the vascular smooth muscle to elicit vasoconstriction.

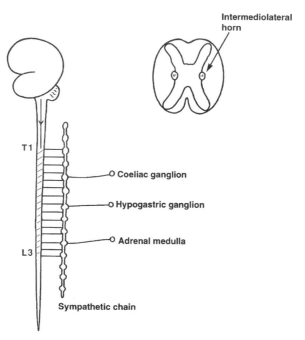

Figure 1.10 Anatomy of the sympathetic nervous system showing the outflow from T1–L3. Preganglionic fibres are short, ending in the sympathetic chain in front of the vertebra, which extends above and below T1–L3. Some preganglionic fibres do pass through to the coeliac and hypogastric ganglia and the adrenal medulla. Descending fibres pass in the intermediolateral horn of the spinal cord.

Vasoconstrictor fibres. Under normal resting conditions, there is activity in the sympathetic nervous system causing vasoconstriction, which is important for the maintenance of blood pressure. Similarly, a fall in sympathetic tone is important in the face of a rise in blood pressure and is part of the baroreceptor reflex. Pharmacological blocking of sympathetic activity, for example with a spinal anaesthetic, will also cause vasodilatation. Increases in vasoconstrictor activity reduce peripheral blood volume and help to maintain central blood volume and therefore blood pressure in the face of haemorrhage.

Vasodilator fibres. These innervate skeletal muscle and sweat glands, causing vasodilatation by the action of acetylcholine and vasoactive intestinal peptide (VIP). They are only activated transiently as part of the 'fight or flight' response, and perhaps act to reduce the large surge in blood pressure which would otherwise occur.

Adrenal medulla. This can be thought of as a large mass of postganglionic sympathetic neurones, receiving innervation from preganglionic fibres running in the splanchnic nerve. Adrenaline and noradrenaline are secreted into the bloodstream from the adrenal medulla in a ratio of 3:1 in response to hypotension, exercise, hypoglycaemia and fear.

Noradrenaline. This causes increased peripheral vascular resistance due to $alpha_1$-stimulation, resulting in a rise in blood pressure. This rise in blood pressure stimulates the baroreceptor reflex, eliciting a fall in heart rate and cardiac output from increased parasympathetic tone and decreased sympathetic drive.

Adrenaline. This causes a rise in cardiac output and heart rate due to stimulation of the $beta_1$-receptors in the heart, which act to raise the blood pressure. There is a variable action on the peripheral vascular resistance as it acts both on alpha vasoconstrictor and beta vasodilator receptors. At lower doses the beta vasodilator effect predominates, while vasoconstriction occurs at higher doses. Adrenaline will cause vasodilatation in liver, skeletal muscle and myocardium, due to the preponderance of beta-receptors in these tissues.

The parasympathetic system

In contrast to the sympathetic system, which has a thoraco-lumbar outflow usually with short preganglionic and long postganglionic fibres, the parasympathetic nervous system has a craniosacral outflow with relatively long preganglionic fibres synapsing with short postganglionic fibres in ganglia close to, or inside, the effector organ (Figure 1.11). The cranial outflow leaves in the oculomotor, facial, glossopharyngeal and vagal nerves (III, VII, IX, X). The first three of these innervate muscles and glands in the head, producing pupillary and ciliary muscle constriction, tears and saliva. The vagus nerve leaves the skull and carries parasympathetic fibres down as far as the large intestine. Vagal stimulation of the heart causes bradycardia, in the lungs it causes bronchoconstriction and increased secretions, and in the gastrointestinal tract it causes increased tone and relaxation of sphincters. The sacral outflow occurs from segments S2–4 to form the sacral nerves. These increase tone in the lower gastrointestinal tract and detrusor muscle of the bladder while relaxing sphincters. Both the pre- and postganglionic neurotransmitter in the parasympathetic system is acetylcholine.

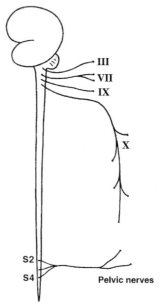

Figure 1.11 The parasympathetic nervous system showing the craniosacral outflow. Preganglionic fibres are long, and terminate in ganglia close to the organ they innervate. III, oculomotor nerve supplying the eye via the ciliary ganglion; VII, facial nerve supplying the lachrymal and salivary glands; IX, glossopharyngeal nerve supplying the parotid glands; X, vagal nerve supplying the heart, bronchi, upper gastrointestinal tract and intestinal organs. The pelvic nerves supply the lower gastrointestinal tract and organs of the pelvis.

Effects of anaesthetics on the cardiovascular system

Both intravenous and inhalational anaesthetics exert their effects on the cardiovascular system by changes in central sympathetic outflow, myocardial contraction, peripheral vascular resistance and the baroreceptor reflex. The extent to which an individual drug will produce changes depends upon the dose and the pharmacodynamics of that drug.

Intravenous agents

- Barbiturates reduce sympathetic output from the central nervous system and cause venodilatation. They also cause direct depression of myocardial contractility, but to a lesser extent than inhalational agents. There is a reflex increase in heart rate via the baroreceptors in response to the resultant drop in blood pressure.
- Benzodiazepines generally only produce a slight decrease in blood pressure due to a small drop in peripheral vascular resistance.
- Propofol produces significant drops in blood pressure due to venodilatation, reduction in peripheral vascular resistance and direct myocardial depression. Vasodilatation is due to decreased sympathetic drive and direct effects on the peripheral vasculature.

- Ketamine is unusual in that blood pressure, heart rate and cardiac output are increased, with a resultant increase in myocardial oxygen demand. This is probably due to a centrally mediated increase in sympathetic output.
- Etomidate has only a small depressant effect on arterial blood pressure, with little effect on the baroreceptor reflex.

Inhalational agents

These agents depress myocardial contractility by decreasing the availability of intracellular calcium ions. The effect is dose-dependent, and is much more marked with halothane and enflurane than with isoflurane. There is also inhibition of the baroreceptor reflex, which leads to a reduced blood pressure and an impaired cardiovascular response to hypovolaemia. Isoflurane has much less of an inhibitory action on the baroreceptor reflex than halothane or enflurane, but much more of a peripheral vasodilatory effect. Nitrous oxide is a direct myocardial depressant, but this is partly offset by an increase in central sympathetic output.

Coronary circulation

Anatomy

The coronary circulation comprises the right and left coronary arteries, arising from the aorta behind the cusps of the aortic valve. They travel over the surface of the heart, sending branches down through the myocardium (Figure 1.12). The right artery supplies the right ventricle and, in 90% of people, sends branches to the inferior surface of the heart, the so-called 'right dominant' system. The left coronary artery divides into the left anterior descending artery, which descends in the anterior interventricular groove

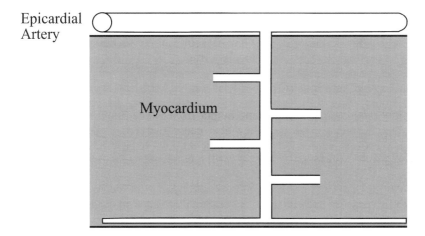

Figure 1.12 Cross-section of myocardial wall, showing epicardial vessels sending perforating branches through the myocardium and down to the subendocardium.

down to the apex of the heart, supplying the septum and anterior left ventricle; and the circumflex artery, which supplies the lateral and, in 10% of people, the inferior surface of the heart. Coronary arteries are essentially end arteries, with only a few small connections. Obstruction will therefore lead rapidly to myocardial hypoxia and infarction, although over time, if the obstruction is gradual, collaterals can develop and help preserve blood flow distally. Blockages of these three main arteries define the territory of an infarct, and correspond to inferior, anterior and lateral myocardial infarcts.

The venous drainage of the heart is mainly into the right atrium (95%), via the coronary sinus. The rest drains via the anterior coronary vein, or directly into the ventricles via the Thebesian veins.

Physiology

At rest the heart receives about 4% of the cardiac output (250 ml/min for an average heart), but this can be increased by three to four times during exercise. The heart extracts about 65–70% of the oxygen from its blood supply, compared to an average of 25% for the rest of the body. This can increase slightly to about 90%, but the majority of increased oxygen needed must be provided by increased blood flow. Coronary blood flow does increase almost linearly with myocardial oxygen consumption due to direct vasodilatation, but the exact mechanism is still not completely understood. It is probably metabolic vasodilatation due to hypoxia or adenosine production in the working myocardium. This outweighs any sympathetic vasoconstrictor impulses.

In the left ventricle during systole, the pressure generated in the myocardium starts to close the coronary arteries and blood flow slows or even stops (Figure 1.6). Most blood flow (80%) therefore occurs during diastole, and it is reduced if diastolic times shorten, as occurs during tachycardia.

Cerebral circulation

The brain receives 14% of the resting cardiac output and uses 20% of the resting oxygen consumption while comprising only 2% of the body weight. This is due to the large amount of oxygen utilized by the grey matter. Maintenance of cerebral perfusion is essential for human life, as loss of cerebral blood flow will cause loss of consciousness in a few seconds and irreversible neuronal death in 3–4 minutes.

Anatomy

The arterial supply of the brain comprises the two vertebral arteries, which join to form the basilar artery, and the two internal carotid arteries, which form an arterial ring at the base of the brain called the circle of Willis (shown in Figure 1.13). This anastamosis helps to maintain cerebral blood flow in the case of obstruction of one of the arteries, but is subject to atheromatous change and may not be patent in the vascular patient. From this, the three major blood vessels–the anterior, middle and posterior cerebral arteries–

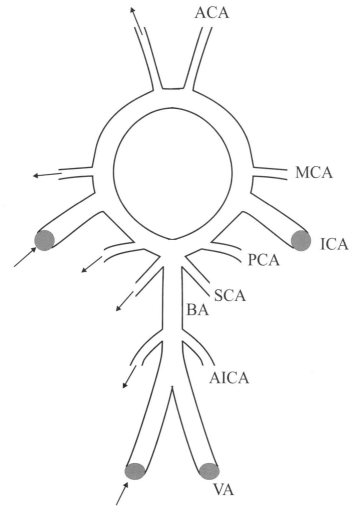

Figure 1.13 The circle of Willis at the base of the brain; not all branches are shown. ACA, anterior cerebral artery; MCA, middle cerebral artery; ICA, internal carotid artery; PCA, posterior cerebral artery; SCA, superior cerebellar artery; BA, basilar artery; AICA, anterior inferior cerebellar artery; VA, vertebral artery. Arrows denote direction of blood flow.

arise. Venous drainage is via the cerebral sinuses into the sigmoid sinus, and then the internal jugular veins.

Physiology

Cerebral blood flow depends on perfusion pressure, arterial P_{O_2} and P_{CO_2}, and neuronal metabolic rate. Although innervated by the autonomic nervous system, this plays little role in controlling cerebral blood flow under normal circumstances. The brain can also act to protect its own blood supply via cardiovascular reflexes, and reduced blood flow causes intense sympathetic

Cerebral
blood flow

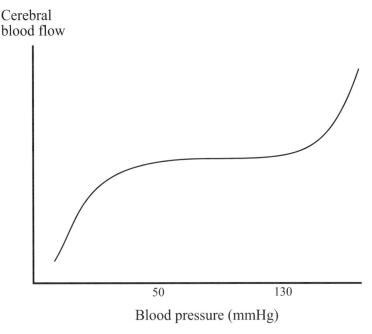

Blood pressure (mmHg)

Figure 1.14 Graph of cerebral blood flow versus blood pressure, showing autoregulation of cerebral blood flow. Cerebral blood flow changes in response to mean arterial blood pressure, showing little change within the range 50–130 mmHg. The curve in a chronically hypertensive patient may be shifted to the right.

stimulation leading to a rise in blood pressure in an attempt to perfuse the brain. The rise in blood pressure is detected by the peripheral baroreceptors, and a reflex bradycardia elicited (the Cushing response) which is characteristic of reduced cerebral blood flow.

Autoregulation. Cerebral blood flow is kept constant over a large range of blood pressures by autoregulation, as seen in Figure 1.14. Rises in blood pressure elicit cerebral vasoconstriction and falls elicit cerebral vasodilatation to keep blood flow constant. This is partly due to increased vessel vasoconstriction in response to an increase in intraluminal pressure, the so-called 'myogenic' response, which seems to be an intrinsic property of vascular smooth muscle. It is also due partly to high blood flow causing increased 'washout' of intrinsic vasodilators produced by the vessels, which leads to vasoconstriction and reduced flow, the 'metabolic' response. Autoregulation occurs in many organs, notably the brain, heart and kidney, but at extremes of blood pressure it will ultimately fail to keep blood flow constant and blood flow will become pressure-dependent. Cerebral autoregulation can become ineffective in head injury, subarachnoid haemorrhage, around cerebral tumours and in conditions of high Pa_{CO_2}. Inhalation anaesthetic agents and other cerebral vasodilators will also impair autoregulation. Isoflurane is the least damaging volatile agent in this respect.

Cerebral
blood flow

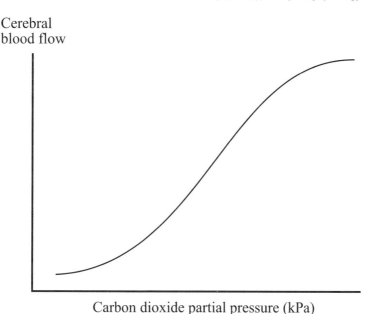

Carbon dioxide partial pressure (kPa)

Figure 1.15 Cerebral blood flow in response to changes in the arterial partial pressure of carbon dioxide. Note the almost linear relationship within normal physiological ranges.

Pa_{CO_2}. Carbon dioxide readily penetrates the blood–brain barrier and combines with water to produce carbonic acid, which disassociates into hydrogen ions. These hydrogen ions cause cerebral vasodilatation and an increase in cerebral blood flow (Figure 1.15). Conversely, lowering the Pa_{CO_2} will cause cerebral vasoconstriction.

Pa_{O_2}. Changes in Pa_{O_2} have little effect on cerebral blood flow until it falls to about 8 kPa. Below this, level cerebral blood flow increases markedly (Figure 1.16). High levels of Pa_{O_2} will cause an insignificant amount of cerebral vasoconstriction.

Cerebral neuronal activity. Local cerebral blood flow is intimately linked to neuronal activity in an almost linear fashion, as shown in Figure 1.17. This may be due to vasodilatation produced by the products of metabolism, probably potassium or hydrogen ions.

Renal circulation

Anatomy

The kidney receives a large proportion of the cardiac output for its size (20–25%). This is mainly directed at the cortex, with the medulla only receiving about 1% of renal blood flow. The renal arteries branch inside the kidney into interlobar arteries, which branch again to form arcuate arteries running along the cortico-medullary junction (Figure 1.18). Inter-lobular arteries then arise at right angles, and at regular intervals give rise

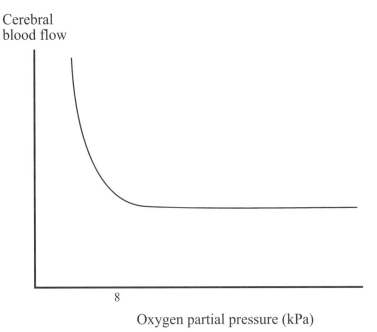

Figure 1.16 Changes in cerebral blood flow in response to changes in the arterial partial pressure of oxygen. Little change is seen until arterial P_{O_2} drops below 8 kPa.

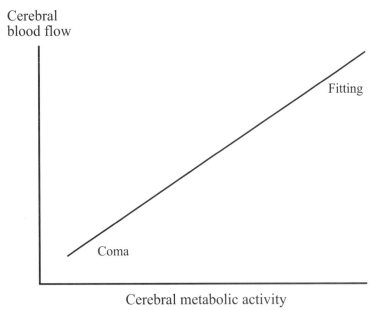

Figure 1.17 Cerebral blood flow in response to increasing cerebral metabolic rate. There is a linear relationship between neuronal activity and cerebral blood flow.

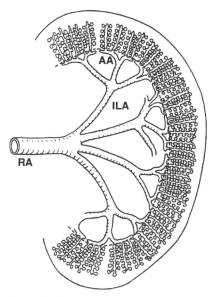

Figure 1.18 Arterial supply to the kidney, showing the division of the renal artery (RA) into interlobar arteries (ILA) and the arcuate arteries (AA) at the junction of the cortex and medulla.

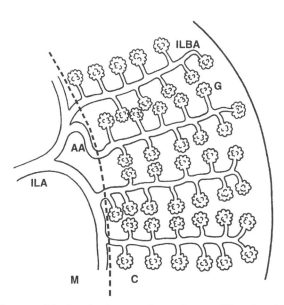

Figure 1.19 Close-up of the junction between the renal cortex (C) and medulla (M). The arcuate arteries (AA) are branches of the interlobar arteries (ILA), and run along the cortico-medullary junction. They branch to form the interlobular arteries (ILBA), from which the glomeruli (G) arise.

to the afferent arteriole of the glomerulus (shown in Figure 1.19). Efferent arterioles of the glomerulus then split into another capillary network, and become the peritubular capillaries into which fluid is reabsorbed from the tubules. There are two different classes of nephrons, cortical (with short loops of Henle) and juxtamedullary (with long loops of Henle), and their accompanying capillary network, the vasa recta. These dip down into the medulla and are responsible for urinary concentration.

Physiology

Autoregulation. As in the brain, there is well-developed autoregulation of renal blood flow (and therefore glomerular filtration) between mean blood pressures of 80 and 180 mmHg. This is due to changes in resistance of the interlobular arteries and afferent and efferent arterioles.

Sympathetic innervation. The kidney is densely innervated with sympathetic vasoconstrictor fibres. Activation of the sympathetic nervous system will cause renal vasoconstriction, which will reduce renal blood flow.

Renin–angiotensin system. Renin is an enzyme produced by specialized cells of the afferent arteriole. It acts on angiotensinogen, a circulating protein produced by the liver, to produce angiotensin I. This is then further degraded to angiotensin II in the lungs by angiotensin-converting enzyme. Angiotensin II is a potent systemic vasoconstrictor, and in the kidney preferentially constricts the efferent arteriole to help maintain the glomerular filtration rate. It also acts to increase production of aldosterone from the adrenal cortex, which increases reabsorption of sodium from the distal tubule. Secretion of renin is triggered by decreases in renal perfusion pressure, sensed by afferent arteriole baroreceptors. Sympathetic stimulation and high levels of circulating catecholamines will also cause renin secretion via stimulation of beta-receptors. The macula densa is an area of modified cells of the ascending loop of Henle in intimate contact with the glomerulus. These cells 'taste' the composition of the tubular fluid, and will cause increased secretion of renin if a decreased sodium or increased chloride concentration is detected.

Pathophysiology

Pathology of atherosclerosis

Atheroma

Atheroma is a disease of the intimal layer of the arterial wall of medium to large sized arteries. Discrete lesions are formed, caused by intimal thickening due to proliferation of smooth muscle and the production of proteins (especially collagen) by this smooth muscle. Varying amounts of lipid are also present in the form of cholesterol, both intracellularly and extracellularly. The composition of these lesions varies from those composed mainly of protein to those composed mainly of lipid with a connective tissue cap, and all the combinations in between (Figure 1.20).

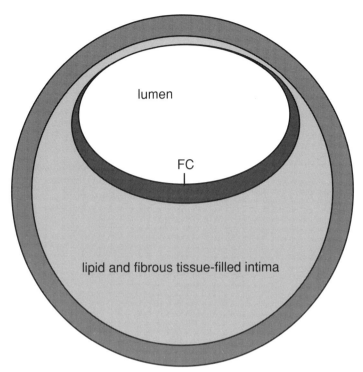

Figure 1.20 Cross-section of an atheromatous artery showing normal media but greatly enlarged intima filled with lipid and fibrous tissue with a cap of fibrous tissue, causing a reduction in size of the lumen. FC, fibrous tissue cap.

Pathology

There is still uncertainty over the initial cause and natural history of atheromatous lesions. It is likely to be multifactorial in origin, but probably involves the alteration of vascular smooth muscle cells from their normal contractile state to a synthetic state in which they can produce collagen, proteoglycans and growth factors. This may be initiated by platelet-derived growth factor (PDGF), which is mitogenic and chemoattractant and is produced from platelets, the vascular endothelium and macrophages. Connective tissue proliferation leads to the formation of a greatly increased intimal thickness. Lipid accumulation also occurs because circulating cholesterol in the low-density lipoprotein form (LDL) is incorporated into the vessel wall as lipid-laden monocytes attach to the endothelium and migrate subendothelially. Here they transform into macrophages. There are also often areas of necrosis within the plaque, and they are often capped by a layer of fibromuscular tissue. Calcification of the lesions can occur, as can haemorrhage into the plaque, causing a rapid increase in size and sudden development of occlusive symptoms.

The initial stimulus to the formation of these lesions is unknown but may be due to 'damage' to the endothelium, which stimulates the endothelium to release growth factors and leads to smooth muscle proliferation. This 'damage' may be caused by hypercholesterolaemia, hypertension, diabetes or cigarette smoking[3].

Two types of lesion are seen;

1 *Fatty streaks.* Intracellular deposits of lipid in the intimal layer are common, and occur from early life. In 40% of children coming to post mortem there is evidence of fatty streaks in the aorta. They are distributed along the artery in the direction of the blood flow, and arise at areas where the velocity of blood in contact with the wall is low. The exact significance and fate of these lesions is unknown, but it seems likely that some may progress to more serious lesions while others may regress.
2 *Fibrolipid plaques.* As mentioned above. these can vary in consistency from the predominantly connective tissue plaques to those containing a small amount of connective tissue with a large amount of lipid and a cap of fibrous tissue. These lesions can protrude into the lumen of the vessel and obstruct blood flow (Figure 1.20). Significant stenosis is said to occur when the diameter of the blood vessel is reduced by 50%.

Lesions containing a large amount of lipid and necrotic tissue with a thin cap are at risk of tearing open and exposing the highly thrombogenic interior to the circulation. Thrombosis can occur and lead to a sudden reduction in vessel luminal diameter, or even total occlusion. This is thought to be the mechanism underlying the sudden development of unstable angina and myocardial infarction. Lesions composed mainly of connective tissue seem to be more stable, and lead to a gradual occlusion more in keeping with the clinical picture of chronic stable angina. The course of the disease is unpredictable, however, and the growth rate of the plaques can not be foreseen.

Ischaemic heart disease

Ischaemia of the heart is an imbalance between the oxygen supply and demand of the myocardium. Atheroma narrows arteries and reduces blood flow and oxygen supply. The natural history of the disease is very variable, as the lesions may remain stable for many years or suddenly fissure and ulcerate and initiate clot formation. A patient can present with chronic stable angina, unstable angina, myocardial infarction or even sudden death, with no previous history.

Angina pectoris is the pain of myocardial ischaemia, and is described as a tightness, discomfort or choking feeling across the chest, down the left arm, down both arms, or up into the neck and jaw. It characteristically occurs on exertion, with stress or on going out into the cold, and is relieved by rest. Myocardial ischaemia can occur without pain, when it is known as 'silent ischaemia'. In the right coronary artery a stenosis of 50% is probably needed to cause ischaemia, while in the left anterior descending or circumflex arteries, 70% stenosis is probably needed. Physiologically, ischaemia causes slowing of ventricular contraction and of the phase of isovolaemic relaxation. End diastolic pressures rise because of increased wall stiffness (decreased compliance). If ischaemia continues, the ST segments of the ECG will fall and the patient may then experience pain. Arrhythmias and acute ventricular failure may also be precipitated by the ischaemia.

Variant angina. In 1959, Printzmetal described a group of patients who developed angina at rest associated with ST segment elevation. This was due to spasm of the coronary arteries, but the exact mechanism is unclear. It can be precipitated by changes in acidity and temperature of the oesophagus, and can occur at night when the resting tone of the coronary arteries is high. It is usually treated with calcium antagonists.

Risk factors for angina or atherosclerosis

- *Age.* Increasing age is associated with increased risk of atheroma and coronary artery disease (CAD).
- *Diet.* Epidemiological studies show that there is an increased prevalence of coronary artery disease in societies that have a high saturated fat intake.
- *Cholesterol.* The higher the serum cholesterol, the higher the risk of that individual developing coronary artery disease. As with hypertension there is no definite cut-off, but an upper limit of 5.2 mmol/l has been quoted. The amount of low-density lipoprotein cholesterol is the important factor, with high-density lipoproteins being seen as protective. Various genetic disorders can predispose to hypercholesterolaemia, and these patients develop coronary artery disease early on in life.
- *Diabetes.* This increases the incidence of atheroma. It is not known if this is due to the high sugar levels or to the associated high lipid levels in this condition.
- *Obesity.* Obesity is associated with hypertension and abnormal lipids, but may not be a risk factor in itself.
- *Blood pressure.* High systolic or diastolic pressures predispose to development of coronary artery disease.
- *Smoking.* This increases the incidence of coronary artery disease.
- *Alcohol.* A moderate alcohol intake is probably slightly protective, but heavy drinkers increase their risk of developing coronary artery disease.
- *Family history.* Patients with relatives developing coronary artery disease early are more likely to do so themselves. This is probably a genetic predisposition.
- *Clotting factors.* Increased levels of fibrinogen and factor VII increase the risk of coronary artery disease.

Management of ischaemic heart disease

Prevention

Patients should be advised to give up smoking, reach a normal body weight, eat healthily and take regular exercise. Hypertension should be controlled; although there is little evidence that treating hypertension will reduce coronary artery disease, it will reduce strokes, renal failure and heart failure. If the serum cholesterol is high it should be reduced, by diet (generally poor results) or drug treatment.

Treatment

Drug treatment of angina is essentially symptom control. It has not been shown that this modifies the disease in terms of reduced mortality.

- Nitrates cause smooth muscle relaxation, resulting in dilatation of coronary arteries and a reduction in preload and afterload, leading to reduced myocardial wall tension and oxygen requirements. This is despite the usual increase in heart rate that occurs.
- Beta blockers block the receptor sites for the activation of adenylate cyclase, and reduce the production of cyclic AMP from ATP. They reduce contractility, heart rate and blood pressure, thereby reducing myocardial oxygen consumption.
- Calcium antagonists block the influx of calcium in the slow calcium channel. Myocardial contractility is reduced, and systemic and coronary artery vasodilatation occurs.

These drugs can be used singularly or in combination if necessary.

Further management and assessment of patients for coronary angiography are detailed on p. 101.

Coronary artery angiography. Started in the 1950s, angiography is used to assess ventricular function and outline the exact anatomy of the coronary arteries prior to surgery. There is a mortality of about 0.2%, usually in patients with severe disease or very poor ventricular function.

Surgical management of ischaemic heart disease. The first saphenous vein bypass grafts were done in the USA in the 1960s. They are very good for controlling symptoms, and overall mortality is about 3%, but most patients slowly redevelop angina. Re-operations can be done, but there is a higher mortality and reduced symptomatic relief. There are subgroups of patients who will benefit from coronary artery surgery with improved long-term survival. Patients with left main stem disease, triple vessel disease, impaired left ventricular function and, perhaps, those with a proximal lesion in the left anterior descending artery will all do better than similar patients on medical management only. It is also recommended for those patients with severe symptoms uncontrolled by medical therapy.

Percutaneous transluminal coronary angioplasty. This was first performed in 1977. A catheter is introduced into a peripheral artery and passed back to the heart, along the coronary artery and through the stenosis. A balloon is then inflated to press the atheroma back against the wall and relieve the obstruction. It is suitable for localized proximal lesions of the coronary arteries. There is a restenosis rate, and occasionally a need for emergency coronary artery bypass grafting due to acute coronary occlusion. However, mortality is low (about 0.5%) and the patient only has a brief hospital stay.

Cardiac failure

Cardiac failure is present when the myocardium is unable to provide the body with the circulation it needs. It has to be distinguished from other conditions, such as hypovolaemia, sepsis, and anaphylaxis, where there is also circulatory failure with reduced oxygen delivery to the tissues. If the problem is essentially a cardiac one, the patient is said to have cardiac failure. This is an extremely significant factor in the development of serious perioperative cardiac complications.

Pathophysiology

The essential problem is decreased contractility of the myocardium, usually due to ischaemia. Reduced cardiac output and poor peripheral circulation to the tissues and, especially, the kidneys set up compensatory mechanisms, which act to retain fluid and increase the circulating volume. From Starling's law and looking at ventricular function curves (Figure 1.4), it can be seen that by increasing the end diastolic pressure and therefore stretch of the myocardium an adequate cardiac output can be achieved, up to a point. Predominantly left-sided failure will lead to symptoms and signs of pulmonary venous and capillary congestion and pulmonary oedema. Right-sided failure will lead to systemic venous and capillary congestion, peripheral oedema and ascites. Circulatory overload and poor myocardial function can cause dilatation of the ventricle. From Laplace's law, this will increase the work needed to produce a similar cardiac output to that of a smaller ventricle and further stress the heart.

Compensatory mechanisms. Neurohumeral mechanisms involved in the process include:

- Increased activity of the sympathetic nervous system and increased circulating levels of catecholamines. This causes generalized arterial and venous vasoconstriction and increased inotropy in the short term. In the long term, there is 'down regulation' of the beta-receptors of the heart and a reduced response to adrenaline. Venous constriction shifts blood from the periphery of the circulation and increases filling pressure of the heart.
- Poor renal blood flow activates the renal renin–angiotensin system, leading to increased levels of circulating angiotensin II. This is one of the most potent vasoconstrictors known, and also increases the production of aldosterone, which acts on the kidney to induce salt and water retention.
- Atrial myocytes secrete atrial natriuretic peptide in response to stretching caused by the increase in circulating blood volume. This hormone causes an increase in sodium excretion, a diuresis and a decrease in vascular resistance that helps to offset the other compensatory mechanisms.

Symptoms and signs

Patients present with reduced exercise tolerance, the extent of which can indicate the severity of the failure. Breathlessness and tiredness are common. Faintness on exertion probably indicates a drop in blood pressure on exercising, and is a serious sign. Orthopnea can be due to respiratory disease, but is usually more a sign of cardiac disease. Paroxysmal nocturnal dyspnoea is a sign of increased pulmonary capillary pressure, and night sweats are common. Weight can increase due to oedema collection, but in the late stages cachexia may occur.

On examination the patient may have poor circulation to the peripheries, with cold hands and feet and a weak thready pulse indicating reduced cardiac output. There is likely to be a tachycardia, and atrial fibrillation is common. Pulsus alternans, alternating small and large pulses (in the presence of a normal ECG to exclude ectopics), is a sign of ventricular disease. The jugular venous pressure, measured from the sternal angle and looking at the internal jugular vein, may be raised above 5–6 cm, indicating volume overload. The 'a' wave in the venous pulse precedes the carotid pulsation and indicates atrial contraction. This may be large if there is right ventricular hypertrophy. The 'v' wave shows blood accumulating in the atrial cavity, and may be increased if there is tricuspid incompetence. The apex beat is displaced if the ventricle is enlarged, and a parasternal heave can be a sign of volume overload or right ventricular hypertrophy. A third heart sound is low-pitched, and occurs after the second sound. It signifies rapid ventricular filling. A fourth sound occurs before the first, and is a sign of normal atria contracting against a stiff ventricle. The normal slight splitting of the second heart sound that occurs on inspiration is reversed in left ventricular disease and left bundle branch block, and splitting occurs on expiration. Blood pressure may be normal; an inappropriately low blood pressure indicates more severe disease, and below 100 mmHg it is a sign of cardiogenic shock. Respiratory rate may be increased, with an increase in the work of breathing signifying pulmonary congestion. Basal crackles that do not clear on coughing can be due to cardiac or pulmonary disease. Peripheral oedema and ascites can occur, but could also be due to renal or liver disease. An enlarged liver stretching the capsule can cause abdominal pain and tenderness.

Investigations

1 *Chest X-ray.* This may show an enlarged heart and upper lobe blood diversion. Kerley B lines are small horizontal lines in the costophrenic angles indicating oedema in the interlobular fissures. Pulmonary oedema is symmetrical, and spreads out from the lung hilar.
2 *ECG.* A tachycardia is common. Left atrial hypertrophy is seen as a bifid P wave or a negative P wave in V_1.
3 *Echocardiography.* This can show ventricular wall movement during systole and, by outlining areas of hypokinesia, akinesia and dyskinesia, indicates increasingly poor myocardial function. The ejection fraction can be measured in a good subject, and pulmonary artery pressures can be estimated. Dilated or hypertrophied hearts can be identified, and valvular anatomy seen.

Treatment

The main aims of treatment are to reduce cardiac work, decrease the volume of the circulation and improve myocardial contractility. The main drugs used for this are therefore vasodilators, diuretics and inotropes respectively.

Arterial vasodilatation will reduce blood pressure and afterload, thereby decreasing myocardial wall tension. Venodilators and diuretics reduce end diastolic pressure and move the myocardium back down the Starling curve. This will potentially reduce cardiac output, but the overloaded heart in cardiac failure is usually operating on a flat portion of the Starling curve and a reduction in filling pressure is usually beneficial. Of the inotropic agents, digoxin is probably the most useful (even if there is no atrial fibrillation), as it helps slow the heart. The combination of diuretics and digoxin is potentially dangerous in that arrhythmias can easily be precipitated by digoxin in the presence of a low potassium.

Angiotensin-converting enzyme inhibitors (ACE inhibitors) have recently been shown to improve survival not only in severe heart failure, but also in heart failure following a myocardial infarction. They are the only drugs that modify the prognosis of the condition.

Hypertension

There is no discrete population of hypertensive patients. Systolic and diastolic blood pressures exhibit a continuous, normal distribution. The risk of developing complications rises with the blood pressure and therefore the exact level at which treatment is required is arbitrary, but guidelines have been formulated. Complications of hypertension include myocardial infarction, heart failure, strokes and renal failure. The risk of developing these complications increases when other risk factors are present, especially smoking and hyperlipidaemia.

Measurement of blood pressure

Care must be taken in the manual measurement of blood pressure, in order to avoid errors. The patient should be relaxed, sitting, with an appropriately sized cuff placed at the level of the heart. A cuff that is too narrow will give a falsely high reading of blood pressure; this is more likely to occur in obese patients. Similarly, a cuff that is too wide will underestimate the blood pressure. On blowing up the cuff, the pulse should be continuously palpated until it disappears. This will prevent hurting the patient, and avoids the problem of missing the auscultatory gap that sometimes exists between Korotkoff sounds I and II. The level of the mercury should be let down at 2–3 mmHg per second, especially in a patient with a slow heart rate. The column of mercury should be observed at right angles in order to minimize parallax error, and reading the blood pressure to the nearest 2 mmHg can reduce observer digit preference. There is sometimes confusion as to which Korotkoff sound to take as the diastolic pressure, Korotkoff sound IV (muffling) or V (disappearance of the sound). If there is any doubt both should be recorded, together with the systolic. In hypertensive patients the pressure should be taken in both arms, as there is often a slight difference.

Causes of hypertension

Blood pressure rises independently with age, salt intake, weight and alcohol consumption. Black populations have a higher prevalence of hypertension than white populations. Moderate exercise and a diet high in potassium may help to lower blood pressure.

Pathology

If no cause or abnormality can be found in the patient, then the hypertension is called 'essential' hypertension. This is true in 95% of cases. In these patients the hypertension is caused by an increase in peripheral vascular resistance with a normal cardiac output. This occurs at the level of the arterioles, and may be due to increased calcium in the smooth muscle of these vessels, leading to vasoconstriction. Over a period of time the muscular layer of the arterioles can increase in thickness, leading to a further increase in peripheral vascular resistance. In essential hypertension, neither the renin–angiotensin system nor increased levels of catecholamines are thought to be the major cause.

In the remaining 5% of cases there is an underlying medical condition which is usually renal, but may be vascular or endocrine.

- *Renal causes*: nephritis, chronic pyelonephritis, polycystic kidneys and diabetes.
- *Endocrine causes*: Cushing's disease, Conn's syndrome, acromegaly and phaeochromocytoma.
- *Vascular causes*: renal artery stenosis, coarctation of the aorta.

Clinical features

The hypertensive patient often has no symptoms, and hypertension is picked up on routine examination. Headaches are no more common than in a normal patient; in fact, the only symptom that is more common is shortness of breath. Symptoms may be due to end organ damage, for example chest pain if coronary artery disease has developed, or polyuria if renal damage has occurred. There is often a family history of high blood pressure.

On examination, the body mass index (BMI) should be measured (weight (kg)/height^2 (m^2)). A BMI greater than 30 is classed as obese, 25–29 as overweight and less than 25 as normal. The cardiovascular system should be examined for signs of heart failure and left ventricular hypertrophy. Carotid, femoral or renal artery bruits should be listened for, and a delayed femoral pulse may indicate coarctation of the aorta. The characteristic features of Cushing's disease and acromegaly may occasionally be evident, and abdominal palpation may reveal palpable kidneys in polycystic disease.

Investigations

1 All patients should have urinalysis to look for proteinuria and haematuria, which may indicate renal damage. Glycosuria will indicate diabetes.

2 Electrolytes. Serum sodium may be high in Conn's syndrome; low serum sodium may be due to diuretic therapy. High potassium levels may due to renal failure, ACE inhibitor treatment or potassium-sparing diuretics.
3 Urea and creatinine levels may be raised due to renal damage from hypertension, or hypertension may be due to primary renal disease.
4 ECG. This allows the assessment of left ventricular hypertrophy which, if present, indicates end organ damage and increases mortality by 3–4 times for any given level of blood pressure. Left ventricular hypertrophy will regress to some extent with successful blood pressure treatment.
5 Further tests. In younger patients, or patients with hypertension that is resistant to treatment, further tests may be indicated. These may include renal ultrasound, renal angiography, and the plasma hormone levels of aldosterone, growth hormone and cortisol. If phaeochromocytoma is suspected, it is best detected by 24-hour urine analysis and plasma noradrenaline levels.

Treatment

Successful treatment of hypertension produces dramatic patient benefits. Before treatment the 2-year mortality from malignant hypertension was 80%; nowadays in treated patients the 2-year survival is 85%. Blood pressure reduction is extremely effective in reducing the stroke rate, and this applies to patients up to the age of 80 years. A beneficial effect on the incidence of cardiac disease is much harder to show, but there is probably a small reduction in mortality. Consensus now is that patients under 80 years of age with systolic blood pressures consistently above 160 mmHg and diastolic pressures greater than 100 mmHg should be treated. Patients with blood pressures close to these values should be followed up regularly[4]. Successful treatment of an isolated systolic hypertension greater than 160 mmHg will also reduce mortality, even if the diastolic pressure is below 100 mmHg. In patients older than 80 years, blood pressure reduction probably increases mortality unless hypertension is very severe.

Obesity should be corrected, a reduced salt diet started, alcohol intake should be moderated and the patient encouraged to take some exercise.

Drug treatment. The first line drugs are beta blockers and thiazide diuretics. ACE inhibitors, calcium channel blockers and alpha blockers can also be used if more appropriate; for example, patients with heart failure are better treated with ACE inhibitors than with beta blockers.

- *Thiazides* are cheap, well tolerated and especially suitable for elderly patients. They should be avoided in diabetes, as they can cause hyperglycaemia and may also cause hypokalaemia and hyperuricaemia.
- *Beta blockers* are useful for young patients with coronary artery disease. They are contraindicated in patients with asthma and cardiac failure, and should be used carefully in patients with peripheral vascular disease.
- *Calcium channel blockers* can be useful in asthma and in patients with angina. In patients with peripheral vascular disease they may improve the symptoms of claudication.
- *ACE inhibitors* are best suited to patients with heart failure, and are of proven benefit in diabetics with proteinuria. Black patients have low

plasma renin levels and do not respond well to ACE inhibition. In renal artery stenosis and in combination with diuretic therapy they may produce a large drop in blood pressure on first dosing, which may cause renal impairment. If blood pressure drops are avoided, they can be beneficial in reducing the decline in renal function in hypertensive patients.

- *Alpha blockers* such as doxazosin, (a long-acting alpha blocker) are becoming increasingly popular in patients with asthma, peripheral vascular disease and prostatism. They also lower blood lipid levels.

Combination therapy. Some combinations of anti-hypertensive treatment seem logical and complement one another. These include beta blockers and thiazides, ACE inhibitors and diuretics, beta blockers and calcium-channel blockers, and beta blockers and alpha blockers.

Suggested further reading

Despopoulos A, Silbernagl S. *Color Atlas of Physiology.* Georg Thieme, 1991.
Foex P. The heart and the autonomic nervous system. In Nimmo W, Robotham D, Smith G eds. *Anaesthesia.* Blackwell Scientific, 1994.
Patterson D, Treasure T. *Disorders of the Cardiovascular System.* Edward Arnold, 1993.
O'Brien ET, Beevers DG, Marshall HJ. *ABC of Hypertension.* BMJ Publishing Group, 1995.
Priebe HJ, Skarvan K. *Cardiovascular Physiology.* BMJ Publishing Group, 1995.
Levick JR. *An Introduction to Cardiovascular Physiology.* Butterworth-Heinemann, 1991.

References

1 Allen DG, Kentish JC. The cellular basis of the length–tension relation in cardiac muscle. *J Mol Cell Cardiol* 1985; **17**: 821–40.
2 Robotham JL, Takata M, Berman M, Harasawa Y. Ejection fraction revisited. *Anesthesiology* 1991; **74**: 172–83.
3 Ross R. The pathology of atherosclerosis–an update. *New Engl J Med* 1986; **314**: 488–500.
4 Sever P, Beevers G, Bulpitt C, *et al.* Management guidelines in essential hypertension: report of the second working party of the British Hypertension Society. *BMJ* 1993; **306**: 983–7

2

Pharmacology of drugs for vascular anaesthesia

Introduction

This chapter aims to review the pharmacology of anaesthetic agents, analgesics and adjuvant drugs commonly used in the perioperative period, in addition to that of acute and chronic cardiovascular medications, which is particularly relevant to the patient presenting for vascular surgery.

Most vascular surgery patients take a number of medications for their cardiovascular problems, e.g. beta-adrenergic blocking drugs, calcium channel blockers, angiotensin-converting enzyme inhibitors, antiplatelet agents and anticoagulants. These drugs may interact with one another and cardiovascular effects may be enhanced by anaesthetic agents, thereby influencing anaesthetic requirements and perioperative management.

Inhalation anaesthetics

Introduction

The inhaled anaesthetics in current use include the weakly potent inorganic gas nitrous oxide and the volatile anaesthetics halothane, enflurane, isoflurane, desflurane and sevoflurane.

Pharmacokinetics

Dosages of inhalational anaesthetics are expressed as MAC, the minimal alveolar concentration at 1 atmosphere at which 50% of patients do not move in response to a surgical stimulus (Table 2.1). MAC reflects the brain partial pressure of the agent because the alveolar partial pressure is in equilibrium with the brain. In practice, a MAC of 1.2–1.3 is necessary to prevent movement in 95% of patients. Duration of anaesthesia and changes in $Paco_2$ do not influence MAC.

MAC is decreased by:

- combinations of inhaled anaesthetics (1% reduction for every 1% nitrous oxide)

Table 2.1 Properties of inhalation anaesthetics

Anaesthetic	Vapour pressure mmHg, 20°C	Blood–gas partition coefficient 37°C	Fat–blood partition coefficient 37°C	MAC % atm in O_2	MAC % atm in 60% N_2O	F_A/F_I at 30 min
Halothane	241	2.3	60	0.77	0.29	0.58
Enflurane	175	1.91	36	1.7	0.6	0.65
Isoflurane	238	1.4	45	1.15	0.5	0.73
Desflurane	673	0.42	18.7	6	2.8	0.91
Sevoflurane	162	0.59	53.4	1.71	0.66	0.85
Nitrous oxide	39 000	0.47	2.3	104		0.99

- central nervous system depressants, e.g. opioids and benzodiazepines
- increasing age
- hypothermia
- alpha$_2$ agonists, e.g. clonidine.

MAC is increased by:

- hyperthermia
- monoamine oxidase inhibitors
- ethanol abuse
- ephedrine.

Induction of anaesthesia occurs when an anaesthetizing partial pressure has been achieved in the brain, after a series of concentration gradients in partial pressures. The aim of inhalational anaesthesia is maintenance of an optimum brain partial pressure of the agent (depth of anaesthesia). This is reflected by the alveolar partial pressure. The rate of induction of anaesthesia with a volatile anaesthetic agent is determined by the rate of increase in the alveolar partial pressure, which depends on the alveolar gas concentration.

Many factors determine the partial pressure of a volatile anaesthetic in tissues.

Inspired anaesthetic concentration (F_I) depends on:

- the circuit size relative to the fresh gas flow
- the fresh gas inflow rate
- solubility in tubing and soda lime.

The alveolar gas concentration (F_A) relative to the inspired anaesthetic concentration (F_A/F_I) determines the speed of induction (Table 2.1). The F_A/F_I is determined by the rate of anaesthetic delivery to the alveoli and by the rate of uptake from them.

Delivery to the alveoli is influenced by:

- alveolar ventilation, which is more pronounced with agents with higher blood gas partition coefficients (Table 2.1)
- the concentration effect of the anaesthetic remaining in the alveoli, which increases the rate of rise of the alveolar concentration
- the second gas effect, which increases the alveolar concentration of a second gas once the first gas has been taken up by the blood.

Uptake of the anaesthetic from the alveoli by the blood is influenced by:

- cardiac output; an increase in cardiac output will increase anaesthetic uptake and decrease the rate of rise in alveolar concentration
- anaesthetic solubility; increasing solubility in blood (Table 2.1) increases uptake and slows the rate of rise in F_A/F_I and in the gradient between alveolar and venous blood.

The rate of equilibration of anaesthetic partial pressure between blood and various tissues is dependent on:

- tissue blood flow, with the vessel rich group (brain, kidney, heart and liver) equilibrating rapidly since they receive approximately 75% of cardiac output
- tissue solubility (Table 2.1); highly soluble agents are slower to equilibrate
- the gradient between arterial blood and tissues; rate of uptake will decrease as the gradient decreases.

Elimination of anaesthetic agents occurs predominantly by exhalation, following the same concentration gradients by which they initially increased in reverse. To a lesser extent, the rate of recovery from anaesthesia is also influenced by metabolism. Dehalogenation and O-dealkylation are carried out by mixed function oxidases in the liver.

Table 2.2 demonstrates onset and emergence times for volatile anaesthetic agents.

Table 2.2 Volatile anaesthetics: onset and duration

Drug	Onset loss of eyelash reflex (MAC) minutes	Emergence obeys command 1 MAC + 66% N_2O minutes
Halothane	dose-dependent	dose-dependent
Enflurane	(2.4) 2.9	15.1
Desflurane	(2.5) 1.2	8.8
Isoflurane	(2) 2–3	15.6
Sevoflurane	(1.8) 1.6	14.3

Pharmacodynamics

Cardiovascular system[1]

Volatile agents produce dose-dependent:

- myocardial depression
- decrease in arterial blood pressure, due to decreased cardiac output and/or systemic vasodilatation
- attenuation of baroreceptor and vasomotor reflexes.

Table 2.3 Cardiovascular effects of volatile anaesthetics

Drug (1 MAC)	Myocardial contractility	Mean arterial pressure	Cardiac output	Systemic vascular resistance	Heart rate
Halothane	↓↓↓	↓↓	↓↓↓	↓↓	↓
Enflurane	↓↓	↓↓↓	↓↓↓	↓↓↓	0/↑
Desflurane	↓	↓	↓	↓↓	0/↑
Isoflurane	↓↓	↓↓	↓↓	↓	↑
Sevoflurane	↓	↓↓	↓↓	↓↓	0
Nitrous oxide (combined with other agent)	↓	↑	↓	↑	0

Mean arterial pressure. The mean arterial pressure is reduced by desflurane, isoflurane and sevoflurane principally through vasodilatation, and by enflurane and halothane as a consequence of depression of myocardial contractility and cardiac output. Using equipotent doses, mean arterial pressure is preserved more by desflurane than by isoflurane. However, cardiac output is preserved by isoflurane, since decreases in stroke volume are offset by increased heart rate.

Heart rate. Desflurane causes little change in heart rate at lighter levels of anaesthesia, and transient increase at deeper levels as plasma catecholamine levels increase. Enflurane also produces dose-dependent increases in heart rate. Isoflurane increases the heart rate 20% above waking levels, and independently of dose above 1 MAC. Sevoflurane has little effect on heart rate. Halothane frequently decreases the heart rate (reversible with atropine or glycopyrrolate), and suppression of sinus node activity may produce a junctional rhythm. Halothane slows conduction through the atrioventricular node and the His-Purkinje system. This increases the likelihood of re-entrant cardiac arrhythmias. Sinoatrial node conduction is depressed least by isoflurane.

Reflexes. Attenuation of the baroreceptor reflex response (tachycardia) to hypotension and of the vasomotor reflex responses (increased peripheral resistance) to hypovolaemia is produced by desflurane, enflurane, halothane and sevoflurane, but is less pronounced with isoflurane.

Contractility. Equipotent doses of isoflurane and sevoflurane produce equivalent direct decreases in myocardial contractility. However, equipotent doses of desflurane are less depressant to the myocardium.

Myocardial irritability. Sensitization of the myocardium to the effects of circulating catecholamines causing dysrhythmias is not as likely with the newer volatile agents, compared to halothane.

Coronary blood flow. Isoflurane produces intramyocardial arteriolar vasodilatation and, in the presence of reduced coronary perfusion pressure and critical location of coronary artery stenosis, could divert blood away from areas of myocardium supplied by pressure-dependent collaterals (coronary artery 'steal'). Thus, isoflurane may uncouple the normally close relationship between coronary artery blood flow and myocardial oxygen requirement more than other agents. This is only of clinical significance in doses greater than 1 MAC. Coronary artery vasodilatation does not occur with desflurane, enflurane, halothane or sevoflurane. However, there is no evidence of different outcomes for coronary artery revascularization using isoflurane compared with enflurane, halothane or sufentanil.

Central nervous system

Central nervous system effects of particular interest in vascular anaesthesia include the effects on cerebral haemodynamics and metabolism, and on neurological monitoring techniques.

Cerebral blood flow is increased in a dose-dependent fashion due to cerebral vasodilatation by desflurane, enflurane (40% increase at 1.1 MAC), sevoflurane, to a greater extent with halothane (200% increase at 1.1 MAC), and least with isoflurane.

Elevation of intracranial pressure parallels the increase in cerebral blood volume. The increase in cerebral blood flow with desflurane, halothane, isoflurane (>1.1 MAC) and sevoflurane is attenuated with time (approximately 2 hours), reflecting a return of cerebral vascular autoregulation.

Reactivity of the cerebral vasculature to carbon dioxide (i.e. ventilation producing a $Paco_2$ of 4 kPa or less decreases cerebral blood flow and intracranial pressure) is preserved with desflurane, isoflurane, and halothane, but not with enflurane.

Decreased cerebral metabolic rate is linked to electrical activity. Cerebral metabolic oxygen requirements are decreased with desflurane, isoflurane and sevoflurane (decreased EEG wave frequency and increased voltage with electrical silence at high concentrations), enflurane (decreased EEG wave frequency and increased voltage but electrical silence does not occur) and halothane (electrical silence at >3 MAC), with the greatest decrease produced by isoflurane (isoelectric EEG at 2 MAC). Enflurane produces a high voltage repetitive spiking activity at high doses. Hyperventilation combined with enflurane anaesthesia increases the risk of seizure activity, thereby increasing cerebral oxygen requirements.

Isoflurane may have a cerebral-protecting effect, by decreasing the cerebral blood flow level necessary to produce ischaemia. In addition, it maintains the relationship between cerebral blood flow and cerebral oxygen requirements.

Desflurane, isoflurane, sevoflurane and, to a lesser degree, halothane cause a dose-dependent increase in latency and a decrease in amplitude of the cortical somatosensory evoked potentials. The greatest changes, however, are seen with enflurane.

Respiratory system

Dose-dependent respiratory depression occurs with volatile agents. In spontaneously breathing patients:

- tidal volume is decreased
- respiratory rate is increased but does not compensate
- alveolar ventilation is reduced
- Pa_{CO_2} rises
- the ventilatory response to hypercapnoea is decreased
- the ventilatory response to hypoxaemia is abolished (0.1 MAC)
- the hypoxic pulmonary vasoconstrictor response is abolished.

Bronchodilator potency, produced by a direct effect, by reductions in afferent nerve traffic or by medullary depression of bronchoconstriction reflexes, is similar, with equipotent doses of volatile agents. However, airway irritability (precipitating coughing, laryngospasm and bronchospasm) may occur, particularly in light levels of anaesthesia. This is less problematic with halothane and sevoflurane.

Renal system

Renal blood flow is decreased during inhalational anaesthesia, due to a decrease in mean arterial pressure or an increase in renal vascular resistance. This is associated with a decrease in glomerular filtration rate and urine output. The metabolism of enflurane and sevoflurane produces fluoride ions, which are nephrotoxic. Although serum levels are measurable, the threshold for renal dysfunction ($>50\,\mu mol/l$) is not exceeded.

Liver

Hepatic perfusion is decreased by inhalation anaesthetics; the greatest decrease is seen with halothane.

Muscle

Potentiation of the effects of neuromuscular blocking agents by volatile anaesthetics involves desensitization of the postjunctional membrane and/or changes in muscle blood flow.

Intravenous anaesthetics

Intravenous anaesthetic agents are used as a bolus for induction of anaesthesia, or are administered by infusion for maintenance of anaesthesia.

This group of drugs includes the ultra short-acting barbiturates methohexitone and thiopentone, etomidate, propofol, benzodiazepines and ketamine.

Mechanism of action

Following administration of standard induction doses (Tables 2.4 and 2.5), the sensory cortex is depressed, motor activity is decreased, cerebellar function is altered and dose-dependent drowsiness, sedation and hypnosis occur. Proposed theories for the mechanism of action of these drugs are biophysical, involving action on cell membranes or transmitter theories describing interaction with neurotransmitters.

Table 2.4 Doses of intravenous anaesthetic agents

	Induction dose (mg/kg)	Infusion (mg/kg per min)
Thiopentone (2.5%)	3–5	
Etomidate	0.2–0.3	
Propofol (1%)	1.5–2.5	0.1
Ketamine	1–2	
Methohexitone (1%)	1–1.5	0.1–0.3

Table 2.5 Intravenous anaesthetic agents

Drug	Induction (seconds)	Redistribution $T_{1/2\alpha}$ (minutes)	Elimination $T_{1/2\alpha}$ (hours)
Thiopentone	30	2–5	12
Etomidate	30	2–4	3
Propofol	30–45	2–4	4
Ketamine	30	10–15	3
Methohexitone	30	2–5	4
Midazolam	2–3		2–4

Modification of inhibitory gamma aminobutyric acid (GABA) transmission may be important in actions of barbiturates, benzodiazepines and etomidate. Barbiturates bind to a receptor that decreases the rate of dissociation of GABA from its receptors, thereby increasing the duration of GABA-activated chloride ion channel opening and hyper-polarization (inhibition) of the postsynaptic neurone. Benzodiazepines bind to a receptor that facilitates the action of GABA at its receptors, thereby increasing the frequency of chloride channel openings produced by GABA. Etomidate increases the number of available GABA receptors. The mechanism of action of ketamine may be due to effects on noradrenaline, serotonin and acetylcholine receptors and/or M-methyl aspartate receptor antagonism.

Pharmacokinetics

Speed of induction with intravenous anaesthetic agents depends on:

- the speed of injection
- the volume of distribution
- cardiac output.

Most of the agents (except ketamine and benzodiazepines) act in one arm–brain circulation time. Onset of unconsciousness is facilitated by prior administration of opioids, and delayed by slow circulation times. The duration of action of these agents is approximately 3–5 minutes.

Termination of the effects of intravenous anaesthetic agents depends on:

- redistribution, and
- clearance.

Elimination half-time ($T_{1/2\beta}$) of intravenous anaesthetic agents is directly dependent on the volume of distribution, and inversely related to clearance.

Termination of the hypnotic action of an induction dose of intravenous anaesthetic is determined by redistribution ($T_{1/2\alpha}$) of the drug to inactive tissue sites. This rapidly reduces plasma drug concentration and the concentration at active receptors. Subsequently, clearance is the dominant influence on the plasma drug concentration and termination of drug effect.

Greater hepatic clearance contributes to a shorter duration of action if repeated doses are administered. However, if multiple doses or infusions saturate inactive tissue sites, the redistribution phase becomes more important in the termination of drug effect. Reduced hepatic blood flow or metabolism caused by volatile anaesthetic agents could delay clearance and prolong the elimination half-time of large or repeated doses of the intravenous agents that are most dependent on hepatic extraction (etomidate, methohexitone). Redistribution is of less significance with benzodiazepines compared with the other intravenous agents.

Elderly patients require lower induction doses of intravenous agents due to slow passage into peripheral compartments or altered distribution of cardiac output.

Time to recovery is fastest with propofol, followed by methohexitone, etomidate, thiopentone benzodiazepines and ketamine.

Pharmacodynamics

Central nervous system

Cerebral blood flow, cerebral metabolic oxygen requirements and intracranial pressure are reduced by intravenous agents. These responses may be helpful in the management of patients requiring neurological protection, e.g. those undergoing carotid endarterectomy.

Cerebral perfusion pressure (the balance between mean arterial pressure and intracranial pressure) is maintained with etomidate and barbiturates, but may be decreased by propofol as a result of mean arterial pressure reduction.

Etomidate and barbiturates in low doses produce an increase in the alpha activity amplitude of the EEG, followed by a progressive decrease in activity and burst suppression at high doses. Thiopentone (8 mg/kg) and etomidate (> 0.3 mg/kg) produce maximum decreases in cerebral oxygen requirements (flat EEG). These doses are associated with a reduction in infarct size in patients with cerebral emboli and temporary focal ischaemia. Conversely, ketamine increases cerebral blood flow, metabolic rate and intracranial pressure, and increases EEG activity (except beta waves). High-dose methohexitone is associated with refractory seizures.

Effects on neurological monitoring may influence the management of patients undergoing vascular surgical procedures. Low doses of thiopentone do not affect somatosensory evoked potentials; higher doses cause depression of non-specific late latency waves. Etomidate can alter the waveforms to mimic ischaemia. Maintenance doses of propofol produce dose-dependent decreases in the amplitude.

These agents do not produce analgesia (except ketamine), and may be hyperalgesic in low doses (barbiturates).

Cardiovascular system

In general, intravenous agents (except ketamine) have depressant effects on the cardiovascular system, reducing mean arterial pressure, cardiac output, systemic vascular resistance and coronary perfusion pressure and causing venodilation (Table 2.6). Hypotensive effects are exaggerated by hypovolaemia.

Etomidate (0.2–0.3 mg/kg) produces the least detrimental cardiovascular changes (minimal effects on myocardial function, cardiac output and peripheral or pulmonary circulation), and may be considered for induction of anaesthesia in hypovolaemic patients or in patients who are potentially haemodynamically unstable.

Propofol (1.5–2.5 mg/kg) produces similar hypotensive effects to thiopentone (3–5 mg/kg).

Ketamine increases the heart rate and systemic and pulmonary artery pressures, and is sometimes used for these sympathomimetic effects in haemodynamically compromised patients (but not those with coronary artery disease). However, myocardial depression may still occur in combination with hypovolaemia, autonomic block and maximum sympathetic stimulation.

Benzodiazepines produce a mild systemic vasodilatation and reduction in cardiac output without changes in heart rate.

The predominant effect of barbiturates such as thiopentone is to reduce cardiac output by:

- myocardial depression
- decreased venous return
- decreased sympathetic outflow.

Heart rate increases with thiopentone induction due to baroreceptor reflex activity. This can be blunted by volatile agents and/or beta agonist medication, thereby exaggerating the myocardial depressant effect.

Table 2.6 Cardiovascular effects of intravenous anaesthetics

Drug (induction dose)	Mean arterial pressure	Cardiac output	Systemic vascular resistance	Heart rate
Thiopentone	↓	↓	0	↑
Etomidate	0	0	0	0
Propofol	↓	0	↓	0/↑
Ketamine	↑↑	↑	↑	↑↑
Methohexitone	↓	↓	↑↑	

Respiratory system

Depression of ventilation characterizes all the intravenous induction agents, and apnoea commonly occurs after administration. Increased airway irritability (asthma, smoking) may lead to bronchoconstriction if the airway is instrumented during light anaesthesia with these agents. Conversely, ketamine causes bronchodilation due to its sympathomimetic effects, but it also increases oral secretions, which may require an antisialagogue.

Liver and kidney

The liver and kidney are indirectly affected due to decreased blood pressure causing decreased hepatic blood flow and urinary output.

Endocrine system

Etomidate decreases the adrenocortical response to stress for up to 8 hours after the induction of anaesthesia. Following induction doses of thiopentone and propofol, plasma cortisol levels are decreased due to adrenal cortical suppression; however, this effect is transient.

Adrenergic agonists

Adrenergic agonists include inotropic drugs[2] (catecholamines) and vasopressor drugs (sympathomimetics). Most of the adrenergic drugs activate both alpha and beta receptors. The dominant effect is due to the combination of receptor activation (Table 2.7). Side-effects reflect excessive alpha or beta activity.

Haemodynamic effects produced by the adrenergic agonists include effects on

- heart rate (chronotropism)
- cardiac output (inotropism)
- conduction velocity of the cardiac impulse
- cardiac rhythm

Table 2.7 Adrenergic agonists: sites of action

Drug	Alpha₁ (arterial)	Alpha₂ (venous)	Beta₁	Beta₂	Dopamine₁	Bolus dose
Adrenaline	+++	+++	++++	++++	0	2–8 µg
Dopamine	+	++++	+++	++++	+++++	
Dobutamine		?	++++	++	0	
Dopexamine				++++	++++	
Ephedrine	++	+++	+++	++	0	3–9 mg
Methoxamine	++++		0	0	0	5–10 mg
Phenylephrine	++++	+++++	0	0	0	50–100 µg
Noradrenaline	+++	+++	0	0	0	
Clonidine	+++					

- systemic vascular resistance
- venous capacitance (venous return).

Adrenaline

Dose:

- as a continuous infusion to improve cardiac output, 0.1–1.0 µg/kg per min
- to check for intravascular administration of epidural test dose, 2–3 ml of 1:200 000 concentration added to local anaesthetic; increase in heart rate (>10 beats per minute) occurs within 45 seconds if administered intravascularly
- to prolong regional anaesthesia, 0.2 mg added to local anaesthetic for spinal block, 1:200 000 concentration for epidural block
- during cardiac arrest, 1–10 mg i.v.
- for allergic reactions. 0.1–0.5 mg
- as a bronchodilator, 10 mg in 3 ml normal saline by nebulizer 2–6-hourly.

Onset of action: 30–60 seconds i.v.
Peak effect: within 3 minutes i.v.
Duration of action: 5–10 minutes i.v.
Elimination: hepatic, renal and gastrointestinal enzymatic degradation

Adrenaline is an endogenous catecholamine with both alpha and beta effects. At therapeutic doses beta effects predominate, producing increased myocardial contractility and heart rate, bronchodilation, increased skeletal muscle blood flow and decreased total peripheral resistance. Alpha effects are more evident in the renal and cutaneous vasculature, resulting in decreased blood flow. Alpha₂ effects include a decrease in onset time and increase in duration of local anaesthetic effects and analgesic effects at the spinal cord.

Interaction/toxicity: enhanced effect with tricyclic antidepressants and bretylium, excess beta stimulation may induce arrhythmias if the myocardium is sensitized by volatile anaesthetics (especially halothane) or digitalis, decreased renal blood flow.

Adverse reactions: hypertension, pulmonary oedema, hyperglycaemia, transient potassium shifts.

Dopamine

Dopamine, a naturally occurring catecholamine, acts directly on alpha, $beta_1$ and dopaminergic receptors (Table 2.7), and indirectly by releasing noradrenaline.

Dose:

Low doses, 1–3 µg/kg per min, produce dopaminergic effects:

- increased renal, mesenteric, coronary and cerebral blood flow
- increased glomerular filtration rate
- increased sodium excretion.

3–10 µg/kg per min stimulates $beta_1$ receptors, causing:

- increased myocardial contractility
- increased stroke volume and cardiac output.

> 10 µg/kg per min stimulates alpha receptors, causing:

- increased peripheral resistance
- decreased renal blood flow
- increased arrhythmia risk
- increased pulmonary artery pressure.

Onset of action: 2–4 minutes
Peak effect: 2–10 minutes
Duration of action: < 10 minutes
Elimination: hepatic

Interaction/toxicity: seizures, hypotension and bradycardia with concomitant use of phenytoin, increased risk of ventricular and supraventricular arrhythmias with volatile anaesthetics.

Adverse effects: angina, arrhythmias (infrequent), hypertension, risk of ischaemia with occlusive vascular disease (e.g. Raynaud's disease), contra-indicated in right heart failure as pulmonary artery pressure is increased, hyperglycaemia due to inhibition of insulin release, nausea and vomiting.

Dobutamine

Dose: 0.5–15 µg/kg per min continuous infusion
Onset of action: 1–2 minutes
Peak effect: 1–10 minutes
Duration of action: < 10 minutes
Elimination: hepatic

Dobutamine, a synthetic beta$_1$-adrenergic agonist derived from isoprenaline, increases myocardial rate and force of contraction. Systolic blood pressure may be increased as a result of increased cardiac output. However, effects on heart rate and systemic vascular resistance are less than with isoprenaline, and dobutamine is therefore used clinically to improve cardiac output in patients with poor myocardial contractility. Atrioventricular conduction is augmented (a rapid ventricular response may be precipitated with atrial fibrillation), but the arrhythmogenic effects are less than that of dopamine, isoprenaline or the catecholamines. In therapeutic doses it also has mild beta$_2$- and alpha$_1$-adrenergic agonist effects, and decreases peripheral and pulmonary vascular resistance. Higher cardiac output and lower pulmonary artery occlusion pressure result if dobutamine is combined with nitroprusside administration.

Interaction/toxicity: increased risk of arrhythmias with bretylium and with volatile anaesthetics, caution in patients with atrial fibrillation.

Dopexamine[3]

Dose: 500 ng/kg per min i.v. infusion, increased at 15-minute intervals by 1 µg/kg per min to maximum of 6 µg/kg per min
Onset of action: 1–2 minutes
Peak effect: 1–10 minutes
Duration of action: 6–11 minutes
Elimination: hepatic

Dopexamine, a synthetic analogue of dobutamine, acts on beta$_2$ receptors in cardiac muscle to produce positive inotropic effects and on peripheral dopamine receptors to increase renal and gastrointestinal blood flow. It also indirectly activates beta$_1$ receptors by noradrenaline actions (due to baroreflex activation and neuronal uptake inhibition). Dopexamine is primarily a vasodilator. Heart rate and cardiac output are increased and systemic vascular resistance is decreased, with little change in mean arterial pressure, preload, or pulmonary artery pressure. Dopexamine has less arrhythmogenic risk than dopamine or dobutamine, and may help preserve renal and gastrointestinal function after ischaemia.

Adverse effects: tachycardia, arrhythmias, vomiting, tremor.

Ephedrine

Dose: 100–200 µg/kg i.v., approximately 3–9 mg
Onset of action: immediate
Peak effect: 2–5 minutes
Duration of action: 10–60 minutes
Elimination: hepatic and renal

Ephedrine, a noncatecholamine sympathomimetic with mixed direct and indirect actions, is administered intravenously as a bolus for its vasopressor effects (venoconstriction is greater than arterial vasoconstriction). It is, however, much less potent than adrenaline, with a longer duration of action.

Effects include increases in cardiac output, arterial pressure and heart rate by alpha- and beta-adrenergic stimulation, and increases in coronary artery blood flow and bronchodilation by beta$_2$ receptor stimulation. Ephedrine is resistant to metabolism by monoamine oxidases and catechol-O-methyl transferases, resulting in a duration of action of 10 minutes or longer.

Interaction/toxicity: increases MAC of volatile anaesthetics, potentiated by tricyclic antidepressants.

Adverse effects: central nervous system stimulation, pulmonary oedema, hyperglycaemia, transient hyperkalaemia and hypokalaemia.

Isoprenaline

Dose: 2–20 µg/kg per min i.v. infusion
Onset of action: immediate
Peak effect: 1 minute
Duration of action: 1–5 minutes
Elimination: hepatic

Isoprenaline is a synthetic sympathomimetic amine, related to adrenaline, but it acts exclusively on beta$_1$- and beta$_2$-adrenergic receptors. It produces inotropic and chronotropic effects, decreases systemic and pulmonary vascular resistance, and increases coronary and renal blood flow in addition to bronchodilation. Cardiac output is increased due to the increase in heart rate and in contractility, whereas myocardial oxygen delivery may be concomitantly reduced due to vasodilatation and decreased diastolic blood pressure (decreased coronary perfusion pressure). It is administered by intravenous infusion for treatment of bradyarrhythmias, long Q-T syndrome, carotid sinus hypersensitivity, heart block and pulmonary hypertension.

Interaction/toxicity: arrhythmias with other sympathomimetics and volatile anaesthetics.

Adverse effects: exacerbation of myocardial ischaemia and hypotension, paradoxic bronchoconstriction, pulmonary oedema.

Phenylephrine

Dose: 0.15–4 µg/kg per min infusion, or 50 –100 µg i.v. bolus
Onset of action: < 1 minute
Peak effect: 1 minute
Duration of action: 15–20 minutes
Elimination: hepatic

Phenylephrine activates alpha-adrenergic receptors with virtually no beta activation, producing intense peripheral vasoconstriction (greater veno-constriction than arterial constriction), increased venous return, increased systolic and diastolic blood pressure and reflex bradycardia. It is used for treatment of hypotension, including that associated with regional anaesthesia. Renal, splanchnic and cutaneous blood flows are reduced, but coronary blood flow is increased in response to increased myocardial work. Pulmonary artery pressure is increased. Phenylephrine in clinical doses does not have significant effects on cerebral vascular resistance, cerebral blood flow or intracranial pressure. Cerebral perfusion pressure is increased when phenyl-ephrine is used to treat hypotension.

Interaction/toxicity: potentiation of pressor effects with monoamine oxidase inhibitors, tricyclic antidepressants, bretylium, other sympatho-mimetics.

Adverse effects: bradycardia, acute pulmonary oedema, risk of myocardial ischaemia in patients with coronary artery disease, renal hypoperfusion, hepatic necrosis, nausea.

Methoxamine

Dose: 1–5 mg i.v.
Onset of action: immediate
Peak effect: 0.5–2 minutes
Duration of action: 15–60 minutes
Elimination: hepatic

Methoxamine is a selective alpha$_1$ receptor agonist, causing a rapid increase in arterial pressure by increasing peripheral resistance. The duration of action is prolonged because methoxamine is not metabolized by monoamine oxidase inhibitors and is already O-methylated, and therefore cannot be inactivated by catechol-O-methyl transferase. Methoxamine has no direct cardiac effects, but reflex bradycardia may occur due to increased arterial pressures. A reduction in cardiac output may occur in response to increased afterload in patients with cardiac dysfunction.

Interaction/toxicity: potentiation of pressor effects with other sympathomi-metics, monoamine oxidase inhibitors and tricyclic antidepressants, risk of cardiac arrhythmias with volatile anaesthetics, severe hypertension with beta blocking agents.

Adverse effects: bradycardia, hypertension, respiratory distress, seizures.

Metaraminol

Dose: 0.01 mg/kg i.v., approximately 0.5–5 mg
Onset of action: 1–2 minutes
Peak effect: > 2 minutes
Duration of action: 20–90 minutes
Elimination: tissue uptake, renal

Metaraminol, a potent sympathomimetic, acts directly on alpha-adrenergic receptors and on beta$_1$ receptors in the heart (but has no effect on beta$_2$ receptors), and also acts indirectly by release of noradrenaline from storage sites. Prolonged infusions may cause depletion of noradrenaline from sympathetic nerve endings. Overall, alpha effects are greater than beta effects. Intense vasoconstriction causes an increase in arterial blood pressure and reflex bradycardia, which may reduce cardiac output. Coronary blood flow is increased, while renal, cutaneous and splanchnic flows are reduced. Pulmonary artery pressure is elevated. Metaraminol has no effect on cerebral vascular resistance or cerebral blood flow, but may increase cerebral perfusion pressure in hypotensive patients.

Interaction/toxicity: potentiation of pressor effects with other sympathomimetics, monoamine oxidase inhibitors and bretylium, decreased pressor effects with tricyclic antidepressants.

Adverse effects: reflex bradycardia, hypotension with prolonged infusion, acute pulmonary oedema, renal hypoperfusion, hepatic necrosis, nausea.

Noradrenaline

Dose: 0.04–0.4 µg/kg per min
Onset of action: < 1 minute
Peak effect: 1–2 minutes
Duration of action: 2–10 minutes
Elimination: enzymatic degradation, pulmonary

Noradrenaline, a catecholamine which stimulates alpha-adrenergic and beta$_1$-adrenergic receptors, is less potent than adrenaline and isoprenaline. It has no beta$_2$ effects. Arterial blood pressure and coronary artery blood flow are increased, and renal, hepatic, cerebral and muscle blood flow are reduced. Cardiac output increases in patients with hypotension when blood pressure increases to optimal levels. Conversely, increased baroreceptor activity may reduce heart rate and cardiac output.

Interaction/toxicity: arrhythmia risk with volatile anaesthetics, bretylium, hypoxia and hypercarbia, pulmonary extraction is decreased by halothane and nitrous oxide, pressor effects potentiated by monoamine oxidase inhibitors and tricyclic antidepressants.

Adverse effects: bradycardia, tachyarrhythmias, hypertension.

Nonadrenergic sympathomimetics

Nonadrenergic sympathomimetics are substances other than catecholamines that increase intracellular cyclic adenosine monophosphate (cAMP) in myocardial cells, either by stimulating adenyl cyclase via receptors or by inhibiting phosphodiesterase enzymes (which normally degrade cAMP). The adenyl cyclase stimulators include glucagon, histamine, forskolin and the cAMP analogue dibutyryl-cAMP. Phosphodiesterase inhibitors include the methylxanthine, theophylline, the bipyridine derivatives, amrinone[4] and milrinone[5], and the imidazolone derivatives, enoximone[6] and piroximone. The more commonly used drugs are discussed below.

Aminophylline

Dose: 5–6 mg/kg i.v. over 20 minutes, then 0.5–1 µg/kg per min infusion (decreased doses in the elderly, in cor pulmonale or in congestive heart failure)
Onset of action: 2–3 minutes
Peak effect: 1 hour
Duration of action: 4–8 hours
Elimination: hepatic

Aminophylline is converted to theophylline, a methylxanthine which exerts its effects by inhibiting phosphodiesterase (thereby increasing the levels of intracellular cAMP), blocking adenosine receptors, antagonizing prostaglandin E_2, stimulating endogenous catecholamine synthesis and release, or by a direct effect in reducing intracellular calcium re-uptake.

Aminophylline is used to treat bronchospasm associated with asthma and chronic obstructive pulmonary disease, as a renal protective agent in patients undergoing angiographic examinations, and in the treatment of postdural puncture headache. Each 0.5 mg/kg of theophylline (from 0.6 mg/kg aminophylline) will increase serum levels by 1 µg/ml. Theophylline increases cardiac output, decreases peripheral resistance and reduces diaphragmatic fatigue. The effects on postdural puncture headache may be due to blockade of adenosine receptors and increases in intracellular cAMP in the choroid plexus, thereby enhancing cerebrospinal fluid secretion.

Interaction/toxicity: increased serum levels with cimetidine, beta blockers, erythromycin, oral contraceptives, cardiac failure and liver dysfunction, decreased serum levels with phenytoin and in smokers, potentiated effect of sympathomimetics, arrhythmia risk with volatile anaesthetic agents (especially halothane), seizures with high plasma levels.

Adverse effects: sinus tachycardia, ventricular arrhythmias, nausea and vomiting, hyperglycaemia, inappropriate antidiuretic hormone secretion.

Amrinone

Dose: 0.75 mg/kg i.v., 2–20 µg/kg per min infusion
Onset of action: 5 minutes
Peak effect: 10 minutes
Duration of action: 30 minutes–1 hour
Elimination: renal, hepatic

Amrinone is a bipyridine derivative inotropic agent that inhibits the myocardial specific phosphodiesterase (F.III), thereby increasing intracellular cAMP, which potentiates delivery of calcium ions to the myocardial contractile system. The net result is a dose-dependent positive inotropic effect. Peripheral vasodilatation occurs, which may reduce arterial pressure. The combined inotropic and vasodilator effects produce an increase in cardiac output in congestive heart failure. Response to amrinone occurs even with alpha and beta blockade or depletion of catecholamines.

Interaction/toxicity: potentiates responses to catecholamines and theophylline.

Adverse effects: hypotension, thrombocytopaenia, hepatic dysfunction.

Enoximone

Dose: 0.5–1.0 mg/kg over 5–10 minutes, then 5–20 µg/kg per min
Onset of action: 5 minutes
Peak effect: 10 minutes
Duration of action: 30 minutes–2 hours, possible sustained benefit after administration ceases
Elimination: renal, hepatic

Enoximone is an imidazolone derivative, which acts as a positive inotropic agent by increasing cAMP in myocardial cells due to inhibition of phophodiesterase. Effects include an increase in cardiac output and decrease in filling pressures and systemic vascular resistance without major heart rate or arterial pressure alteration, i.e. with minimal increases in myocardial oxygen demand. Enoximone is rapidly metabolized, but the metabolite is active and therefore its cardiovascular effects may persist for some hours.

Interaction/toxicity: risk of ventricular tachycardia or supraventricular arrhythmias (especially in patients with pre-existing arrhythmias), potentiation of effects with renal impairment, relatively contraindicated in hypertrophic cardiomyopathy, stenotic valvular disease or other outlet obstruction.

Adverse effects: hypotension, limb pain, urinary retention.

Milrinone

Dose: 50 µg/kg over 10 minutes, then 375–750 ng/kg per min
Onset of action: 5 minutes
Peak effect: 10 minutes
Duration of action: 30 minutes–1 hour, sustained benefit after administration ceases
Elimination: renal, hepatic

Milrinone, a bipyridine derivative that is more potent than amrinone, increases intracellular cAMP levels by phosphodiesterase inhibition. This results in a marked increase in cardiac output and substantial reductions in filling pressures and systemic vascular resistance, with little change in heart rate or arterial pressure. The inotropic and vasodilator effects occur without adverse effects on the myocardial oxygen demand–supply ratio, and with a lower incidence of side-effects compared to amrinone. Clinical use of milrinone is, in the short term, for treatment of congestive heart failure that is unresponsive to conventional therapy or in acute heart failure. Because of its potent vasodilator effects, its use is precluded in circulatory failure associated with peripheral vasodilatation.

Interaction/toxicity: risk of ventricular tachycardia or supraventricular arrhythmias, potentiation of effects with renal impairment and with hypokalaemia.

Adverse effects: hypotension, nausea and vomiting, diarrhoea, limb pain.

Digoxin

Dose: 0.5–1 mg i.v. in divided doses over 24 hours
Onset of action: 5–30 minutes
Peak effect: 1–4 hours
Duration of action: 3–4 days
Elimination: renal

Digoxin is a cardiac glycoside composed of a sugar and a cardenolide. Direct inotropic action occurs due to inhibition of the sodium–potassium adenosine triphosphatase ion transport system. Myocardial contractility is increased and myocardial oxygen requirements are reduced in the failing heart. An indirect vagomimetic effect also occurs, causing decreased sinoatrial node activity and delayed conduction through the atrioventricular node (Class V anti-arrhythmic, Table 2.9). Digoxin is used in the treatment of supraventricular arrhythmias and as an inotrope in cardiac failure. The therapeutic level is 0.5–2 ng/ml.

Interaction/toxicity: enhanced toxicity in hypokalaemia, hypomagnesae-mia, hypercalcaemia; increased serum levels with calcium channel blockers, esmolol, amiodarone, captopril, benzodiazepines, anticholinergics, erythro-mycin; suxamethonium may cause arrhythmias in digitalized patients, excess serum level may cause atrioventricular block, ventricular tachycardia or ventricular fibrillation.

Alpha antagonists

Alpha blocking drugs are used in the chronic treatment of hypertension and benign prostatic hypertrophy (doxazosin, indoramin, terazosin), in the preoperative preparation of patients with phaeochromocytoma (prazosin, phenoxybenzamine), in Raynaud's syndrome (prazosin) and, occasionally, for intraoperative control of hypertension (phenoxybenzamine, phento-lamine).

Patients taking the oral medications doxazosin, indoramin, prazosin and terazosin are at increased risk of hypotension on induction of anaesthesia. Other adverse effects include neurological symptoms such as extra pyramidal effects, increased incidence of nausea and vomiting and increased somno-lence, all of which may significantly impact on recovery from anaesthesia.

Prazosin is a selective postsynaptic alpha$_1$ antagonist. Therefore the negative feedback for noradrenaline release mediated by presynaptic alpha$_2$ activity remains intact, and prazosin does not cause tachycardia.

The intravenous preparations phentolamine and phenoxybenzamine are occasionally used in the perioperative treatment of hypertension, but more often in the management of phaeochromocytoma or hypertensive crises resulting from excess sympathomimetics or monoamine oxidase inhibition.

Phentolamine

Dose: 0.05–0.1 mg/kg i.v. (approximately 2.5–5 mg); 10–20 µg/kg per min infusion
Onset of action: 1–2 minutes
Peak effect: 2 minutes
Duration of action: 10–15 minutes
Elimination: hepatic, renal

Phentolamine is an imidazoline which blocks peripheral alpha$_1$ receptors (producing vasodilatation) and presynaptic alpha$_2$ receptors (causing enhanced neuronal release of noradrenaline from adrenergic neurones). This may enhance the beta stimulant effects of phentolamine producing inotropic and chronotropic effects. Overall, effects on arterial pressure depend on the relative contribution of the vasodilating and cardiac stimulating effects. At usual doses the vasodilating effects predominate, decreasing blood pressure and masking the inotropic effects. Pulmonary vascular resistance and pulmonary artery pressure are decreased. Cerebral blood flow is generally maintained; however, cerebrovascular spasm may occur. Hypotension caused by phentolamine must be treated with noradrenaline.

Interaction/toxicity: potentiation of the beta$_2$ vasodilating effects of adrenaline, ephedrine, dobutamine and isoprenaline.

Adverse effects: prolonged hypotension, myocardial ischaemia risk, cerebrovascular occlusion.

Phenoxybenzamine

Dose: 1 mg/kg over 2 hours
Onset of action: 2–3 minutes
Duration of action: 24 hours
Elimination: renal

Phenoxybenzamine is a powerful alpha blocker, causing a marked decrease in arterial blood pressure and a compensatory tachycardia.

Interaction/toxicity: prolonged duration of effect with renal impairment, contact hypersensitivity.

Adverse effects: myocardial ischaemia risk with coronary artery disease, contraindicated in patients with porphyria, cerebrovascular disease and following myocardial infarction.

Beta antagonists

Beta antagonists block the beta adrenoceptors in the heart, peripheral vasculature, bronchi, pancreas and liver. In addition, baroreceptor reflex sensitivity is altered, and some beta blockers decrease renin secretion. Myocardial contractility, heart rate and blood pressure are decreased, reducing myocardial oxygen requirements. Beta blockers may cause more severe myocardial depression and precipitate cardiac failure. Antiarrhythmic effects occur due to attenuation of the effects of the sympathetic stimulation on automaticity and conduction in the heart.

Beta antagonists are distinguished by differing pharmacokinetic (beta$_1$ selectivity, lipid or water solubility) and pharmacodynamic (membrane stabilizing activity, intrinsic sympathomimetic activity, vasodilating action) characteristics.

Intrinsic sympathomimetic activity (oxprenolol, pindolol, acebutolol, celiprolol) is the capacity to stimulate some adrenoceptors, causing less bradycardia and less extremity coldness.

Water soluble beta blockers (atenolol, celiprolol, nadolol, sotalol) are less likely to enter the brain and cause sleep disturbance, but also have the most tendency to accumulate in renal impairment.

Beta$_1$ selectivity, i.e. cardioselectivity (atenolol, betaxolol, bisprolol, metoprolol, acebutolol), confers greater safety in patients with obstructive airways disease, diabetes and peripheral vascular disease, as beta$_2$ activity is maintained.

Arteriolar vasodilatation occurs with some beta blockers (celiprolol, carvedilol), causing a decrease in peripheral resistance.

Beta-adrenergic blocking agents are used:

- to treat hypertension
- to prevent the hypertensive response to intubation and extubation
- as anti-anginal therapy (by decreasing cardiac work and therefore myocardial oxygen consumption)
- following acute myocardial infarction in selected patients (atenolol and metoprolol)
- as antiarrhythmics (by reducing sympathetic activity and by decreasing automaticity and conduction velocity) to control the ventricular response in atrial fibrillation, and in the treatment of supraventricular tachycardia and ventricular tachycardia (sotalol)
- to treat anxiety
- as migraine prophylaxis (inhibition of arteriolar spasm in pial vessels)
- in the preoperative preparation of patients with thyrotoxicosis and phaeochromocytoma.

Side-effects include heart block, worsening of congestive heart failure, bronchospasm, coronary artery vasoconstriction and inhibition of insulin release. Excessive sympathetic activity may occur following abrupt withdrawal, reflecting up-regulation of beta receptors due to chronic suppression. Generally beta blocker therapy is avoided in patients with bronchospastic disease, or a cardioselective agent is used with caution.

Most of these agents are administered orally as maintenance therapy. In the past, concern about additive depressant effects of the anaesthetic technique and beta blocking agents led to discontinuation of therapy in the preoperative period. Now, however, these drugs are usually continued during the perioperative period, since the combination of anaesthesia and beta blockade does not produce excessive depression of the non-failing heart. In addition, beta blockers may protect the ischaemia-prone myocardium, and withdrawal may produce arrhythmias, angina and myocardial infarction[7,8].

The beta blocking agents most commonly used in the perioperative period (usually intravenously), as well as the mixed antagonist labetalol, are considered below.

Atenolol

Dose: 5 mg over 5 minutes i.v., 5 mg 10 minutes later, 150 µg/kg infusion over 20 minutes, repeated 12-hourly, 50–200 mg p.o.
Onset of action: < 5 minutes i.v., < 1 hour p.o.
Peak effect: 5 minutes i.v., 2–4 hours p.o.
Duration of action: 12 hours i.v., 24 hours p.o.
Elimination: renal

Atenolol is a cardioselective (not cardiospecific) beta blocker, without membrane stabilizing or intrinsic sympathomimetic properties. However, in high doses the drug blocks beta$_1$ and beta$_2$ receptors. It is occasionally administered some hours prior to anaesthesia, to attenuate haemodynamic responses during induction of anaesthesia and during the perioperative period[9].

Interaction/toxicity: potentiation of hypotension by volatile anaesthetics and calcium channel blockers, prolonged elevation of plasma potassium after suxamethonium administration.

Adverse effects: hypotension, bradyarrhythmias, bronchospasm, nausea and vomiting, pancreatitis, thrombocytopaenic purpura, arthralgia.

Esmolol

Dose: 500 µg/kg i.v., 50–200 µg/kg per min infusion
Onset of action: 1–2 minutes
Peak effect: 5 minutes
Duration of action: 3–10 minutes
Elimination: esterases (cytosol of red blood cells)

Esmolol is a cardioselective beta blocker with a rapid onset and short duration of action. At high doses, selectivity is reduced and inhibition of beta$_2$ receptors in bronchial and vascular smooth muscle occurs.

Interaction/toxicity: potentiation of myocardial depression with volatile and intravenous anaesthetics, increases serum levels of digoxin, esmolol levels are increased with concomitant use of morphine and warfarin, prolongs suxamethonium neuromuscular blockade and may enhance actions of nondepolarizing neuromuscular blockers.

Adverse effects: confusion, depression, nausea and vomiting, cutaneous erythema.

Labetalol

Dose: 0.25 mg/kg over 2 minutes i.v., 0.5–2 mg per min infusion to a maximum dose of 4 mg/kg
Onset of action: 2–5 minutes
Peak effect: 5–15 minutes
Duration of action: 2–4 hours
Elimination: hepatic, urine and faeces

Labetalol is an adrenergic blocking agent with mild alpha$_1$ and predominant beta-adrenergic receptor blocking actions (alpha:beta blockade ratio, 1:7). A dose-dependent decrease in blood pressure occurs without profound decrease in heart rate or reflex tachycardia.

Interaction/toxicity: bioavailability is increased by cimetidine, blunts reflex tachycardia caused by nitroglycerin, potentiated by volatile anaesthetics.

Adverse effects: headache, drowsiness, tremor, cholestasis.

Metoprolol

Dose: 15 mg i.v. (5 mg over 2 minutes × 3)
Onset of action: immediate
Peak effect: 20 minutes
Duration of action: 5–8 hours
Elimination: hepatic

Metoprolol is a cardioselective beta blocker, which can inhibit $beta_2$ receptors in high doses. The antihypertensive effects may be due to a combination of reduction in cardiac output, decreased renin release and a central action.

Interaction/toxicity: potentiation of hypotensive effects by volatile anaesthetics, potentiation of all muscle relaxants, increased serum levels of digoxin and morphine.

Adverse effects: pancreatitis, nausea and vomiting, bronchospasm.

Propranolol

Dose: 10–30 µg/kg every 2 minutes to a maximum of 10 mg
Onset of action: <2 minutes
Peak effect: within 1 minute
Duration of action: 1–6 hours
Elimination: hepatic, pulmonary

Propranolol is a non-selective beta blocker without intrinsic sympathomimetic activity. Decreases in heart rate and cardiac output ($beta_1$ block) are greater if sympathetic nervous system activity is increased at the time of administration. $Beta_2$ receptor blockade may increase peripheral and coronary vascular resistance.

Interaction/toxicity: potentiation of hypotension by inhaled and intravenous anaesthetics and calcium channel blockers, antagonizes sympathomimetic cardiac stimulation and bronchodilation, potentiation of vasoconstriction by ephedrine, increased serum levels with concomitant use of chlorpromazine and cimetidine, increased serum levels with enzyme inducers (e.g. barbiturates), potentiation of digoxin, all muscle relaxants, hypoglycaemia.

Adverse effects: congestive heart failure, AV block, bronchoconstriction, disorientation, nausea and vomiting, mesenteric thrombosis, agranulocytosis, thrombocytopaenic purpura.

Vasodilators

Vasodilators[2] decrease arterial blood pressure by dose-related direct effects on vascular smooth muscle independent of alpha or beta receptors. These drugs frequently produce baroreceptor-mediated tachycardia, and combination with a beta antagonist may be required.

Sodium nitroprusside

Dose: 0.25–5 µg/kg per min
Onset of action: 30–60 seconds
Peak effect: 1–2 minutes
Duration of action: 1–10 minutes
Elimination: hepatic (rhodanase)

Sodium nitroprusside is a potent peripheral vasodilator, which acts on arterial and venous smooth muscle. This may result from generation of nitric oxide. Baroreceptor-mediated reflex tachycardia is activated in response to the decrease in arterial blood pressure. Pulmonary ventilation:perfusion ratios may be altered by nitroprusside (increased shunt). Cerebral blood flow is increased. Nitroprusside is metabolized to cyanide, which is converted to thiocyanate by liver rhodanase, a slow rate limiting process. Some thiocyanate combines with vitamin B_{12} to form cyanocobalamin. Tachyphylaxis occurs due to secretion of renin and increased angiotensin II formation.

   Interaction/toxicity: increased cyanide toxicity risk in B_{12} deficiency, cyanide toxicity causes elevated mixed venous Po_2 (cellular hypoxia when cyanide binds to cytochrome oxidase) and metabolic acidosis, potentiation of hypotension by anaesthetics and other antihypertensives, thiocyanate toxicity (>10 mg per 100 ml) produces muscle weakness, confusion and hypothyroidism.

   Treatment of cyanide toxicity comprises B_{12} administration (1 g per 50 mg nitroprusside) over 30 seconds, sodium nitrite 5 mg/kg to convert haemoglobin to methaemoglobin, then sodium thiosulphate (150 mg/kg over 15 minutes) to speed the conversion of cyanide to thiocyanate.

   Adverse effects: tachycardia, raised intracranial pressure, nausea, vomiting, disorientation, anti-platelet effect.

Nitroglycerin

Dose: 0.5–2 µg/kg i.v. bolus, 0.1–5 µg/kg per min infusion
Onset of action: 1–2 minutes
Peak effect: 1–5 minutes
Duration of action: 3–5 minutes
Elimination: hepatic (glutathione organic nitrate reductase), renal

Nitroglycerin is an organic nitrate that produces a vasodilator effect, principally on venous capacitance vessels, by induction of nitric oxide. Nitric oxide activates guanylate cyclase in the smooth muscle cells, inducing cyclic GMP production. This causes phosphorylation of myosin light chains and smooth muscle relaxation. The end results are decreased venous return and reduced left ventricular end diastolic pressure (preload) and ventricular size, which decrease cardiac work. At higher doses, systemic vascular resistance (afterload) is also reduced. These effects improve myocardial oxygen supply–demand ratio. In addition, nitroglycerin causes redistribution of flow to ischaemic subendocardium, and may decrease the area of muscle damage following myocardial infarction. Cerebral blood flow is increased.

Interaction/toxicity: potentiation of hypotension by phenothiazines, calcium channel blockers and other nitrates, antagonism of the anticoagulant effect of heparin, methaemoglobinaemia at high doses.

Adverse effects: tachycardia, nausea and vomiting, decreased splanchnic blood flow.

Hydralazine

Dose: 0.1–0.2 mg/kg i.v.
Onset of action: 5–20 minutes
Peak effect: 10–80 minutes
Duration of action: 2–4 hours
Elimination: hepatic acetylation

Hydralazine, a phthalazine derivative, has a direct relaxant effect on arteriolar smooth muscle by interfering with calcium ion transport. The resulting decrease in afterload is frequently accompanied by an increase in heart rate, stroke volume and cardiac output. Cerebral and renal blood flow is maintained or increased. Plasma renin activity is increased.

Interaction/toxicity: enhanced hypotensive response with concomitant use of diuretics, other hypotensives and monoamine oxidase inhibitors; reduction in pressor response to adrenaline, lower bioavailability in rapid acetylators, systemic lupus erythematosis with doses > 200 mg/kg.

Adverse effects: paradoxic pressor response, tachycardia, myocardial ischaemia risk, peripheral neuritis, allergic reactions, leukopaenia, splenomegaly, agranulocytosis.

Drugs used in Raynaud's syndrome

Management of patients with Raynaud's syndrome who develop severe symptoms may require vasodilator treatment, and this may influence anaesthetic management if surgery is also required. Nifedepine (calcium channel blocker), prazosin (alpha antagonist) and thymoxamine have been shown to be beneficial. Other agents which are of unproven effectiveness include cinnarazine (antihistamine), naftidrofuryl (which may cause hepatic dysfunction), nicotinic acid derivatives and oxpentifylline (which may precipitate angina, thrombocytopaenia or cholestasis).

Calcium channel blockers

Calcium channel blockers[10] interact with the cell membranes to interfere with inward movement of calcium through the slow channels (transition between resting, activated and inactivated states is delayed compared to fast sodium channels).

They influence:

- myocardial cells (reduced contractility)
- the conducting system cells (depressed formation and propagation of electrical impulses)

- vascular smooth muscle cells (decreased coronary or peripheral vascular smooth muscle tone).

The calcium channel blockers are a heterogeneous group, with differing structures and properties. The therapeutic effects (antiarrhythmic, anti-anginal, antihypertensive) are disparate, since the drugs differ in their predilection for the various sites of action.

Verapamil reduces heart rate and cardiac output and impairs atrioventricular conduction. It is therefore used for treatment of angina, hypertension and supraventricular tachycardia. The hydropyridine calcium channel blockers such as nifedepine and nicardipine have more influence on coronary and peripheral vessels and less on the myocardium, and have no antiarrhythmic effects. Amlodipine and felodipine have similar activity to nifedepine, but a longer duration of action. All are used in the treatment of hypertension and in angina associated with coronary artery spasm. Isradipine and lacidipine predominately affect the peripheral vasculature, and are only used as antihypertensives. Diltiazem has myocardial and peripheral vascular effects, but causes less myocardial depression than verapamil. Nimodipine acts preferentially on cerebral artery smooth muscle, and is confined to treatment of vascular spasm following intracerebral haemorrhage.

Anaesthesia requirements may be altered in patients receiving calcium channel blockers:

- halogenated anaesthetic agents and calcium channel blockers exert additive effects on calcium ion flux in the myocardium and vascular smooth muscle
- combination therapy with calcium channel blockers and beta-adrenergic blockers has been associated with profound bradycardia and asystole during induction with high doses of opioids
- neuromuscular blockade is potentiated.

However, although titration of anaesthetic drugs is prudent, preoperative withdrawal of calcium channel blockers is not necessary–particularly since this may be associated with coronary artery spasm.

Calcium channel-blocking drugs most commonly used in the perioperative period are described below.

Verapamil

Dose: 0.075–0.25 mg/kg i.v. over 2 minutes (5–10 mg)
Onset of action: 2–5 minutes
Peak effect: within 10 minutes
Duration of action: 30–60 minutes
Elimination: renal

Verapamil is a calcium channel blocker that slows AV conduction and prolongs the effective refractory period in a rate-related manner. It reduces ventricular rate in atrial flutter and fibrillation, interrupts re-entry at the AV node and restores sinus rhythm in paroxysmal supraventricular tachycardia. Occasionally anterograde conduction across accessory bypass tracts may result in an increase in the ventricular response rate (e.g. Wolff–Parkinson–White). Myocardial contractility, systemic vascular resistance and arterial pressure are reduced, thereby reducing myocardial oxygen demand. Intracranial pressure is increased.

Interaction/toxicity: additive cardiovascular effects with volatile anaesthetics, angiotensin-converting enzyme inhibitors and venodilators; increased toxicity of digoxin, benzodiazepines, hypoglycaemics and theophylline; AV conduction disturbances with concurrent use of beta blockers; hypotension and bradycardia with bupivacaine; decreased clearance with cimetidine; competition for binding sites with oral anticoagulants and other protein-bound drugs.

Adverse effects: excessive AV block, worsening of cardiac failure in left ventricular dysfunction, bronchospasm, seizures, urticaria.

Nifedipine

Dose: contents of 10 mg capsule placed sublingually
Onset of action: 5 minutes
Peak effect: 20–45 minutes
Duration of action: 4–12 hours
Elimination: hepatic, renal

Nifedepine is a dihydropyridine calcium channel blocker with greater coronary and peripheral arterial vasodilator properties than verapamil, minimal effects on venous capacitance, and little or no effect on SA node or AV node activity. The antihypertensive effect may be somewhat offset by reflex increases in heart rate and cardiac output and fluid retention. Myocardial oxygen supply–demand balance is improved. Nifedepine is a cerebral vasodilator, increasing cerebral blood flow and intracranial pressure and decreasing cerebral perfusion pressure.

Interaction/toxicity: additive cardiovascular effects with volatile anaesthetics, angiotensin-converting enzyme inhibitors and venodilators; increased toxicity of digoxin, benzodiazepines, hypoglycaemics and theophylline; AV conduction disturbances with concurrent use of beta blockers; hypotension and bradycardia with bupivacaine; decreased clearance with cimetidine; competition for binding sites with oral anticoagulants and other protein bound drugs.

Adverse effects: relatively contraindicated in acute myocardial infarction, hypovolaemia, aortic stenosis, obstructive cardiomyopathy, myocardial depression or raised intracranial pressure; bronchospasm, pulmonary oedema, nausea, diarrhoea, pruritus.

Sympatholytics

Sympatholytics block noradrenaline release from presynaptic neurones or central sympathetic system outflow, resulting in an antihypertensive effect. This group includes methyl dopa, clonidine[11] and moxonidine. Methyldopa is converted in the brain by dopa decarboxylase to alpha-methylnoradrenaline, which activates alpha$_2$ adrenergic receptors. Methyldopa produces a paradoxic hypertensive response to propranolol, and dementia symptoms with butyrophenones. These drugs reduce anaesthetic requirements for inhaled and injected agents. The sympatholytic most commonly administered in the perioperative period is clonidine (described below).

Clonidine

Clinical uses of clonidine include premedication, treatment of hypertension, supplementation of anaesthesia, epidural and spinal anaesthesia, and prolongation of duration of local anaesthetics.

Dose:

- premedication, 3–5 µg/kg p.o.
- hypertension, 0.15–0.3 mg i.v. over 5 minutes
- supplementation of anaesthesia, 2–4 µg/kg i.v. bolus over 5 minutes, 1–2 µg/kg per hour infusion
- epidural, 2–10 µg/kg in 10 ml normal saline or local anaesthetic, 0.2–0.8 µg/kg per hour infusion
- spinal, 0.3–3 µg/kg.

Onset of action: 30–60 minutes p.o., <5 minutes i.v., epidural/spinal <15 minutes
Peak effect: 2–4 hours p.o., 30–60 minutes i.v.
Duration of action: 8 hours p.o., >4 hours i.v., 3–4 hours epidural/spinal
Elimination: renal, hepatic

Clonidine is a selective alpha$_2$-adrenergic receptor agonist (alpha$_1$:alpha$_2$ ratio, 1:200) which inhibits sympathetic outflow through activation of these receptors in the medullary vasomotor centre. This results in a decrease in arterial pressure, heart rate and cardiac output. Clonidine also produces dose-dependent sedation and minor respiratory depression (which does not enhance opioid-induced respiratory depression).

The symptoms and signs of opioid withdrawal are suppressed by clonidine, as it replaces opioid-mediated inhibition of central nervous system sympathetic outflow by alpha$_2$-mediated inhibition.

Clonidine also acts on alpha$_2$ adrenoceptors in the dorsal horn neurones of the spinal cord. This produces local effects, including inhibition of the release of substance P (presynaptic first order neurones) and decrease in the rate of depolarization (postsynaptic second order neurones). These effects (which are separate from opioid-mediated analgesia) are not inhibited by opioid antagonists (e.g. naloxone), but are blocked by alpha$_2$ blocking agents (e.g. phentolamine).

As an adjunct to anaesthesia, clonidine attenuates the haemodynamic response to laryngoscopy and intubation, reduces opioid and volatile agent requirements (50% reduction in MAC), prolongs regional blockade and enhances postoperative analgesia.

Interaction/toxicity: augmentation of pressor response to ephedrine.

Adverse effects: cardiac failure, AV block, depression, urinary retention, angioneurotic oedema, sudden withdrawal of chronic therapy may produce severe rebound hypertension and left ventricular failure with a marked rise in plasma catecholamine levels.

Anticoagulants

Heparin (standard/unfractionated)

Dose: 50–75 units/kg i.v. loading, approximately 5000 units; 20 units/kg per hour infusion, approximately 20 000–40 000 units over 24 hours
Onset of action: immediate
Peak effect: immediate
Duration of action: 1–3 hours (half-life), dose-dependent
Elimination: hepatic

Heparin, a mucopolysaccharide organic acid (present in the liver and granules of mast cells and basophils), is used for anticoagulation during vascular surgery and in the prophylaxis and treatment of venous and arterial thrombosis. It is obtained from beef lung and from porcine intestinal mucosa. Heparin combines with antithrombin III (heparin cofactor) and inhibits thrombus formation by inactivating activated factors IX, X, XI, XII, inhibiting the conversion of prothrombin to thrombin. It also forms complexes with thrombin, resulting in thrombin inactivation, and prevents the formation of a stable fibrin clot by inhibiting the activation of fibrin stabilizing factor.

The therapeutic effect is monitored by measurement of the activated coagulation time and/or activated partial thromboplastin time (1.5–2 times control for full anticoagulation).

Interaction/toxicity: increased risk of bleeding with aspirin, dipyridamole; reduced effect with digoxin, propranolol, nicotine and antihistamines.

Adverse effects: bleeding or hyperheparinaemia (treated with protamine sulphate: 1 mg neutralizes approximately 100 units heparin), thrombocytopaenia (6–10 days), elevated liver enzymes, erythema, hypersensitivity.

Low molecular weight heparins

The low molecular weight heparins certoparin, dalteparin, enoxaparin and tinazaparin are effective in the prevention of venous thromboembolism. They have a longer duration of action compared with unfractionated heparin, and are usually administered by once-daily subcutaneous injection. The standard prophylactic regimen does not require monitoring.

Heparinoids

Danaparoid is a heparinoid, used for prophylaxis of deep vein thrombosis in surgical patients. It may have a role to play in patients who develop thrombocytopaenia in association with heparin (although there may be cross-sensitivity).

Warfarin

Dose: 2–10 mg per day p.o. (can be administered i.v. or i.m.)
Onset of action: 8–12 hours
Peak effect: 1–5 days

Duration of action: 2–10 days
Elimination: renal, hepatic

Warfarin, a derivative of 4-hydroxy coumarin, is used in the prophylaxis or treatment of thromboembolism associated with atrial fibrillation or prosthetic heart valves, or after myocardial infarction. It depresses liver synthesis of vitamin K-dependent clotting factors II, VII, IX and X, and also inhibits thrombus formation when stasis is induced. It does not affect established thrombus, but may prevent extension. The therapeutic effect is monitored by measurement of prothrombin time, which is reported as the international normalized ratio, INR (the ratio of the patient's prothrombin time to the control prothrombin time is standardized to account for laboratory variability and the tissue thromboplastin used). Therapeutic ranges are: INR 2 for venous thrombosis prophylaxis, and INR 3–4.5 for recurrent pulmonary embolism and prosthetic heart valves.

Interaction/toxicity: increased risk of haemorrhage with concomitant use of platelet aggregation inhibitors (aspirin, non-steroidal anti-inflammatory agents), enhanced anticoagulation with cimetidine, regional anaesthesia is contraindicated.

Adverse effects: frank bleeding (treatment is vitamin K 5 mg i.v., factors II, IX and X if available, or fresh frozen plasma); other adverse effects include agranulocytosis, eosinophilia, leukopaenia, neuropathy, nephropathy and release of atheroma plaque emboli.

Anti-platelet drugs

These drugs, by inhibiting platelet aggregation, may inhibit thrombus formation on the arterial side of the circulation (anticoagulants have little effect on platelet aggregation). Patients presenting for vascular surgery are often on maintenance therapy, or have recently received anti-platelet agents as part of their preoperative evaluation/preparation. The additive effect of these drugs and anticoagulants administered intraoperatively must be considered as part of the anaesthetic management. This group includes:

- aspirin, 75–300 mg p.o. daily is effective in the secondary prevention of cardiovascular and cerebrovascular disease
- dipyridamole, used as an adjunct to anticoagulation with prosthetic heart valves and to induce coronary vasodilatation as part of the evaluation of coronary artery disease (dipyridamole–thallium scan)
- abciximab, a monoclonal antibody occasionally used as an adjunct to heparin and aspirin during transluminal coronary angioplasty
- epoprostenol (prostacyclin), given by infusion to inhibit platelet aggregation during haemodialysis, also a potent vasodilator.

Anticoagulant antagonists

Aminocaproic acid

Dose: 4–5 g i.v. over 1 hour, then 1–1.25 g/hour for approximately 8 hours
Onset of action: immediate

Peak effect: 1–3 hours
Duration of action: 3–5 hours
Elimination: renal

Aminocaproic acid is an inhibitor of plasminogen activators and plasmin, thereby enhancing haemostasis when fibrinolysis is contributing to bleeding. It is administered as an adjunct to therapy (blood transfusion, fibrinogen, clotting factors) in life-threatening situations and in combination with heparin when there is evidence of intravascular coagulation.

Interaction/toxicity: arrhythmia risk with rapid infusion, thrombus formation in disseminated intravascular coagulation.

Adverse effects: hypotension, bradycardia, myopathy, rhabdomyolysis, renal failure.

Aprotinin

Dose: 2 000 000 units over 20 minutes, 500 000 every hour until the end of surgery
Onset of action: immediate
Duration of action: 2–3 minutes

Aprotinin is a proteolytic enzyme inhibitor acting on plasmin and kallikrein. It inhibits fibrinolysis by inhibiting plasmin, and may also protect platelet membrane receptors responsible for platelet adhesion. Its efficacy outside cardiac surgery has not been proven, but it may also be useful during vascular surgery for bleeding caused by fibrinolysis.

Adverse effects: allergy, renal failure, activation of the extrinsic coagulation pathway.

Desmopressin (DDAVP)

Dose: 0.3 µg/kg i.v. in 50 ml saline over 30 minutes
Onset of action: 15–30 minutes
Peak effect: 1.5–3 hours
Duration of action: 6–20 hours
Elimination: renal

Desmopressin is a synthetic analogue of 8-arginine vasopressin (antidiuretic hormone). In addition to the treatment of diabetes insipidus, it is used to maintain haemostasis after cardiac surgery and in the treatment of haemophilia A and von Willebrand's disease. Desmopressin releases von Willebrand's factor, which is necessary for adequate activity of factor VIII and optimal function of platelets.

Interaction/toxicity: water intoxication and hyponatraemia.

Adverse effects: vasoconstriction, myocardial ischaemia, allergy, platelet aggregation and thrombocytopaenia.

Vitamin K

Dose: 2.5–25 mg i.v., 1 mg/min
Onset of action: 1–2 hours

Peak effect: 3–6 hours
Duration of action: variable
Elimination: hepatic

Vitamin K, used for the treatment of hypoprothrombinaemia and to reverse the effects of oral anticoagulants, is an aqueous solution of vitamin K_1, which is necessary for the hepatic synthesis of factors II (prothrombin), VII, IX and X. The onset of action is slow, and administration of plasma and blood transfusion is necessary for severe bleeding.

Interaction/toxicity: anaphylaxis.

Adverse effects: overcorrection of prolonged prothrombin time may precipitate thromboembolic phenomena, cardiac or respiratory arrest.

Protamine sulphate

Dose: 1 mg i.v. neutralizes approximately 100 units of heparin (not > 50 mg over 10 minutes)
Onset of action: 30 seconds–1 minute
Peak effect: < 5 minutes
Duration of action: 2 hours
Elimination: hepatic

Protamine is a low molecular-weight protein prepared from fish sperm or testes, which neutralizes heparin by combining with it to form a stable complex with no anticoagulant properties.

Interaction/toxicity: rapid intravenous injection causes histamine release, hypotension and increased pulmonary vascular resistance.

Anti-arrhythmics

Anti-arrhythmic drugs can be classified according to their effects on the electrical activity of myocardial cells (see Table 2.8), or more simply into:

- those that act on supraventricular arrhythmias (e.g. adenosine, verapamil)
- those that act on both supraventricular arrhythmias and ventricular arrhythmias (e.g. amiodarone, disopyramide)
- those that act on ventricular arrhythmias (e.g. lignocaine).

In general, the negative inotropic effects of anti-arrhythmics are additive and particularly detrimental in impaired myocardial function. Most of these drugs can also be pro-arrhythmic, and this effect is enhanced with hypokalaemia.

The anti-arrhythmics which are most likely to be used perioperatively in the vascular surgery patient are described below.

Supraventricular arrhythmias

Adenosine is usually the treatment of choice for terminating paroxysmal supraventricular tachycardias. Intravenous digoxin is used for rapid control

Table 2.8 Anti-arrhythmic drugs: Vaughan Williams classification

Class	Drugs	Mechanism	Action
I		Membrane stabilizing	
Ia	Quinidine Procainamide Disopyramide	Na^+ channel block (phase 1 upstroke)	Atrial, AV node, ventricular
Ib	Lignocaine	Na^+ channel block (selective for ischaemic tissue)	Ventricular
Ic	Flecainide	Na^+ channel block	Conduction system
II	Propranolol Esmolol etc.	Beta receptor block	Atrial, AV node, ventricular
III	Amiodarone Bretylium	K^+ channel block (delays phase 3 repolarization)	Primarily ventricular
IV	Verapamil Diltiazem Adenosine	Ca^{++} channel block (indirect Ca^{++} block, direct K^+ channel opening)	Atrial, AV node
V	Digoxin	Na^+–K^+ adenosine triphosphate transport system inhibition	SA node AV node

of the ventricular rate in atrial fibrillation and atrial flutter. Verapamil is also effective for supraventricular tachycardia, but should not be used when the QRS complex is wide or in Wolff–Parkinson–White syndrome.

Adenosine

Dose: 6–12 mg i.v. rapidly, may repeat within 1–2 minutes
Onset of action: < 20 seconds
Peak effect: 20–30 seconds
Duration of action: 3–7 seconds
Elimination: cellular uptake and metabolism (deamination, phosphorylation)

Adenosine is an endogenous nucleoside which slows conduction and interrupts re-entry pathways through the AV node, thereby restoring sinus rhythm in acute supraventricular tachycardia (including that in Wolff–Parkinson–White syndrome). It does not convert atrial flutter, atrial fibrillation or ventricular tachycardia to sinus rhythm.

Interaction/toxicity: prolonged bradycardia with calcium channel block, antagonized by theophylline, potentiated by dipyridamole.

Adverse effects: may produce a short first-, second-, or third-degree heart block, bronchoconstriction.

Supraventricular arrhythmias and ventricular arrhythmias

Drugs used for both supraventricular arrhythmias and ventricular arrhythmias include amiodarone, beta blockers, disopyramide, flecainide and quinidine.

Disopyramide is used to control arrhythmias following myocardial infarction, but it impairs contractility. Flecainide has similar actions to lignocaine, and is indicated for junctional re-entry tachycardias (e.g. paroxysmal atrial fibrillation). It may precipitate serious arrhythmias in a minority of patients. Quinidine effectively suppresses supraventricular and ventricular arrhythmias, but may precipitate rhythm disorders.

Amiodarone

Dose: 5 mg/kg over 20–120 minutes
Onset of action: <2–24 hours
Duration of action: 20–100 days
Elimination: hepatic

Amiodarone is a benzofuran derivative with mixed Class Ic and Class III anti-arrhythmic effects. It increases the refractory period and prolongs the action potential duration in all cardiac tissues, including accessory pathways. It impairs sinus node function, is an alpha and beta receptor antagonist and a potent vasodilator (including coronary artery dilatation with long-term therapy).

Interaction/toxicity: increases serum levels of digoxin; potentiates warfarin anticoagulants; bradycardia/sinus arrest may occur with concomitant beta blocker, calcium channel or lignocaine therapy; long-term therapy may cause altered thyroid function, pulmonary fibrosis, hepatitis, peripheral neuropathy and corneal deposits.

Adverse effects: arrhythmias, cardiac failure.

Ventricular arrhythmias

This group includes bretylium (used only in resuscitation), lignocaine and moracizine.

Lignocaine

Dose:

- anti-arrhythmic, 1 mg/kg i.v. bolus, then 0.5 mg/kg every 2 minutes to maximum of 3 mg/kg in 1 hour; 20–50 µg/kg per min infusion
- attenuation of pressor response to intubation, 1–1.5 mg/kg i.v. 1–2 minutes before laryngoscopy, or 2 mg/kg translaryngeally just before intubation.

Onset of action: 45–90 seconds i.v.
Peak effect: 1–2 minutes
Duration of action: 10–20 minutes
Elimination: pulmonary, hepatic

Lignocaine, in addition to its local anaesthetic properties, is a Class Ib anti-arrhythmic that suppresses automaticity and shortens the effective refractory period and action potential duration of the Purkinje system and of ventricular muscle. Lignocaine also attenuates the pressor response to intubation by an analgesic and local anaesthetic effect. Cerebral vascular resistance and cerebral blood flow are decreased, causing a decrease in intracranial pressure. Therapeutic doses do not decrease systemic arterial pressure, myocardial contractility or cardiac output.

Interaction/toxicity: may antagonize or potentiate effects of phenytoin, propranolol or quinidine; potentiates suxamethonium-induced neuromuscular blockade; reduced clearance with beta blockers, cimetidine; high plasma levels may cause seizures, respiratory and circulatory depression.

Anticholinergics

Anticholinergics interfere with the muscarinic actions of acetylcholine (ACh) as a neurotransmitter by competitive inhibition at cholinergic postganglionic nerves. They decrease salivary, bronchial and gastric secretions, and reduce gastrointestinal tone and motility. Intraocular pressure increases due to pupillary dilatation (not significant at premedicant doses). Peripheral vagal blockade of the sinus and AV node increases heart rate. Drugs that cross the blood−brain barrier (tertiary amines) stimulate and then depress the medullary centre.

The anticholinergics are used for:

- sinus bradycardia
- antagonism of muscarinc effects of anticholinesterases during reversal of neuromuscular blockade
- premedication: antisialogogue, sedative, amnesic and vagolytic effects
- prevention of vomiting with epidural opioids (transdermal scopolamine).

This group includes atropine, glycopyrrolate and scopolamine. Sensitivity at different muscarinic sites shows marked variation among drugs. Scopolamine is the most potent antisialogogue, and also has the most sedative and amnesic effects. Atropine is associated with the greatest increase in heart rate, and scopolamine has the least effect. Glycopyrrolate is a better antisialogogue than atropine, has no central nervous system actions and causes less tachycardia. All three cause relaxation of gastro-oesophageal sphincter tone.

Side-effects include confusion and restlessness, especially in the elderly (not with glycopyrrolate), increased intraocular pressure, relaxation of bronchial smooth muscle causing increased physiological dead space, inhibition of sweating and tachycardia.

Atropine

Dose:

- bradycardia, 0.6–1.2 mg i.v. repeated every 3 minutes to a maximum of 40 µg/kg
- premedication, 0.3–0.6 mg i.v. or i.m.

● reversal of neuromuscular blockade, 0.015 mg/kg i.v. with anti-
cholinesterase.

Onset of action: 45–60 seconds
Peak effect: 2 minutes
Duration of action: vagolysis 1–2 hours, antisialogogue effect 4 hours
Elimination: hepatic, renal

Interaction/toxicity: additive effects with antihistamines, phenothiazines, MAO inhibitors, procainamide, quinidine, benzodiazepines, major tranquillizers; intraocular pressure increases enhanced with nitrates, steroids, disopyramide; potentiates sympathomimetics; antagonizes metoclopramide, may produce central anticholinergic syndrome.
Adverse effects: tachycardia, CNS effects, urinary retention, blurred vision.

Glycopyrrolate

Dose:

● premedication, 4–6 µg/kg (0.1–0.2 mg) i.v. or i.m.
● reversal of neuromuscular blockade, 0.01 mg/kg i.v. with anti-
cholinesterase.

Onset of action: < 1 minute i.v.
Peak effect: 5 minutes i.v.
Duration of action: vagal blockade 2–3 hours, antisialogogue effect 7 hours
Elimination: renal, hepatic

Glycopyrrolate is a semisynthetic quaternary ammonium anticholinergic; therefore it does not cross the blood–brain barrier and, unlike atropine and scopolamine, does not have CNS effects.

Scopolamine

Dose:

● premedication, 0.006 mg/kg
● transdermal patch (mastoid area), 0.5–1.5 mg every 72 hours.

Onset of action: immediate i.v., 30 minutes t.d.
Peak effect: 50–80 minutes i.v., 3 hours t.d.
Duration of action: 2 hours i.v., 72 hours t.d.
Elimination: hepatic, renal

Scopolamine is an ester of the organic base scopine (tertiary amine) and readily crosses the blood–brain barrier, producing marked and long-lasting sedative and amnesic effects. It also inhibits the vestibular input to the CNS and has a direct action on the vomiting centre.
Interaction/toxicity and *adverse effects* are similar to atropine.

Anticholinesterases

Reversible cholinesterase inhibitors (neostigmine, pyridostigmine, edrophonium) inhibit the action of the enzyme acetyl cholinesterase, which normally destroys ACh by hydrolysis. This results in accumulation of ACh at muscarinic and nicotinic receptors, which facilitates transmission of impulses across the neuromuscular junction, increases gastrointestinal motility and causes a decrease in heart rate. These drugs are used for reversal of non-depolarizing muscle relaxants, treatment of myasthenia gravis and post-operative ileus.

During reversal of neuromuscular blockade, the simultaneous administration of anticholinergic medication protects against undesired muscarinic effects (bradycardia, salivation and increased bronchial secretions, peristalsis, bronchospasm) without preventing nicotinic effects (reversal of non-depolarizing blockade). Neostigmine is the drug most commonly used for this purpose.

Neostigmine

Dose: reversal, 0.05 mg/kg i.v. to a maximum of 5 mg (with atropine 0.015 mg/kg or glycopyrrolate 0.01 mg/kg)
Onset of action: <3 minutes
Peak effect: 3–14 minutes >20% twitch height, up to 30 minutes <20% twitch height
Duration of action: 40–60 minutes
Elimination: hepatic, plasma esterases

Interaction/toxicity: may prolong depolarizing phase I block, reduced effect with aminoglycosides, hypothermia, hypokalaemia, acidosis, cholinergic crisis in overdosage.

Diuretics

This group of drugs includes thiazides, loop diuretics, potassium-sparing diuretics and osmotic diuretics.

Diuretics are used for:

- hypertension
- peripheral and pulmonary oedema due to cardiac failure
- renal protection during aortic cross clamping
- oliguria due to renal failure
- oedema due to hepatic cirrhosis
- primary aldosteronism
- cerebral oedema.

Thiazides (bendrofluazide, chlorothiazide. indapamide, xipamide, metolazone) are moderately potent diuretics; they inhibit sodium reabsorption at the distal convoluted tubule. Thiazides are used in the treatment of cardiac failure and, in low doses, for control of hypertension. They act within 1 hour of oral administration, and most have a duration of action of up to 24 hours. Adverse effects include changes in plasma potassium, uric acid and glucose.

Loop diuretics (frusemide, bumetanide, ethacrynic acid, torasemide) inhibit sodium and chloride resorption from the loop of Henle (medullary portion), and are powerful diuretics which can produce hypokalaemia. They are used in the treatment of hypertension, oedema associated with cardiac failure, hepatic cirrhosis and nephrotic syndrome, and in the initial treatment/diagnosis of acute oliguria. Large doses can cause deafness and myalgia.

Potassium-sparing diuretics (amiloride, triamterene) are sometimes used as alternative therapy in patients who develop hypokalaemia with thiazides or loop diuretics, although their diuretic activity is weaker. Spironolactone, which antagonizes aldosterone, is used to treat oedema associated with cardiac failure or hepatic cirrhosis and for primary aldosteronism.

Mannitol, an osmotic diuretic, is used for renal protection during aortic aneurysm surgery and in the treatment of increased intracranial pressure.

Diuretics most likely to be administered in the perioperative period in vascular surgery patients are described below.

Frusemide

Dose: 5–40 mg i.v. over 1–2 minutes, larger doses by infusion < 4 mg/min
Onset of action: 5–15 minutes
Peak effect: 20–60 minutes
Duration of action: 2 hours
Elimination: renal

Frusemide is the diuretic of choice in acute fluid overload. It may reduce pulmonary artery occlusion pressure even before diuresis occurs. It may be useful in the management of oliguria associated with vascular surgery, but should only be used if intravascular volume is adequate. Frusemide also decreases intracranial pressure by mobilizing oedema fluid and altering sodium movement in glial tissue.

Interaction/toxicity: ototoxicity is associated with rapid infusion of large doses; renal impairment with concomitant use of aminoglycosides, potentiates antihypertensives and adrenergic blockers; hypokalaemia may predispose to digoxin toxicity and prolonged action of neuromuscular blockers; may precipitate hepatic encephalopathy in liver disease.

Adverse effects: hypotension, pancreatitis, gastric irritation, hyperglycaemia, hyperuricaemia, hypokalaemia, hypochloraemic alkalosis.

Mannitol

Dose: 0.25–1 g/kg i.v.
Onset of action: diuresis 15–60 minutes, decreased intracranial pressure < 15 minutes
Peak effect: 1 hour
Duration of action: 3–8 hours
Elimination: renal

Mannitol is an inert sugar that is not metabolized. It is freely filtered at the glomerulus, thereby raising the osmolarity of the renal tubular fluid and inhibiting tubular reabsorption of water and electrolytes. Mannitol increases urinary excretion of water, sodium, bicarbonate and chloride, but does not alter urinary pH. Intravascular volume is acutely expanded, and renal blood flow may increase.

Adverse effects: hypertension, pulmonary oedema, hypernatraemia, hyponatraemia, hyperkalaemia, acidosis, dehydration.

Angiotensin-converting enzyme inhibitors

Angiotensin-converting enzyme (ACE) inhibitors[12] (captopril, enalapril, cilazapril, fosinopril, lisinopril, trandolapril, quinapril) are commonly administered orally in the treatment of hypertension and cardiac failure. They have a higher affinity for ACE than angiotensin I (e.g. x200 000 for enalapril), thereby inhibiting the conversion of angiotensin I to angiotensin II, which is a potent vasoconstrictor and releases aldosterone. Bradykinin inactivation (by ACE) is decreased, causing vasodilatation. This results in a decrease in systemic vascular resistance and arterial pressure, with a slight increase or no change in heart rate, stroke volume and cardiac output. Natriuresis occurs due to inhibition of water and salt retention and specific renal vasodilatation. Venous dilatation also occurs. Therefore, preload and afterload are reduced. Cerebral blood flow and intracranial pressure are increased.

Adverse effects include hypotension (additive effects with other antihypertensive drugs and volatile anaesthetics), possibility of hyperkalaemia (especially if combined with potassium-sparing diuretics), bronchospasm, persistent cough (caused by bradykinin), progressive renal dysfunction (especially with renovascular disease and in cardiac failure when renal function is dependent on the renin–angiotensin–aldosterone system) and haematological dysfunction (neutropaenia, thrombocytopaemia, haemolytic anaemia).

Angiotensin II receptor antagonists (losartan and valsartan) have similar properties to the ACE inhibitors. However, they do not inhibit the breakdown of bradykinins and are therefore used as alternatives when persistent cough limits the use of ACE inhibitors.

Since major aortic surgery is associated with activation of the renin–angiotensin system and reduction in renal cortical blood flow, there has been some interest in acute preoperative treatment with ACE inhibitors to protect the kidney from ischaemic injury. However, no beneficial effect has yet been demonstrated. In addition, severe intraoperative hypotension (MAP <60 mmHg) has been reported in patients receiving ACE inhibitors, and therefore in some vascular surgery patients preoperative discontinuation of these drugs may be appropriate.

Opioids

Opioids include all natural and synthetic drugs that bind to morphine receptors; agonists (e.g. morphine, fentanyl), agonist-antagonists (pentazocine) and antagonists (naloxone). Opioids interact with specific receptors

Table 2.9 Opioid receptors

Mu	Kappa	Sigma
Supraspinal analgesia (μ_1)	Spinal analgesia	Dysphoria
Respiratory depression (μ_2)	Respiratory depression	Hallucinations
Euphoria dependence	Sedation	Vasomotor stimulation

(Table 2.9) in the central nervous system and elsewhere, e.g. the gastrointestinal tract. The greatest density of receptors mediating analgesia are found in the periaqueductal grey matter of the midbrain and in the substantia gelatinosa of the spinal cord. Endogenous opioid receptor ligands (endorphins) include beta-endorphins from the pituitary, met- and leu-enkaphalin and dynorphins.

The opioid agonists are used for:

- intraoperative analgesia
- postoperative analgesia (parenteral, patient-controlled analgesia, neuraxial, oral, transdermal)
- induction and maintenance of anaesthesia (sole drug or adjuvant)
- premedication
- adjuvant therapy to facilitate mechanical ventilation and tolerance of endotracheal intubation.

Pharmacokinetics

After i.v. administration opioids undergo rapid redistribution, and all have large volumes of distribution. Onset of action and duration of clinical effect are dependent on lipid solubility, e.g. morphine has a longer duration of clinical effect (relatively lipid-insoluble and distributed to hydrophilic tissues such as skeletal muscle) than fentanyl (high lipid-solubility and rapid redistribution). Elimination is primarily by the liver, and is somewhat dependent on hepatic blood flow and enzyme activity.

During continuous infusion, the terminal half-lives do not adequately reflect the overall concentration decay curves for opioids that are metabolized according to a three-compartment pharmacokinetic model, since the duration of action and biological half-life increases with the duration of infusion as a result of accumulation in the second and third compartments. Therefore, the context-sensitive half-time (effective biological half-life) has been developed to explain the discrepancy between the terminal half-life and the time for the blood concentration to fall by 50%. It is defined as the time for the effect-site concentration to fall to 50% after a variable-length infusion. The context-sensitive half-times of fentanyl and alfentanil increase with the duration of infusion, whereas that of remifentanil is constant[13].

Pharmacodynamics

Central nervous system

The onset of action is within minutes after i.v. administration; higher lipid-solubility is associated with more rapid onset, e.g. only 10% of morphine is non-ionized/lipid-soluble and can cross the blood–brain barrier, whereas the extreme lipid solubility of fentanyl causes respiratory depression within 2 minutes. Sedation and analgesia occur in a dose-dependent manner, euphoria is also common. As doses increase, the MAC of volatile anaesthetic agents is reduced. In large doses, amnesia and loss of consciousness may occur (except with high-dose pethidine, which may produce CNS excitation and seizures). Opioid analgesia does not affect sensory and motor modalities, i.e. the patient is aware of the stimulus but describes it as less or not painful.

Stimulation of the chemoreceptor trigger zone causes emesis, with a similar incidence for all opioid agonists at equianalgesic doses. Cerebral blood flow, cerebral metabolic rate and intracranial pressure are usually reduced.

Cardiovascular system

At usual clinical doses, opioids have little effect on myocardial contractility (except for pethidine, which is a direct myocardial depressant) but may enhance myocardial depressant effects of volatile agents. Systemic vascular resistance is usually moderately decreased due to reduced medullary sympathetic outflow and arteriolar and venous dilation. However, if histamine release occurs (e.g. with morphine), a greater decrease occurs. Bradycardia is dose-dependent, and is due to stimulation of the vagal nucleus in the medulla (except for pethidine, which produces an increase in heart rate).

Respiratory system

Opioids produce dose-dependent respiratory depression. This is equivalent for all opioids at equianalgesic doses, although peak effect and duration depend on the pharmocokinetics of each drug. A decrease in respiratory rate is followed by decrease in tidal volume and decrease in ventilatory response to Pa_{CO_2}. Apnoea may occur with large doses or rapid administration. Responses are accentuated in the elderly and by concomitant administration of other CNS depressants. Depression of the cough reflex is due to a direct effect on the medulla. Additional respiratory impairment may be due to muscle rigidity, which is dependent on dose, rate of administration and presence of nitrous oxide.

Other effects

Miosis occurs due to stimulation of the Edinger–Westphal nucleus. Gastrointestinal secretions increase, gastric emptying is delayed and intestinal motility is reduced. Biliary tract tone also increases, which may cause biliary colic or mimic angina. Vesical sphincter stimulation may cause urinary retention. High doses of opioids block the metabolic stress response to surgery (catecholamine and adrenocorticoid release, suppression of phagocytosis, antibody production and T-lymphocyte function), and may therefore reduce the incidence of postoperative immunosuppression and ischaemic events. Allergic phenomena are rare due to similarities with endogenous endorphins. Flushing, urticaria and weals in the injection area reflect localized drug-induced histamine release, rather than allergy. Pruritus after epidural/intrathecal administration is due to altered sensory modulation, which occurs with direct binding of opioids to opiate receptors in the medulla.

Interactions

Combinations of opioids and nitrous oxide may produce significant negative inotropic effects, especially in patients with poor left ventricular function. Benzodiazepines and opioid combinations cause decreases in cardiac output and arterial pressure that do not occur with either drug alone. The effect of diuretics in patients with cardiac failure may be decreased by opioids. CNS depression is potentiated by sedatives, antihistamines and phenothiazines, and effects are exaggerated and prolonged by monoamine oxidase inhibitors and by tricyclic antidepressants.

Analgesia is enhanced by alpha$_2$ agonists (clonidine, adrenaline). Addition of adrenaline to intrathecal/epidural opioids results in increased side-effects (e.g. nausea) and prolonged motor block. Opioids enhance the action of local anaesthetics as they have weak local anaesthetic properties (depression of nerve conduction) and effects on peripheral nerve opiate receptors.

Coexisting disease

The elderly demonstrate decreases in clearance and increased intensity and prolongation of effects of opioids.

Renal disease has a limited impact on dosage requirements, since only a small amount of most opioids is excreted unchanged in the urine. Exceptions include norpethidine (the major metabolite of pethidine), which may accumulate, causing respiratory depression and seizures, and morphine glucuronide (the major metabolite of morphine) which, if present at high plasma concentration, may cross an altered blood–brain barrier associated with uraemia.

Liver disease predictably increases the $T_{1/2\beta}$ of opioids, and accumulation can occur with repeated doses.

Obesity may be associated with increased volume of distribution and prolonged $T_{1/2\beta}$. Doses should be based on ideal body weight. Large or repeated doses may result in accumulation.

The opioids most commonly used in the perioperative period are described below.

Morphine

Dose:

- i.v., 0.05–0.2 mg/kg
- epidural bolus, 40–100 µg/kg (2–5 mg) diluted in 10 ml normal saline or local anaesthetic

- epidural infusion, 2–20 µg/kg per hour
- spinal, 4–20 µg/kg
- patient-controlled analgesia, 10–60 µg/kg i.v. bolus.

Onset of action: < 1 minute i.v., 15–60 minutes epidural/spinal
Peak effect: 5–20 minutes i.v., 90 minutes epidural/spinal
Duration of action: 2–7 hours i.v., 6–24 hours epidural/spinal
Elimination: hepatic metabolism to morphine glucuronide, < 15% excreted unchanged in the urine

Plasma levels of morphine do not consistently correlate with the intensity of analgesia or depression of ventilation.

Fentanyl

Dose:

- analgesia, 0.7–2 µg/kg i.v. (give 2–4 minutes before laryngoscopy to attenuate pressor responses)
- induction, 5–40 µg/kg i.v. bolus or 0.25–2 µg/kg per min infusion for up to 20 minutes (with muscle relaxant to avoid muscle rigidity)
- anaesthetic supplement, 2–20 µg/kg i.v. bolus or 0.025–0.5 µg/kg per min infusion
- sole anaesthetic, 0.25–0.5 µg/kg per min (average 50–150 µg/kg)
- epidural bolus, 1–2 µg/kg per min in 10 ml saline or local anaesthetic, or 0.5–0.7 µg/kg per hour infusion
- spinal bolus, 0.1–0.4 µg/kg
- patient-controlled analgesia, 0.2–1.0 µg/kg i.v. bolus.

Onset of action: within 30 seconds i.v., 4–10 minutes epidural/spinal
Peak effect: 5–15 minutes i.v., < 30 minutes epidural/spinal
Duration of action: 30–60 minutes i.v., 1–2 hours epidural/spinal
Elimination: extensive hepatic metabolism (N-dealkylation), pulmonary

Fentanyl, a phenylpiperidine derivative, is up to 125 times as potent as morphine, with a rapid onset and short duration of action due to high lipid-solubility and rapid redistribution from the CNS to inactive tissue sites. Plasma concentration of 15 ng/ml is produced by a loading dose of 50 µg/kg followed by 0.5 µg/kg per min associated with a reduction in MAC of up to 66%. Respiratory depression lasts longer than analgesia, and may recur after apparent recovery as skeletal muscle flow increases. Cardiovascular stability is maintained, even at high doses.

Alfentanil

Dose:

- analgesia, 5–10 µg/kg i.v.
- induction, 50–300 µg/kg i.v. bolus; or 0.5–15 µg/kg infusion over approximately 20 minutes (with muscle relaxant to avoid muscle rigidity)

- anaesthesia supplement, 10–100 µg/kg i.v. bolus; or 0.05–1.25 µg/kg per min infusion
- sole anaesthetic, 1.25–8 µg/kg per min (average total dose 500–2000 µg/kg)
- epidural, 10–20 µg/kg bolus; or 2–5 µg/kg per hour infusion.

Onset of action: 1–2 minutes i.v., 5–15 minutes epidural
Peak effect: 1–2 minutes i.v., 30 minutes epidural
Duration of action: 10–15 minutes i.v., 1–2 hours epidural
Elimination: hepatic

Alfentanil is associated with more hypotension and bradycardia than fentanyl. The pKa of 6.5 results in large proportions of non-ionized drug, which can cross the blood brain–barrier. It is less lipid-soluble than fentanyl, giving a smaller volume of distribution, and more drug is available for hepatic metabolism. The $T_{1/2\beta}$ is shorter than that of fentanyl. These properties are useful for continuous infusion, as they preclude accumulation. Alfentanil produces up to 70% reduction in MAC. It does not produce any clinically significant changes in cerebral blood flow, cerebral metabolic rate or intracranial pressure. Serum levels and effects of alfentanil are increased by concomitant administration of propofol.

Sufentanil

Dose:

- analgesia, 0.2–0.6 µg/kg i.v.
- induction, 2–10 µg/kg i.v. bolus; or 0.1–0.5 µg/kg per min infusion over approximately 20 minutes (with muscle relaxant to avoid muscle rigidity)
- anaesthesia supplement, 0.6–4.0 µg/kg i.v. bolus; or 0.005–0.05 µg/kg per min infusion
- sole anaesthetic, 0.05–0.1 µg/kg per min (average total dose 10–30 µg/kg)
- epidural, 0.2–0.7 µg/kg bolus; or 0.04–0.4 µg/kg per hour infusion
- spinal, 0.02–0.08 µg/kg
- patient-controlled analgesia, bolus 0.08 µg/kg

Onset of action: 1–3 minutes i.v., 4–10 minutes epidural/spinal
Peak effect: 3–5 minutes i.v., <30 minutes epidural/spinal
Duration of action: 30–45 minutes i.v., 2–4 hours epidural/spinal
Elimination: hepatic

Sufentanil is a thiamyl analogue of fentanyl, with up to seven times the analgesic potency and a shorter $T_{1/2\beta}$. Cardiovascular effects are similar to those of fentanyl. The cerebral metabolic requirement for oxygen is decreased, and there is no significant effect on cerebral blood flow or intracranial pressure.

Remifentanil

Dose: anaesthesia supplement, initially 0.5–1.0 µg/kg over 30–60 seconds, then infusion 0.05–2.0 µg/kg per min
Onset of action: 1–1.5 minutes
Peak effect: 1.5 minutes
Duration of action: 3–5 minutes

Remifentanil has a constant context-sensitive half-time of 3–5 minutes, irrespective of the duration of infusion, as there is no significant accumulation[13]. This short dosage-independent effective biological half-life is due to rapid metabolism of its propanoic methyl ester linkage by non-specific esterases in the blood and tissues. This produces a carboxylic acid metabolite, with no µ-opioid receptor activity. The pharmacokinetic profile of remifentanil may be of particular benefit in patients where rapid recovery is desirable and in whom postoperative pain is not a prominent feature, e.g. carotid endarterectomy patients. In other situations, adequate analgesia by alternative means must be established before emergence.

Interaction/toxicity: increased sensitivity in the elderly to µ-opioid receptor agonist effects, no dose adjustment in hepatic or renal impairment, thiopentone/propofol combined with remifentanil produces up to 30% reduction in arterial pressure.

Naloxone

Dose: 10–100 µg/kg i.v., may repeat at 2–3 minute intervals up to maximum 10 mg
Onset of action: 1–2 minutes
Peak effect: 5–15 minutes
Duration of action: 1–4 hours
Elimination: hepatic

Naloxone is a pure opioid antagonist, which inhibits opioid agonists at µ-, δ- and κ-receptor sites and reverses associated respiratory depression, sedation, hypotension, analgesia and biliary spasm. Naloxone also reverses the effects of agonist-antagonists (e.g. pentazocine) and the respiratory depression associated with captopril, clonidine and codeine. It has no pharmacologic activity in the absence of opioids.

Adverse effects: increased sympathetic nervous system activity (tachycardia, hypertension, pulmonary oedema, arrhythmias), nausea and vomiting with rapid i.v. administration, duration of action of opioid may exceed that of naloxone, tremor/seizures in individuals physically dependent on opioids.

Spinal and epidural anaesthesia and local anaesthetics

Regional anaesthesia and analgesia are commonly used in vascular surgery, either alone or in combination with general anaesthesia.

Advantages include:

- attenuation of endocrine and metabolic changes (i.e. increased cate-cholamines, cortisol, glucose, antidiuretic hormone)
- reduced intraoperative blood loss
- reduction in thromboembolic complications due to increased lower limb perfusion, decreased platelet aggregation and improved fibrinolytic function
- reduction in postoperative pulmonary complications
- fewer intraoperative cardiovascular alterations (lower pulmonary artery occlusion pressure, less arrhythmias, less myocardial ischaemia).

Physiological effects of spinal anaesthesia

- Sympathetic nervous system (SNS) blockade is unavoidable, and exceeds sensory blockade by two or more dermatomes. Sensory blockade extends above the level of motor blockade.
- Cardiovascular effects, all due to preganglionic SNS blockade, include bradycardia (T1–4 block), venodilatation and decreased venous return, decreased cardiac output and arterial pressure.
- Nausea during spinal anaesthesia may be due to unopposed vagal activity and increased peristalsis, hypotension or cerebral ischaemia.
- Intercostal muscle paralysis interferes with coughing and ability to clear secretions.
- Bladder atonia results from sacral blockade, and T5–L1 sympathetic efferent block causes an increase in sphincter tone, resulting in urinary retention.
- A decrease in glomerular filtration rate occurs if hypotension reduces renal blood flow.
- Hepatic blood flow decreases with hypotension, T5–L1 block results in parasympathetic predominance and contracted bowel.
- Lower limb vasodilatation predisposes to hypothermia.

Physiological effects of epidural anaesthesia

- SNS blockade is more gradual in onset, and usually develops after sensory analgesia is established.
- Haemodynamic responses depend on level of anaesthesia (above T5), systemic absorption of local anaesthetic, inclusion of adrenaline, intravascular fluid volume and cardiovascular status.
- Increased blood flow to the lower limbs is associated with compensatory vasoconstriction above the level of the block.
- The degree of hypotension determines decreases in cerebral, renal and hepatic blood flow.

Pharmacologic considerations for spinal anaesthesia

- Lignocaine or bupivacaine are usually used based on the site and duration of surgery and desired intensity of motor blockade (Table 2.10).
- Determinants of local anaesthetic distribution in the CSF include baricity (hyperbaric solutions contain glucose to increase density > 1.008), total

Table 2.10 Local anaesthetics for epidural (E) and spinal (S) anaesthesia

Drug	Dose	Onset (minutes)	Duration (+adrenaline) hours	Maximum dose (+adrenaline)
Bupivacaine (0.25–0.75%)	S 7–15 mg E 50–150 mg	<1 min 4–17 min	2–4 (2–4) 1.5–3 (2–4)	2 mg/kg (3 mg/kg)
Lignocaine (1–2% or 5% hyperbaric)	S 50–100 mg E 200–400 mg	1–2 min 5–15 min	1–2 (1–2) 0.5–1.0 (0.75–1.5)	4 mg/kg (7 mg/kg) 5 mg/kg (7 mg/kg)

dose administered, volume of drug, shape of the spinal canal and patient position.

In the supine position, hyperbaric solutions gravitate to the thoracic area T5–6 (assuring adequate anaesthesia for procedures above L1), whereas isobaric solutions remain in the lower dermatomes (providing intense anaesthesia of prolonged duration). Isobaric bupivacaine is usually the local anaesthetic of choice for lower limb vascular procedures.

- Duration of blockade depends on the specific drug and dose, and on the addition of vasoconstrictor. Adrenaline (200–250 µg) or phenylephrine (2–5 mg) prolongs spinal anaesthesia by local vasoconstriction and by direct antinociceptive effects.

Pharmacologic considerations for epidural anaesthesia

The quality of anaesthesia is determined by:

- the local anaesthetic
- the dose, volume (1.6 ml per segment) and concentration of drug injected
- addition of adrenaline (1:200 000) to reduce systemic absorption; the effect is more marked with shorter-acting local anaesthetics, e.g. lignocaine effect is prolonged by 50%. Premixed solutions are buffered at low pH, which reduces the amount of local anaesthetic available and slows the onset of the block. This can be avoided by adding adrenaline immediately before use
- the site of injection (but not speed of injection or patient position). Onset of block occurs first, and is most intense at the level of injection. Spread occurs more rapidly in a cephalad direction, due to the smaller size of the thoracic nerve roots. Spread is greatest 20–30 minutes after injection
- addition of opioid, e.g. fentanyl, shortens the onset, increases the level and prolongs the duration of block

Table 2.11 Spinal anaesthesia: complications

Complication	Prevention	Treatment
1 Hypotension	Hydration (500 ml of crystalloid)	Ephedrine 3 mg increments
2 Bradycardia		Atropine 0.3–1.2 mg
3 Postdural puncture headache	Small gauge needle	Analgesia Bed rest Hydration Epidural blood patch
4 Extensive spread Hypotension Nausea Inadequate tidal volume		i.v. fluid, vasopressors Ventilatory support Intubation if risk of aspiration
5 Backache	Careful positioning	
6 Parasthesia	Withdraw needle before injection of local anaesthetic	

Table 2.12 Epidural anaesthesia: complications

Complication	Prevention	Treatment
1 Toxicity due to local anaesthetic	Restriction of total dose Check for accidental intravascular injection with test dose and adrenaline	See Table 2.14
2 Local tissue toxicity	Check for accidental subarachnoid injection with test dose	
3 Hypotension	Hydration (500 ml of crystalloid)	Ephedrine 3 mg increments Phenylephrine 100 µg increments
4 Accidental subarachnoid injection	Test dose	See Table 2.11
5 Accidental dural puncture and headache		See Table 2.11 Convert to spinal anaesthesia or reposition at higher interspace
6 Epidural haematoma	Check coagulation status, and Interval of 2 hours between epidural and heparinization	Surgery
7 Broken catheter	Never withdraw catheter through epidural needle	Conservative management

- pH adjustment; addition of 8.4% sodium bicarbonate (1 ml per 10 ml of lignocaine, 0.1 ml per 10 ml bupivacaine) decreases the onset time by increasing the amount of local anaesthetic base
- age (local anaesthetic volume should be reduced by 50% in the elderly).

Complications

Complications of spinal and epidural anaesthesia are related to the technique and to local anaesthetic effects (Tables 2.11 and 2.12).

Local anaesthetics

Local anaesthetics are weak bases, comprising an aromatic moiety connected to a substituted amine through an ester or amide link. The pKa values are near physiologic pH, and ionized (hydrophilic) and non-ionized (more lipid-soluble) forms are present. Amide local anaesthetics (lignocaine, bupivacaine) are the most commonly used agents for regional anaesthesia and analgesia during and after vascular surgery, and are described below.

Local anaesthetics are supplied at an acidic pH to enhance chemical stability. Plain solutions are adjusted to a pH of 6, and those containing a vasoconstrictor are adjusted to a pH of 4, because catecholamines are labile at alkaline pH. Lower pH values decrease the non-ionized proportion, and slow the onset of anaesthesia.

Antioxidants (sodium metabisulfite, sodium ethylenediaminetetraacetic acid) and antimicrobial preservatives (parabens derivatives) may be added to multidose vials. Only preservative-free solutions are used in spinal and epidural anaesthesia, to prevent potential neurotoxicity.

Mechanism of action

Local anaesthetics block generation and propagation of the action potential in nerve tissue (also in cardiac muscle and in the brain) by inhibiting ion flux across the channels that specifically conduct sodium (Na^+). They have no effect on the resting or threshold potential, but decrease the rate of rise of the action potential (increase in Na^+ permeability) so that the threshold potential is not reached. Non-ionized molecules interact with Na^+ channels by passing through the lipid axonal membrane, whereas ionized molecules access receptors on the inside of the Na^+ channels through the aqueous Na^+ channel pore.

Factors influencing the local anaesthetic effect include:

- lipid solubility which increases potency
- low pKa which increases the speed of onset of neural blockade
- high protein binding which prolongs the duration of action
- systemic absorption, which influences the amount of drug remaining at the perineural site
- proximity of injection to the nerve
- volume of drug injected

Table 2.13 Classification of nerve fibres

Fibre	Size (microns)	Function
A$_{alpha}$	6–22	Motor efferent, proprioception afferent
A$_{beta}$	6–22	Motor efferent, proprioception afferent
A$_{gamma}$	3–6	Muscle spindle efferent
A$_{delta}$	1–4	Pain, temperature, touch afferent
B	<3	Preganglionic autonomic
C (unmyelinated)	0.3–1.3	Pain, temperature, touch afferent, postganglionic autonomic

- concentration of drug
- type of nerve fibres.

Nerves are classified according to size and function (Table 2.13). Smaller diameter fibres are more easily blocked than larger ones. Myelinated fibres are more readily blocked than unmyelinated ones, because only the nodes of Ranvier need to be blocked. Neural blockade progresses in the order:

1 Sympathetic block with peripheral vasodilatation and increase in skin temperature.
2 Loss of pain and temperature sensation.
3 Loss of proprioception.
4 Loss of touch and pressure sensation.
5 Motor paralysis.

Distribution and metabolism

Local anaesthetics do not depend on blood flow to transport them to their site of action, but uptake into the circulation is important in terminating their action. Local anaesthetic absorbed into the venous system is distributed to the lungs where uptake occurs, limiting the amount that reaches the systemic circulation. Maximum plasma levels are reached within 25 minutes of administration, so surveillance for toxic effects is important during this time. Subsequently, in the liver, the amide linkage is cleaved by initial N-dealkylation followed by hydrolysis. Elimination half-life is approximately 2–3 hours. Decreased cardiac output, by decreasing hepatic blood flow, delays removal of local anaesthetic from the plasma, and liver disease prolongs the $T_{1/2a}$.

Toxicity

Amide local anaesthetics are not allergenic (except for reactions to methylparaben preservative). Neurotoxicity can occur due to unintentional subarachnoid injection of large volumes or high concentrations of local anaesthetics. Systemic toxicity results from accidental intravascular injection or overdose.

Table 2.14 Local anaesthetic toxicity

Central nervous system	Cardiovascular system
Immediate symptoms – light-headedness – tingling of tongue and around lips – numbness – tinnitus – metallic taste – visual disturbances	*Immediate symptoms* – decrease in ventricular contractility, low cardiac output and arterial blood pressure – conduction defects – loss of peripheral vasomotor tone
Later signs – muscle twitching – loss of consciousness – grand mal seizure – coma	*Later signs* – cardiovascular collapse

Management
– oxygen
– for seizure, midazolam 1–2 mg or
  thiopentone 1–4 mg/kg
– suxamethonium if intubation necessary
 	
– prolonged CPR until cardiotoxic
	Management
	– oxygen
	– volume replacement
	– vasopressors
	– large doses of adrenaline may be
	  necessary
	– ventricular tachycardia, DC cardioversion
	– bretylium more effective than lignocaine
	  for bupivacaine-induced arrhythmias
	– effects subside with redistribution

The maximum safe dose of a local anaesthetic is based on the likely peak blood levels that will occur after perineural injection. These are not absolute and, although stated in mg/kg, there is no consistent correlation between the patient's body weight and peak plasma levels. Peak blood levels depend on the total dose of anaesthetic, the vascularity at the site of injection, whether vasoconstrictors are added, local vasodilatation induced by the local anaesthetic, local tissue binding, tissue perfusion and cardiac and liver disease (Table 2.14).

Lignocaine (regional anaesthesia)

Dose: 50–100 mg spinal bolus; 200–400 mg epidural bolus
Onset of action: 1–2 minutes spinal, 5–15 minutes epidural
Peak effect: < 30 minutes
Duration of action: 1–2 hours spinal, 30–90 minutes epidural

Bupivacaine

Dose: 50–150 mg epidural bolus; 7–15 mg spinal bolus
Onset of action: 4–17 minutes epidural, < 1 minute spinal
Peak effect: 30–45 minutes epidural, 15 minutes spinal
Duration of action: 1.5–3 hours epidural, 2–4 hours spinal

References

1. Eger EI. New inhaled anesthetics. *Anesthesiol* 1994; **80**: 906–22.
2. Wyands JE, Nathan H. Inotropes and vasodilators in the management of acute heart failure. *Cardiothoracic Vasc Anesth Update* 1990; **1**: 1–10.
3. Jaski BE, Peters C. Inotropic, vascular and neuroendocrine effects of dopexamine hydrochloride and comparison with dobutamine. *Am J Cardiol* 1988; **62**: 63–7.
4. Royster R, Butterworth J, Prielipp R *et al*. Combined inotropic effects of amrinone and epinephrine after cardiopulmonary bypass in humans. *Anesth Analg* 1993; **77**: 662–72.
5. Feneck RO. The European Milrinone Multicentre Trial Group: Intravenous milrinone following cardiac surgery: II. Influence of baseline hemodynamics and patient factors on therapeutic response. *J Cardiothoracic Vasc Anesth* 1992; **6**: 563–7.
6. Vernon M, Heel R, Brogden R. Enoximone: a review on its pharmacological properties and therapeutic potential. *Drugs* 1991; **42**: 997–1017.
7. Bristow MR, Kantrowitz NE, Ginsburg R. Beta-adrenergic function heart muscle disease and heart failure. *J Mol Cell Cardiol* 1985; **17**: 41–4.
8. Leone BJ, Lehot JJ, Francis CM *et al*. Beta blockade reverses regional dysfunction in ischemic myocardium. *Anesth Analg* 1987; **66**: 607–9.
9. Wallace A, Layag B. Prophylactic atenolol reduces postoperative myocardial ischemia. *Anesthesiol* 1998; **88**: 7–17.
10. Reves JG, Kissin I, Lell WA *et al*. Calcium entry blockers: uses and implications for anesthesiologists. *Anesthesiol* 1982; **57**: 504–8.
11. Maze M, Tranquilli W. Alpha$_2$ adrenoceptor agonists; defining the role in clinical anesthesia. *Anesthesiol* 1991; **74**: 581–5.
12. Colson P, Saussine M, Seguin JR *et al*. Hemodynamics effects of anesthesia in patients chronically treated with angiotensin-converting enzyme inhibitors. *Anesth Analg* 1992; **805**: 74–8.
13. Egan TD, Lemmens HJM, Fiset P *et al*. The pharmacokinetics of the new short-acting opioid remifentanil in healthy male volunteers. *Anesthesiol* 1993; **79**: 881–92.

3

Preoperative assessment

Overview

Peripheral vascular disease is a marker for severe illness and carries a poor long-term prognosis. This was recognized as early as 1960 in a follow-up study by Boyd, in which he found that only 22% of patients were still alive 15 years after presenting with intermittent claudication[1]. This is because atherosclerosis is a systemic illness and many vascular patients have co-existing coronary artery disease, which is the main long-term cause of death and carries a poor prognosis. Coronary artery disease will also predispose to early postoperative myocardial infarction and death in a significant minority of patients. One study looking at coronary angiography in patients with aortic aneurysms found an overall rate of severe, correctable coronary artery disease of 31% in the 302 patients. Patients with clinically suspected coronary artery disease had a 42% chance of severe, surgically correctable disease, while those without clinical symptoms still had a 19% chance[2]. It is notable, however, that many risk factors for the development of coronary artery disease in the general population do not seem to be risk factors for the development of perioperative myocardial infarctions or adverse cardiac events. These include smoking, family history, hyperlipidaemia and obesity. Hypertension and diabetes may be factors in the development of post-operative cardiac disease, but there is conflicting evidence. Many of the aspects of cardiac disease in the perioperative period are controversial, with differing results reported from published studies. This is partly because the number of patients needed to produce meaningful results is very large.

Assessment of risk in vascular patients is important because the relatively high chance of perioperative complications compared to other types of surgery must be balanced against the proposed benefit to the patient, and a net benefit to the patient should be demonstrable. This is especially true for 'prophylactic' operations, such as elective aortic aneurysm surgery or carotid endarterectomy, but becomes less important for more urgent operations in patients with rest pain in the legs or symptomatic/large aortic aneurysms, as the results of delaying surgery may result in limb loss or death. For example, it would be appropriate to defer surgery in an elderly patient with severe heart disease and a 4.5 cm aortic aneurysm, but if, 1 year later, that aneurysm is now 7.5 cm, the surgical risks are probably less than the risk of doing nothing. Also, patients and relatives may want to know the risks that surgery entails, and it is appropriate that a patient with a significant chance of major morbidity or mortality is aware of this fact preoperatively.

Cardiovascular disease is the leading cause of perioperative critical incidents, and will be dealt with first. Adverse cardiac events (ACE) include myocardial infarction, sudden cardiac death, pulmonary oedema and severe dysrhythmias or severe/unstable angina. The role of respiratory disease in postoperative death is less significant although there is a high prevalence of respiratory disease in this population from smoking, and significant morbidity results in the form of chest infections. Renal disease is often overlooked as a significant factor in postoperative morbidity and mortality, and is a marker of poor short- and long-term outcome.

Perioperative myocardial infarction and ischaemia

Myocardial infarction is most likely to occur between the second and fourth postoperative days[3], is often subendocardial, and is painless in about 50% of patients[3,4]. The reason for the lack of pain is unknown. In some patients it may be due to diabetic neuropathy, in others it may be due to concomitant analgesia administration, and in others it may be related to abnormal central processing of peripheral noxious stimuli[5]. The reported incidence of infarction varies, and depends on how rigorous the search with serial ECGs and cardiac enzymes. The mortality is high, approximately 50–70%[6,7], and the exact mechanisms of postoperative myocardial infarction have not been fully elucidated. Important factors in the development of postoperative ischaemia include:

- increased myocardial work: hypertension, tachycardia (including that caused by postoperative pain) and fluid overload
- decreased myocardial oxygenation: hypotension, hypoxaemia (particularly at night because of rebound increase in rapid eye movement (REM) sleep with accompanying airway obstruction)
- increased postoperative coagulability of the blood
- coronary vasospasm or intraplaque haemorrhage in the coronary artery.

Some authors suggest that long duration subendocardial ischaemia is more important in the development of postoperative myocardial infarction than the classically reported pathology of a ruptured atheromatous plague blocking a coronary artery[8]. This is because most cardiac events (85%) are preceded by ST-segment depression. This may open up possible treatment options in the postoperative period, including prolonged ECG monitoring and early anti-ischaemic therapy. However, a pathological analysis of 42 hearts of patients suffering perioperative myocardial infarction showed similar changes to those in 25 hearts of patients suffering non-perioperative infarction. There was a similar incidence of atherosclerotic narrowing (93%) and plaque haemorrhage (45%) in both groups[9]. Left main-stem and three-vessel coronary artery disease were common.

The increased tendency to thrombosis and the surge in catecholamines in the postoperative period may also play a part. Catecholamines increase the tendency for ischaemia in three possible ways:

- increased heart rate and blood pressure
- α_1-coronary vasoconstriction
- increased thrombotic tendency.

Epidural blockade of afferent impulses and reduction of the stress response to surgery may possibly be beneficial. One study showed a reduction in thrombotic and cardiovascular complications in a group of vascular patients undergoing lower extremity revascularization and receiving epidural analgesia postoperatively, compared to a group receiving opioid analgesia[10]. However, not all investigators have found this.

Many important questions need to be answered in the perioperative management of patients with cardiac disease for vascular (and all non-cardiac) surgery:

- Which preoperative factors predispose to adverse cardiac events in the perioperative period?
- Is further testing useful in the management of these patients?
- How can the patient be best prepared for surgery?
- How can postoperative cardiac events be minimized or avoided?

The use of cardiovascular risk indices

The standard medical format of history, examination and special investigations should be followed. Important risk factors for postoperative myocardial infarction or cardiac events have been identified in large prospective studies, such as the work of Goldman et al.[11]. These are based on simple factors identifiable from the history and examination, or from simple tests. They give an indication of the approximate risk group for that patient, classified as high, medium or low. The disadvantage of these purely clinical cardiac risk indices is that patients with severe asymptomatic disease may not be picked up.

Goldman's study looked at 1001 patients who had undergone non-cardiac major surgery, of which only 82 were vascular patients. Nine factors that were associated with a statistically significant increase in postoperative cardiac events were identified. These were then assigned a points value, depending on the degree of increased risk.

Goldman Cardiac Risk Index

- Third heart sound (gallop rhythm) or raised jugular venous pressure: 11 points
- Preoperative myocardial infarction within the previous 6 months: 10 points
- Rhythm other than sinus or premature atrial contractions on electrocardiograph: 7 points
- More than five premature ventricular contractions per minute documented at any time preoperatively: 7 points
- Age >70 years: 5 points
- Emergency operation: 4 points
- Intraperitoneal, intrathoracic, or aortic operation: 3 points

- Important valvular aortic stenosis (>50 mmHg gradient): 3 points
- Poor general condition, any of the following: $Po_2 < 8\,kPa$ or $Pco_2 > 6.6\,kPa$, $K^+ < 3.0$ or $HCO_3 < 20\,mmol/l$, urea $> 18\,mmol/l$ or Cr $> 260\,mmol/l$, abnormal liver enzymes, signs of chronic liver disease, or patient bedridden from non-cardiac cause: 3 points.

Total possible number of points is 53, and any patient with greater than 12 points is considered high-risk.

Interestingly, angina was not found to be a risk factor for postoperative myocardial infarction. This may be because most myocardial ischaemia is silent. Symptomatic cardiac ischaemia is only a small proportion of the total amount of ischaemia occurring, and did not stand out by itself as a separate risk factor. Also, factors important in the long-term development of coronary artery disease, such as diabetes, high blood pressure, smoking, etc., do not feature as individual risk factors for postoperative myocardial infarction. This risk index has been found to underestimate the risk associated with aortic surgery in patients with low overall scores[12], and in vascular patients in general[13]. This may reflect the fact that only a small proportion of the patients was undergoing vascular surgery.

Goldman did not verify his results by using his index to predict adverse cardiac events in a prospective trial. In 1986, Detsky et al.[14] published a modified form of the index which they had tested in 455 patients. Angina was added, minor surgery was included and the clinical signs of heart failure (third heart sound and raised JVP) were altered to 'the prior occurrence of pulmonary oedema'. Only three levels of points (5, 10, or 20) were used to simplify things, and this index proved to be acceptable. It must be said that the specificity of these indices is very low, and it is not possible to rule out serious complications in low-risk patients undergoing major surgery. For example, in Detsky's study, 37% of serious cardiac events took place in patients with low-risk scores.

Detsky Cardiac Risk Index

- Suspected critical aortic stenosis: 20 points
- Angina, Canadian Cardiovascular Society Class (CCSC) III (marked limitation of ordinary activity, i.e. walking 100–200 yards on the level or climbing more than one flight of stairs): 10 points
- Angina CCSC IV (unable to carry on any physical activity without discomfort, anginal symptoms may be present at rest): 20 points
- Myocardial infarction within the last 6 months: 10 points
- Myocardial infarction greater than 6 months ago: 5 points
- Unstable angina within the last 6 months: 10 points
- Alveolar pulmonary oedema, within 1 week: 10 points
- Alveolar pulmonary oedema, ever: 5 points
- Rhythm other than sinus, with or without atrial ectopy: 5 points
- Presence of more than five premature ventricular contractions per minute at any time: 5 points
- Poor general medical status: 5 points
- Age >70 years: 5 points
- Emergency surgical procedure: 10 points.

A high-risk score of more than 15 points is also predictive of poor long-term survival and quality of life[15].

Eagle Cardiac Risk Index

In 1989, Eagle produced a cardiac risk index based on the results of vascular surgery in 200 patients[16]. When the results of dipyridamole-thallium imaging were added to this risk index, a greater sensitivity and specificity for postoperative cardiac events was achieved. This was only applicable to the intermediate-risk patients (those with one or two of the risk factors), and added little information in the high- or low-risk groups.

- Age greater than 70 years
- Diabetes
- Angina
- Q waves on electrocardiogram
- Ventricular arrhythmias.

A high score is classed as the presence of three or more of the above factors.

How can all this be put together to provide an estimate of operative risk for a particular patient undergoing a particular operation? Integrating the results of studies looking at patient cardiac risk index, operation performed and occurrence of complications, Goldman produced a table giving approximate risks for different types of patients undergoing different types of surgery[17]. In Table 3.1, patients are assigned a class number dependent on their cardiac risk index score, and by considering this in combination with the type of surgery undertaken an approximate risk of major cardiac complication can be calculated.

Important factors in the history

A full history can often provide most of the information needed to decide on a patient's cardiovascular risk status preoperatively.

Functional state of the patient

The purpose of preoperative assessment for any type of surgery is to gain an overall impression of the cardiorespiratory capabilities of that patient and to estimate the 'cardiorespiratory reserve'. A rough prediction of that patient's ability to tolerate the stresses of the perioperative period can then be made.

The New York Heart Association (NYHA) has produced a classification based on a patient's ability to exercise before being stopped by cardiac symptoms, such as angina or shortness of breath from congestive cardiac failure[18]. This provides a useful classification of severity of symptoms based on a patient's functional capacity.

Table 3.1 Likelihood of major cardiac complications depending on a patient's cardiac risk index score

Type of patient and surgery	Baseline risk of cardiac complications (%)	Approximate risk of major cardiac complications in this type of patient as justified using the multifactorial index (%)			
		Class I	Class II	Class III	Class IV
Minor surgery	1	0.3	1	3	19
Major surgery and >40 years old	4	1.2	4	12	48
Abdominal aortic surgery, or >40 years old with high-risk medical conditions	10	3	10	30	75

Goldman combined risk table. The table outlines the approximate risk of an adverse cardiac event in patients having the three types of surgery as shown. The approximate risk of cardiac complications in each of the four patient groups has been calculated from the results of studies. The class of patient is derived from the Goldman cardiac risk index, and corresponds to: class I = 0–5 points, class II = 6–12 points, class III = 13–25 points and class IV = >26 points (after Goldman 1988[17]).

New York Heart Association Classification

- *Class 1*: Patients have cardiac disease, but no resulting limitation of physical activity. Ordinary physical activity does not cause undue fatigue, palpitation, dyspnoea or anginal pain.
- *Class 2*: Patients with cardiac disease resulting in slight limitation of physical activity. They are comfortable at rest. Ordinary physical activity results in fatigue, palpitation, dyspnoea or anginal pain.
- *Class 3*: Patients with cardiac disease resulting in marked limitation of physical activity. They are comfortable at rest. Less than ordinary physical activity results in fatigue, palpitation, dyspnoea or anginal pain.
- *Class 4*: Patients with cardiac disease resulting in the inability to carry on any physical activity without discomfort. Symptoms of cardiac insufficiency or of the anginal syndrome may be present, even at rest. If any physical activity is undertaken, discomfort is increased.

Age

Increasing age results in a reduced functional capacity of the 'healthy' heart and an increased incidence of cardiovascular and associated diseases. Arterial Po_2 decreases with increasing age, and glomerular filtration rate and hepatic function are reduced. Physiological age is probably more important than chronological age, and age by itself should not be used as a discriminating factor against patients without evidence of other high-risk conditions or pathology[19]. Good results can be achieved in the otherwise 'fit' elderly patient.

Previous myocardial infarction

Previous myocardial infarction is identified in most studies looking at perioperative cardiac risk as an important risk factor for the development of another myocardial infarction perioperatively. The risk of this occurring depends on the time between the previous infarction and the proposed surgery. Various figures have been quoted (Table 3.2).

The study by Steen *et al.* found a marked correlation between time under anaesthesia and subsequent myocardial infarction for thoracic and upper abdominal surgery, but not for other types of surgery. Generally it can be seen from the earlier studies that the risk of another postoperative myocardial infarction was found to decrease with time, and beyond about 6 months there seemed to be no further decrease in risk, which remained at about 5–6%. Traditionally it has therefore been recommended that elective surgery should be postponed for 6 months following a myocardial infarction, if possible. In vascular surgery, however, postponement of surgery must be weighed against the increased risk of limb loss, stroke or rupture of aortic aneurysm, which may occur if surgery is delayed. In the studies by Rao and Shah[20], however, there was no significant association between the second perioperative myocardial infarction and time elapsed since the first infarction. The use of invasive monitoring and aggressive treatment of blood pressure and heart rate with fluids and vasoactive drugs, associated with a prolonged period in

Table 3.2 Myocardial reinfarction rate after surgery—a comparison of studies

Study	Patients in study	Site of surgery	Rate of myocardial reinfarction (%) from time of previous MI		
			0–3 months	4–6 months	> 6 months
Tarhan 1972[3]	422	Abdominal, aortic, thoracic, orthopaedic, peripheral, urological, head and neck, vertebral	37	16	5–6
Steen 1978[7]	587	Abdominal, aortic, thoracic, urological, other sites	27	11	4–5
Rao 1973–6[21]	364	Abdominal, aortic, thoracic, orthopaedic, urological, eye, peripheral	36	26	5
Rao 1977–82[21]	733	Abdominal, aortic, thoracic, orthopaedic, urological, eye, peripheral	5.7	2.3	<2
Shah 1990[20]	275	Abdominal, aortic, thoracic, peripheral vascular, orthopaedic, urological, eye, ENT	4.3	0	5.7

The study by Rao[21] looked at two groups of patients; one group was operated on between 1973 and 1976 and the other group between 1977 and 1982. Note the improvement in myocardial reinfarction rate with the later studies.

intensive care, may have been a factor in the reduced incidence of re-infarctions reported[21].

It has been suggested that if the patient has recovered well, has no angina and a good exercise tolerance, then perhaps elective surgery may be considered at 6 weeks post-infarction[6,17]. If significant angina, ST segment depression on exercise testing or large reversible perfusion defects on dipyridamole-thallium imaging are present, then referral for coronary angiography and revascularization should be made.

Heart failure

Many studies have shown that the presence of heart failure preoperatively confers a large added risk of perioperative adverse event. Simple clinical information on exercise tolerance, presence of a third heart sound or chest X-ray appearances of pulmonary oedema or cardiomegaly are usually sufficient to predict patients at a high risk of developing pulmonary oedema postoperatively. The symptoms and signs of heart failure are more fully described on p. 27.

Angina

The severity of the angina can be defined by the limitations caused to the patient's lifestyle and the reduction in exercise capacity, as described in the New York Heart Association's guidelines above. Angina may remain stable for years, or start to occur at decreasing intervals or reduced levels of activity. This is then called unstable angina, and may become so severe that the angina occurs at rest. Patients with severe/unstable angina should be referred for cardiological opinion with a view to performing coronary angiography and to revascularizing the heart if anatomically possible. Although missing from the Goldman cardiac risk index, chronic stable angina is probably a factor predisposing to postoperative adverse cardiac events, and the severity of the angina and ease with which it is provoked is important[14]. The medical treatment of angina should be optimized preoperatively, and this involves the use of nitrates, calcium channel blockers and beta blockers. The cardio-selective beta blockers atenolol and metoprolol are probably the best for patients with peripheral vascular disease. Much myocardial ischaemia is silent, however, and evidence exists which suggests that patients with silent myocardial ischaemia preoperatively are also in a high-risk group for postoperative cardiac events[22].

Emergency surgery

Patients presenting for emergency surgery are usually more ill, have had less time for investigation and optimization, and have been found to be at greater risk of an adverse cardiac event.

Important factors in the clinical examination

The cardiovascular system should be examined fully. Specific factors to look for include those that denote significant cardiac disease, which should be optimized preoperatively. Specifically, blood pressure should be measured in both arms, carotid pulse character assessed and bruits listened for, JVP examined, heart and lung fields listened to and peripheral oedema considered.

Hypertension

The level and duration of effective blood pressure control in the pre-operative period for optimal safety during anaesthesia is not known. It is generally thought that blood pressure should be normalized preoperatively because hypertensive patients are more unstable in the perioperative period, especially on induction and laryngoscopy, and myocardial ischae-mia can be precipitated by hypo- or hypertension. Prys-Roberts[23] showed in 1971 that treated hypertensive patients have less blood pressure lability under anaesthesia than untreated patients. If the diastolic blood pressure is above 110 mmHg, increased risks of myocardial ischaemia[23,24], myocardial infarction[7], dysrhythmias[24], transient and permanent neurological events[25] and renal failure[26] have all been reported. Patients with diastolic blood pressures below 110 mmHg seem to have a similar operative course to non-hypertensive patients[26]. The necessary duration of effective pre-operative blood pressure control is controversial and unknown.

Hypertension should be treated according to previously published guidelines[27], with referral to a cardiologist if blood pressure is consistently above 160/100 mmHg. Ideally blood pressure should be controlled within the weeks prior to surgery (aiming for a level of 140/90 mmHg)[28], but if the diastolic is lower than 110 mmHg it is not necessary to cancel surgery and it is probably reasonable to proceed if surgery is needed. Hypertension is likely to be a risk factor in the development of a postoperative adverse cardiac event, although not all workers have found this. It does not appear in the Goldman, Detsky or Eagle indices, but a recently published case-control study has highlighted hypertension as an independent risk factor for the development of ACE[29]. Hypertension (and tachycardia) occurring in the recovery room has been found to be predictive of increased postoperative mortality[30]. Preoperative hypertension, despite treatment, was found to be the only predictive factor in the development of preoperative myocardial ischaemia measured by ambulatory ECG monitor-ing in a study of 325 patients[31]. There is also evidence that hypertension is linked to significant increases in postoperative myocardial ischaemia, detected by ambulatory monitoring[32].

Blood pressure should be measured in both arms, as there may be a significant difference, and radiofemoral delay should be considered to exclude coarctation of the aorta. An abdominal bruit should also be listened for because this may suggest renal artery stenosis, which would have implications for subsequent medication (angiotensin-converting enzyme inhibitors) and the risk of renal failure postoperatively.

Treatment of blood pressure is as described on p. 31. It is essential that preoperative medication be continued throughout the perioperative period, to avoid rebound hypertension.

Heart failure

Signs of heart failure (including third heart sound, tachycardia, raised jugular venous pressure and peripheral oedema) should be sought. Basal crackles in the chest are unreliable, and may be a sign of chest disease. Treatment should be optimized preoperatively, with diuretics, digoxin and angiotensin-converting enzyme inhibitors being the mainstays of treatment. Referral for cardiological opinion and optimization of treatment should be made if any doubt exists as to the adequacy of treatment. Further discussion on heart failure can be found on p. 27.

Hypertrophic cardiomyopathy

Patients with this condition pose special problems in the perioperative period. They tolerate reductions in preload and drops in peripheral vascular resistance poorly, as these may lead to reductions in end-diastolic volume and an increase in the ventricular outflow obstruction. Reductions in preload also cause large drops in stroke volume due to the decreased compliance of the enlarged ventricle, and these patients need to be kept well 'filled-up'. Catecholamines increase contractility, and increase the outflow obstruction. Hypotension should be treated with fluids and vasoconstrictors.

Valve disease

Aortic stenosis. The normal aortic valve area is 2.5–3.5 cm^2, and a reduction in this value to 1.0 cm^2 will usually necessitate valve replacement. A gradient of 50 mmHg across the valve is deemed significant for the Detsky index, and this can be measured by Doppler ultrasound. The ventricle will hypertrophy to force blood through the narrowed valve to maintain a cardiac output which is essentially 'fixed'. The subendocardial layer of the ventricle will be at risk from ischaemia, and the ventricle will be less able to respond to stress by increasing the cardiac output. Symptoms of angina and blackouts are signs of advanced disease and of a ventricle that is becoming unable to cope. Clinically, a harsh pansystolic murmur over the aortic area (often radiating up to the neck), a slow rising pulse and a low pulse pressure may be present. Tachycardia and a reduction in systemic blood pressure are poorly tolerated as coronary blood supply is reduced, and a vicious circle of lower and lower cardiac output with resultant cardiac arrest can occur. Preoperative treatment and investigation are the same as in the non-operative setting, and valve replacement may be advisable.

Mitral stenosis. Almost all mitral stenosis is thought to be due to rheumatic fever, and as such is becoming more rare in this country. Characteristically, the commissures fuse and the valve orifice narrows down to 1×0.5 cm before cusp thickening and calcification occurs. The left atrium hypertrophies and enlarges, and atrial fibrillation is likely. Thrombus may form in the large fibrillating atrium, and systemic emboli can occur.

Clinically, women are more commonly affected, and shortness of breath on exertion, orthopnoea and palpitations due to the onset of atrial fibrillation are common presenting symptoms. On auscultation, the first heart sound is loud and an opening snap may be heard, together with a low, rumbling diastolic murmur. Patients with mitral stenosis tolerate tachycardia poorly due to reduced diastolic filling time, and pulmonary oedema is likely to be provoked. Severe stenosis may warrant valve replacement preoperatively.

Regurgitant valves. Regurgitant valvular disease is generally tolerated better peroperatively than stenotic valve disease. Vasodilatation occurring after induction helps forward flow of blood and reduces the regurgitant fraction of the stroke volume. Any tachycardia developing will also reduce regurgitation by decreasing the diastolic filling time. The exception to this is when ventricular function is poor, and in these cases decompensation can occur perioperatively and preoperative valve replacement should be considered. Significant aortic and mitral regurgitation also may necessitate appropriate antibiotic prophylaxsis for bacterial endocarditis.

Prosthetic valves. Patients with prosthetic valves need antibiotic prophylaxsis, and perioperative control of their anticoagulation. Generally it is recommended to substitute peroperative heparin therapy for oral anticoagulation in patients undergoing major surgery.

Simple preliminary investigations

Blood tests

Important blood tests include:

- full blood count to exclude anaemia and give a baseline haemoglobin
- urea and creatinine to evaluate renal function
- electrolytes, especially if the patient is on drugs that may alter plasma potassium, e.g. diuretics or angiotensin-converting enzyme inhibitors
- blood sugar if patient is diabetic.

ECG

A normal ECG does not exclude the possibility of severe coronary artery disease and, apart from detecting a recent myocardial infarction or third-degree heart block, will probably not alter anaesthetic management. However, it is a simple, non-invasive test, which can serve as a baseline and, if atrial fibrillation or frequent ventricular ectopics are found, will identify a higher risk patient. Q waves may be present, denoting a previous (perhaps silent) myocardial infarction, and ST segment abnormalities may suggest ischaemia. Left ventricular hypertrophy may be present in hypertensive patients, and left bundle branch block usually denotes significant ventricular disease. All patients undergoing vascular surgery should have an ECG performed preoperatively.

Ventricular arrhythmias. Ventricular arrhythmias not associated with structural heart disease have a good prognosis and need no treatment. If associated with heart disease, for example following a myocardial infarction, they are a marker for increased mortality. Amiodarone may be beneficial and improve survival[33], but class I anti-arrhythmic agents (flecanide or encainide) will not, as these lead to increased mortality when compared to no treatment. Beta blockade may also be beneficial, but cardiological opinion should always be sought preoperatively in the patient with frequent ventricular ectopic beats and poor myocardial function. Indications for anti-arrhythmic therapy are the same as in the non-operative setting[6].

Atrial fibrillation. This is a very common arrhythmia with a variety of causes. Efforts should be made to find a precipitating factor (if present), and treat the cause if possible.

Causes of atrial fibrillation include:

- ischaemic heart disease
- hypertension
- valvular heart disease
- alcohol
- chronic pulmonary disease
- electrolyte imbalance
- hypovolaemia (especially postoperatively)
- thyrotoxicosis.

The rate can be controlled with digoxin, diltiazem or sotalol. Cardioversion can be attempted, either by DC shock or pharmacologically, with drugs such as amiodarone. Some patients with atrial fibrillation (especially those over 65 years old) are candidates for anticoagulation to prevent systemic embolus, and aspirin or warfarin can be used[34]. A cardiologist should be involved early in the management of these patients.

Pacemakers

The indications for insertion of a temporary pacemaker are essentially the same as those for the insertion of permanent pacemakers in the non-operative setting. These would include symptomatic or high-degree heart block. Permanent pacemakers are usually checked annually, but can be checked preoperatively. Some pacemakers will need to be reprogrammed (or used with a magnet) to prevent unwanted inhibition by diathermy. Bipolar diathermy is not always totally safe. Implantable defibrillators should be switched off preoperatively and turned on again at the end of the operation to prevent unwanted shocks triggered by diathermy[6].

Chest X-ray

This may show an increase in heart diameter or signs of cardiac failure, upper lobe diversion, Kerley B lines or frank pulmonary oedema.

Further testing of cardiovascular status

It is not possible at present to design specific tests that mimic exactly the stresses of the perioperative period, and to apply these to patients in order to identify those who will develop problems. It is useful in some patients to investigate the cardiovascular system further and, occasionally, to stress the myocardium to assess the response of the patient's heart. Vascular patients may not be able to exercise due to claudication, previous strokes or amputations, and it is sometimes difficult from the history to get an idea of the patient's exercise tolerance. Stress testing may identify patients who become ischaemic when stressed, but the further management of these patients (coronary angiography, coronary angioplasty or even coronary artery bypass grafting (CABG)) is controversial. One meta-analysis of clinical studies on preoperative testing concluded that patients with low- or high-risk scores on the clinical risk indices do not benefit from further investigation, as their status is known. Patients at intermediate risk, however, may benefit from further testing and risk stratification, and dipyridamole-thallium scintigraphy and ambulatory ECG monitoring seem the most useful investigations[35].

Many vascular patients have coronary artery disease, but only a few will go on to develop complications in the perioperative period. The following tests, if positive, are quite sensitive for detecting coronary artery disease, but have a low specificity for predicting which patients will have problems because of the relatively low number of patients suffering an adverse cardiac event in the postoperative period. A negative test is generally good in that it denotes a high likelihood of no complications. Routine testing of every patient and referral for coronary angiography and then CABG is not recommended, as it does not result in overall patient benefit[36]. In general, tests should only be performed if they are likely to influence patient management in terms of a change in surgical procedure, medical treatment or perioperative monitoring[6].

Exercise ECG

Exercise raises the heart rate, stroke volume, myocardial contractility and blood pressure. This will increase myocardial oxygen requirements and allow an assessment to be made of the patient's ability to respond to stress. Maximum heart rate × blood pressure gives the rate pressure product, and this can give a rough estimate of what that patient may tolerate in the perioperative period. If the patient can tolerate 85% of their predicted maximum heart rate, they present a low risk for surgery. Exercise testing also gives an estimate of functional capacity from the length of time patients can manage on the standard test protocols.

Usually the patient is asked to walk on a treadmill at gradually increasing speeds and gradients while their ECG is continually monitored for ST segment changes. A drop in the ST segments is said to correlate to subendocardial ischaemia, while ST-elevation can be due to transmural ischaemia or abnormal wall movements occurring in an area of previous infarction. The blood pressure is also manually read by the attendant, as a fall in blood pressure is a sign of severe heart disease and should lead to the test being stopped. Any symptoms reported are noted, and the patient continues to exercise until a rest is necessary. Criteria for a positive test include:

- \> 1 mm ST segment depression associated with typical angina-like chest pain
- \> 2 mm ST segment depression.

A positive test helps to confirm the clinical impression that coronary artery disease is present. However, a negative test will not totally rule out the presence of coronary artery disease, especially in a patient with a classical history. There is also the possibility of false positive tests, including patients with left ventricular hypertrophy, mitral valve prolapse, Wolff–Parkinson–White syndrome and those taking digoxin. False negative tests can be caused by failure to reach a high enough heart rate, poor exercise tolerance or failure to note drops in blood pressure, which are significant. Beta blocker therapy will reduce the heart rate and confuse the result.

Vascular surgical patients are rarely able to exercise to their full cardiac capacity due to claudication, strokes and amputations, and therefore other tests are often needed as follows.

Echocardiography

The reflections of sound waves from the beating heart can show continuous two-dimensional pictures of the ventricular cavity, allowing non-invasive assessment of ventricular function. An approximate estimate of ejection fraction can be made from the changes in the ventricular cavity between end systole and end diastole (see p. 9 and Figure 4.7). The echocardiogram report will also note increasing degrees of ventricular dysfunction in the form of hypokinesia, akinesia or dyskinesia of the ventricular wall. Assessment of the valves can be made and significant stenosis or regurgitation documented, making this an important investigation if a murmur is heard clinically. Pressure gradients across the valves can also be estimated, and pulmonary artery pressure approximated.

Stress echocardiography

Stress echocardiography involves increasing the heart rate of the patient while performing echocardiography, in order to identify new or worsening wall motion abnormalities. Dobutamine (10–40 μg/kg per min) or atropine (0.25–1.0 mg i.v.) can be used to increase the heart rate to target levels. It is most appropriately used for patients unable to exercise or those who have an abnormal resting ECG. This can provide information on the likely response of the patient to stress in the perioperative period and is useful for predicting patients at high risk of complications, both perioperatively and in the longer term[37]. The data seem to suggest that the larger the area of abnormal movement, the greater the risk of cardiac problems perioperatively, so a quantitative measurement is also possible.

Overall, the results compare well with dipyridamole-thallium scintigraphy for sensitivity and specificity for postoperative complications[38]. One meta-analysis of 20 studies looked at dipyridamole-thallium scintigraphy, ejection fraction estimated by radionuclide ventriculography, ambulatory ECG and dobutamine stress echocardiography, to see which test was the most effective in the detection of postoperative adverse cardiac outcome. No test emerged as the best overall because the confidence intervals overlapped, but dobutamine stress echocardiography fared very well and had the highest predictive value of the tests studied[39]. It has not been as well validated as the other modes of investigation, but shows promise as a cheap and sensitive test for coronary artery disease[40].

Multiple unit gated acquisition angiography (MUGA) scans

A MUGA scan involves injecting radiolabelled albumen or red blood cells intravenously and measuring the radioactivity over the heart with a gamma camera. The camera scans the heart at specific points on the cardiac cycle, as timed from the ECG, and the radiation from the ventricles during systole and diastole are compared. Ejection fraction can be calculated accurately, and areas of poor ventricular contraction can also be outlined.

Studies looking at the predictive value of ejection fraction of the heart have produced conflicting results. While ejection fraction is usually maintained in the normal range until heart disease is severe[41] and is useful for predicting the long-term prognosis after myocardial infarction[42], there is conflicting evidence whether a low ejection fraction is an independent risk factor for cardiac events in the postoperative period. Some studies report that it is[43,44], while others report good results in patients with poor ejection fractions ($<35\%$)[45,46]. The value of routinely measuring ejection fraction pre-operatively is therefore unclear, possibly because ejection fraction may be normal in a heart with severe coronary artery disease until it is stressed. Whatever the overall value of preoperative ejection fraction, similar information can be gained from a two-dimensional echocardiogram at less cost and with no radiation risk.

Ambulatory ECG

A continuous ECG monitor can be attached to the patient preoperatively and the results recorded on a cassette attached to the patient's waist. This is often used by cardiologists to detect arrhythmias in patients reporting palpitations, but ST segment analysis is also possible. Recently it has become recognized that a lot of ischaemia (defined by ST segment depression > 1 mm) is 'silent', in that it causes no symptoms. It is not exactly certain how 'silent' and 'painful' ischaemia are different (if at all) with respect to mechanism and prognosis. Many studies have shown that postoperative myocardial ischaemia is common after anaesthesia for major surgery (30–40% of patients), that it is mainly silent and is significantly associated with an increase in the risk of adverse cardiac events[22]. One study reported a 30% incidence of postoperative ischaemia, which was closely correlated with preoperative ischaemia and postoperative adverse cardiac events[47]. The presence of preoperative silent ischaemia may be an important predictive factor in the postoperative development of an adverse cardiac event[48]. One study of 200 patients undergoing vascular surgery reported preoperative silent myocardial ischaemia at rest to be the only significant predictor of silent myocardial infarction[49]. The absence of preoperative ischaemia is a good predictor of no adverse event (99% specific in the study by Raby et al.[48]). Postoperative ischaemia may be associated with hypoxaemia, especially the longer episodes, but this is not an invariable finding[32]. Postoperative ischaemia is also detectable by continuous bedside ECG monitoring, or by ambulatory devices if facilities are available. As many postoperative cardiac events are preceded by ST segment depression it may be possible (by continuous monitoring in the postoperative period) to identify and then treat this ischaemia and thereby reduce the overall incidence of myocardial infarction, although this has not been proved in practice. In one case report, continuous ECG recordings allowed early detection and treatment of postoperative silent ischaemia in a patient with ST segment depression (up to 4 mm) associated with a tachycardia[50]. This could be a more logical approach than investigating large numbers of patients preoperatively and treating coronary disease with bypass grafting[51]. This would require more intensive post-operative care than is now available on general wards.

Performance of preoperative ambulatory ECG monitoring may be useful if the patient is unable to exercise and the ECG is normal at rest. Detection of silent ischaemia in these patients may be an indication for escalating medical therapy prior to surgery. About 10% of the population have ECG abnormalities that make ST segment monitoring impossible. This includes LBBB, some patients with LVH and some patients on digoxin. Ambulatory ECG monitoring is a very cost-effective method of evaluating vascular patients preoperatively.

Dipyridamole-thallium scintigraphy (DTS)

Following intravenous injection of thallium 201 (a radioactive potassium analogue), it is distributed into myocardium cells in proportion to the blood flow. Areas of ischaemia will be under-perfused and appear as defects in the radiographic image of the heart. Dipyridamole is a vasodilator, and will cause peripheral and coronary vasodilatation and reflex tachycardia. Normal coronary arteries dilate and blood flow will increase through them. Atheromatous coronary arteries will not dilate, and blood flow to the corresponding areas of myocardium supplied by these vessels will be reduced (the 'coronary steal' effect). Ischaemic areas will therefore show a decrease in thallium uptake compared to normal areas of myocardium when thallium is injected with the dipyridamole, and will appear as a filling defect. The dipyridamole infusion is then stopped and further pictures taken a few hours later to see if the thallium has redistributed, thereby implying that the defects are reversible and not the result of previous infarction (which will give a fixed defect because of coronary occlusion). The presence of reversible defects implies ischaemia and has been found to be more sensitive and specific for coronary artery disease than exercise ECG, but gives no information on functional capacity. On the other hand, in vascular patients unable to exercise, dipyridamole-thallium scintigraphy will stress the heart and highlight ischaemic areas. A DTS scan showing redistribution is associated with an increased risk of cardiac events after vascular surgery[52]. Similarly, a large left ventricular cavity as measured on DTS is predictive of postoperative adverse cardiac events[53]. A normal scan with no perfusion defects is associated with a very low incidence of complications[52]. However, the positive specificity of the test is low (10–25%), and if used as a screening test for coronary angiography it will result in large numbers of patients being exposed to invasive testing.

Coronary angiography and coronary bypass grafting

Coronary angiography is the gold standard investigation for the presence of coronary artery disease. Accurate pictures of coronary anatomy are obtained, the site of any atheromatous lesions can be seen and the suitability for surgery can be assessed. Ventriculography is also performed, and useful information about the contractile function of the left ventricle, ejection fraction and end diastolic filling pressures is also obtained. Medical indications for angiography may include:

- angina uncontrolled on medical treatment, or rest pain or severe symptoms
- recent increase in symptoms
- positive exercise test
- reversible defect present on DTS scanning
- abnormal stress echo indicating ischaemia.

The point of coronary angiography is to assess the suitability of the patient for surgical reconstruction of the coronary arteries with vein or internal mammary artery bypass grafts or coronary angioplasty. In large studies, coronary revascularization has been shown to be advantageous to patients with specific types of lesion:

- angina poorly controlled on medical treatment
- left main stem coronary artery stenosis
- disease of three coronary arteries[54], especially with reduced ventricular function.

Patients undergoing vascular surgery have a high prevalence of coronary artery disease, and a proportion may benefit from coronary angiography followed by coronary artery surgery, if appropriate, before vascular surgery. Centres that have promoted the preoperative performance of coronary angiography and coronary artery bypass grafting have shown a reduced mortality for subsequent major surgery of 0.9%, as opposed to 2.4% for those patients without prior grafting[55]. Unfortunately the mortality rate from the coronary artery surgery in vascular patients is about 4.0–5.3%[56], and prior revascularization will not be of overall short-term benefit if morbidity and mortality rates from vascular surgery are kept low. There is however a long-term advantage for patients who survive CABG, as they will have a long-term survival similar to patients with mild or no coronary artery disease[57]. However, this is gained at the expense of increased short-term mortality. If the long-term benefits of CABG surgery are taken into account, then this becomes a more attractive option (Figure 3.1)[6].

Prospective, randomized studies showing an overall reduced mortality from coronary artery bypass grafting prior to vascular surgery have not been performed, and the patients who will benefit from this are difficult to define. If the patient has chronic stable angina and NYHA class II disease or less, then there is no overall benefit in prior cardiac revascularization. Mortality from major non-cardiac surgery in these patients is about 2.4%. Prior coronary artery bypass grafting will reduce this to 0.9%, but there is a 1.4% mortality associated with the cardiac surgery, giving a mortality of 2.3% for the combined procedures[55]. Patients with severe or unstable angina who can wait for their vascular surgery are likely to benefit from angiography and subsequent CABG surgery, as this is probably the best treatment for them in

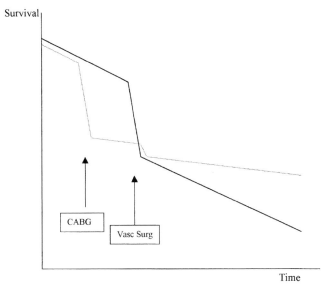

Figure 3.1 Long-term survival after vascular surgery. This theoretical diagram outlines the potential advantages of coronary artery bypass grafting (CABG) before vascular surgery (Vasc Surg) in patients with coronary artery disease needing vascular surgery. All patients have similar initial survival curves. The patients who have CABG before their vascular surgery (dotted line) initially show a drop in survival because a proportion of them will die following CABG, but their subsequent survival curves are less steep than those patients who do not have CABG before vascular surgery (solid line). After the vascular surgery, the total number of patients alive in the short term is about the same because the patients who have undergone prior CABG have a reduced rate of mortality for their subsequent vascular surgery. However, in the long term those patients having a successful CABG will do better than those who have had no CABG (if all patients have appropriate surgically correctable disease).

the long-term irrespective of the vascular surgery. The fact that they will undergo subsequent vascular surgery at a reduced risk of myocardial infarction and death[58,59] should be seen as a bonus, and not as a goal in itself. The overall value of prophylactic CABG for patients of intermediate risk has not been studied in a randomized prospective trial. The problems are the increased mortality of the coronary bypass operation and the delay in having definitive vascular surgery.

Many patients presenting for vascular surgery present with late stage disease, and may not be able to wait long enough to have cardiac surgery performed. The waiting list time for routine cardiac angiography and surgery is up to 2 years in many centres. This is a long time in the natural history of vascular disease, and many patients will not be able to wait that long. Patients needing coronary angiography and possibly CABG before vascular surgery will however by definition have severe or unstable symptoms, and will possibly be able to have their surgery performed as an urgent procedure earlier than this depending on the local situation. Some authors have also recommended postponing all but emergency surgery in the 6 months after CABG because of the increased risk of cardiac complications[60], which will postpone vascular surgery even longer.

Suitable patients to consider recommending for preoperative coronary angiography include those with:

- high-risk results during non-invasive testing
- angina unresponsive to medical therapy
- unstable angina pectoris.

Coronary angioplasty

Percutaneous dilatation of atheromatous lesions of the coronary arteries can be performed. Complications include coronary dissection or occlusion, dysrhythmias and tamponade; a certain proportion require emergency surgery. There are few studies on coronary angioplasty prior to vascular surgery. One reported a 5.6% myocardial infarction rate and a 1.9% mortality rate in 50 patients undergoing non-cardiac surgery a mean of 9 days post-coronary angioplasty[61]. Five patients needed emergency coronary artery bypass grafting after coronary angioplasty, and were excluded from the study. Another study reported a 5.8% myocardial infarction rate in patients undergoing abdominal aortic surgery after coronary bypass grafting, compared to a 0% rate for those having aortic surgery after coronary angioplasty[62].

There is probably a window for surgery in that (over time) the disease progresses and restenosis occurs, necessitating further angioplasty. Surgery may best be performed in the first few months after a successful angioplasty, but there are no controlled trials comparing patients treated with medical therapy with others treated with coronary angioplasty preoperatively. The guidelines recommended are the same as in the non-operative setting[6]. In a recent study comparing coronary angioplasty with medical treatment in patients suitable for either, there was an improvement in symptoms in the angioplasty group but no overall difference in mortality[63].

Summary

The preparation of patients for non-cardiac surgery has recently been reviewed by the American College of Cardiology and the American Heart Association Task Force, and they have produced extensive and comprehensive guidelines for practice[6]. In general, it is recommended that the preoperative treatment for patients undergoing vascular surgery should essentially be the same as for patients in the non-operative environment. Preoperative coronary revascularization is only to be advised for a small minority of patients at high risk of perioperative infarction, and the concept of 'getting a patient through' an operation with a coronary artery bypass graft is to be avoided. Preoperative CABG should be performed if it is the best overall treatment for that patient, and the benefit in terms of performing subsequent surgery at a reduced risk is secondary. The number of patients in which this is appropriate is low. It is felt that the preoperative cardiac assessment of these patients is an opportunity to institute a long-term cardiovascular treatment plan and follow-up.

Clinical predictors of cardiovascular risk are outlined in this report and are subdivided into major, intermediate and minor predictors of adverse cardiac events.

Major clinical predictors

- Recent myocardial infarction with severe/unstable angina.
- Decompensated congestive cardiac failure.
- Significant arrhythmias (high-grade A-V block, symptomatic arrhythmias in the presence of underlying heart disease, supraventricular arrhythmias with uncontrolled ventricular rate).
- Severe valvular disease.

Intermediate clinical predictors

- Mild angina pectoris.
- Prior myocardial infarction.
- Compensated or previous congestive cardiac failure.
- Diabetes mellitus.

Minor clinical predictors

- Advanced age.
- Abnormal ECG.
- Rhythm other than sinus.
- Low functional capacity.
- History of stroke.
- Uncontrolled systemic hypertension.

Functional capacity is also important, and can be measured in terms of the patient's ability to perform the functions of daily living. This is expressed in metabolic equivalent (MET) levels. One MET is defined as the resting oxygen consumption of a 40-year-old 70 kg man, and equals 3.5 ml/kg. Multiples of this basic unit can be used to grade and allow classification of differing activities. Excellent functional capacity is assumed to be the ability to perform activities associated with greater than 7 METs. Moderate functional capacity is 4–7 METs and poor functional capacity is less than 4 METs.

Activities that are associated with less than 4 METs include eating, dressing, using the toilet, walking around inside the house, dusting, washing dishes, baking, slow ballroom dancing, playing a musical instrument, golfing with a cart and walking at 2–3 mph for 50–100 yards. Activities that are associated with more than 4 METs include climbing a flight of stairs, walking up a hill, walking on the level at 4 mph, scrubbing floors, lifting/moving heavy furniture, doubles tennis or golf. Activities that are associated with more than 10 METs include strenuous sports such as swimming, singles tennis, football, running and skiing.

Table 3.3 The Duke Activity Status Index

Activity, can you . . .	Weight
Walk indoors, such as around your house?	1.75
Do light work around the house like dusting, washing dishes?	2.70
Take care of yourself, that is, eating, dressing, bathing, use the toilet?	2.75
Walk 100–200 yards on level ground?	2.75
Do moderate work around the house like vacuuming, sweeping floors, carrying groceries?	3.50
Do gardening such as raking leaves, weeding, pushing a power motor?	4.50
Have sexual relations?	5.25
Climb a flight of stairs or walk up a hill?	5.50
Participate in moderate recreational activities like golf, bowling, dancing, doubles tennis, throwing a baseball or football?	6.00
Participate in strenuous sport like swimming, singles tennis, football, basketball or skiing?	7.50
Do heavy work around the house such as scrubbing floors, lifting and moving heavy furniture?	8.00
Run a short distance	8.00

The Duke Activity Index
This table is based on a series of 12 questions that form the basis of the Duke activity index[64]. Scores can be added up and correlated with maximal oxygen uptake when measured on exercise testing. Although not exactly equal to metabolic equivalents (METs), this scale can give an indication of the energy expended in various activities.

An activity index has been produced in the form of a simple questionnaire containing 12 questions (Table 3.3)[64]. The weighting of each activity is based on the known metabolic cost of that activity in MET units, and a total score of all the activities that the patient can easily perform is calculated. This total correlates significantly with the peak oxygen uptake of the patient when exercised on a bicycle.

Surgery-specific risk

The type of surgery itself also influences the stresses imposed on the patient.

High-risk surgery includes emergency surgery, particularly in the elderly, aortic and major vascular surgery, peripheral vascular surgery and prolonged procedures associated with major fluid shifts/blood loss.

Intermediate surgery includes carotid endarterectomy, head and neck surgery, intraperitoneal and intrathoracic surgery, orthopaedic and prostate surgery.

Low-risk surgery includes endoscopic and superficial procedures, cataract and breast surgery.

These guidelines have been put together in a flow diagram (Figure 3.2).

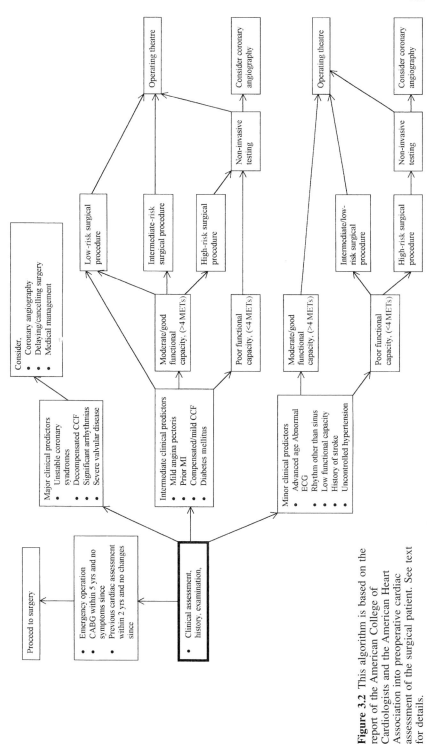

Figure 3.2 This algorithm is based on the report of the American College of Cardiologists and the American Heart Association into preoperative cardiac assessment of the surgical patient. See text for details.

The future

There is at present no consensus of opinion and a great variation in the individual practices of doctors involved in the preoperative preparation of patients for vascular surgery[65,66]. There have been no large scale multicentre studies assessing the clinical and cost-effectiveness of the various algorithms used by clinicians in the preoperative screening and management of patients for vascular surgery[67]. Although relatively large when compared to other types of surgery, the number of adverse cardiac events is in fact quite small, and large numbers of patients are required to provide meaningful results. There is likely to be a large cost involved in such a trial, but overall savings may be possible by the avoidance of unjustified expensive preoperative tests[68].

The postoperative management of patients also needs to be addressed. It could be that looking to surgically correct coronary artery disease, or spending large amounts of money on expensive tests to predict which patient will have an adverse cardiac event, is the wrong way to progress. Perhaps efforts should be directed at understanding the mechanisms of postoperative myocardial ischaemia/infarction, and in monitoring and treating post-operative ischaemia for as long as is necessary.

Physiological optimization

Preoperative placement of pulmonary artery catheters and optimization of filling pressures and cardiac output by the use of fluids and/or inotropes or vasodilators has been used to reduce complications in some types of major surgery. One study reduced the mortality rate of 89 patients undergoing peripheral vascular surgery from 9.5% to 1.5% using pulmonary artery catheters preoperatively to 'optimize' the cardiovascular system with fluids, vasodilators and inotropes[69]. Another study of 107 patients (including 58 vascular surgery patients) used dopexamine to increase oxygen delivery to a target level of 600 ml/min per m^2 perioperatively. This produced a reduction in mortality rate from 22.2% in the 'optimally' treated control group to 5.7% in the dopexamine group, $P = 0.015$[70]. Preoperative loading with 2l of normal saline after pulmonary artery catheterization has also been associated with reduced complications, better intraoperative stability and less need for vasopressors in the perioperative period[71]. These strategies, however, require preoperative treatment in intensive care, a high-dependency unit or in theatre, and facilities (particularly in the United Kingdom) are limited although these procedures could possibly save money overall by reducing complications.

Pharmacological optimization

There is increasing evidence of a cardioprotective effect in oral beta blockers, given preoperatively, in reducing perioperative myocardial ischaemia. Mangano[72] published a study in 1996 in which intravenous atenolol was given to 99 patients before non-cardiac surgery, and was continued for the duration of their hospital stay. Their perioperative course was compared to 101 patients in a placebo group. Mortality on leaving hospital was significantly less in the atenolol group, and this difference was still present up to 2 years postoperatively, mainly due to a reduction in deaths from cardiac causes in the first 6–8 months of the study. In another study of 83 patients undergoing aortic aneurysm surgery, oral metoprolol followed by intravenous metoprolol in the perioperative period produced a significant reduction in postoperative myocardial infarction rate (3% vs. 18%) when compared to a closely matched group. There were also significantly less cardiac arrhythmias[73]. In another case-control study involving vascular patients, 106 patients suffering postoperative myocardial infarction were matched with a control group without postoperative myocardial infarction. The use of beta blockers was significantly less in the group that suffered myocardial infarction (30% vs 50%), and was associated with a 50% decrease in risk[74].

The use of beta blockers before vascular surgery should be considered in any patient with hypertension and/or angina in whom there is no contraindication.

Pulmonary disease

Chronic obstructive airway disease (COAD) is common in vascular patients, as are pulmonary complications after anaesthesia and surgery. These include airway closure, atelectasis, sputum retention and chest infections, ultimately resulting in hypoxia. These are due to the 11% drop in functional residual capacity on induction of anaesthesia that can persist into the postoperative period, especially with abdominal surgery, and lead to hypoxia from ventilation/perfusion mismatch. Factors that increase the likelihood of chest infections occurring include:

● upper abdominal surgery[75]
● previous chest disease (sputum production, wheeze, airflow obstruction)
● smoking
● age greater than 70[76]
● obesity (may have sleep apnoea)
● ? poor postoperative analgesia
● general, compared to regional anaesthesia (Table 7.2).

History

The patient should be asked about cough, dyspnoea, wheeze and sputum production. A history of chest infections and sputum production for 3 months of the year makes the diagnosis of COAD likely. A functional assessment should include an estimate of exercise tolerance limited by chest symptoms, but in the vascular patient claudication often halts exertion first. Note any prescribed medication, namely bronchodilators or steroids. Patients with late onset asthma may have nasal polyps and be allergic to aspirin, and should be asked about their tolerance to other non-steroidal anti-inflammatory drugs. Asthmatic patients should not receive beta blockers, as these can exacerbate bronchospasm.

Examination

Signs of chronic chest disease and respiratory distress include:

- barrel-shaped chest
- expiratory wheeze
- pursed lips, providing expiratory positive end-expired pressure to prevent airway closure
- central cyanosis
- the warm, vasodilated hands of CO_2 retention
- increased respiratory rate
- use of the accessory muscles of respiration
- raised JVP and peripheral oedema, which suggest cor pulmonale.

Investigations

Full blood count. If the haemoglobin is raised, this suggests chronic hypoxia with secondary polycythaemia. A raised white cell count suggests active infection.

Chest X-ray. This is a poor indicator of functional capacity of the lungs. It may be useful as a baseline, if the patient has not been X-rayed in the previous year, or if details of the anatomy are required. It may be justified, if there has been a recent exacerbation of the patient's symptoms, to look for collapse or consolidation, which would require treatment prior to surgery.

Arterial blood gases. Indicated if severe lung disease is suspected. Baseline levels are useful, and detection of patients dependent on hypoxic respiratory drive ('blue bloaters') is possible. Although rare, this condition has profound effects on anaesthetic management, as these patients are extremely likely to suffer respiratory depression in the postoperative period after a general anaesthetic. A period of ventilatory support or a regional technique will be required. Hypoxia with a normal or low $Paco_2$ can be due to diffuse parenchymal disease or an acute problem such as chest infection or pulmonary embolus.

Respiratory function tests. These are easy to perform, and allow a quantitative assessment of the patient's respiratory function. Nomograms are available to compare the patient with a predicted value for the same age, height and sex. Forced expiratory volume in 1 second (FEV_1) and forced vital capacity (FVC) is measured. In obstructive disease, expiration is obstructed and the FEV_1 is reduced to a greater extent than the FVC so the ratio FEV_1/FVC is reduced to below the normal value of $>70\%$. In restrictive disease both FEV_1 and FVC are reduced, but by a similar amount, so the FEV_1/FVC ratio remains normal.

The lower the value recorded the greater the severity of the chest disease, and values less than 50% of the normal define serious disease[77]. An FEV_1 of 1.5 litres will probably result in a serious reduction in the ability of the patient to cough postoperatively.

Preoperative optimization

If possible, surgery should be performed at the best time of year for that patient, i.e. when chest symptoms are minimal. The patient should be admitted a few days early for preoperative physiotherapy and to learn breathing exercises that can be used postoperatively. Other factors for consideration include:

- stopping smoking, preferably for 8 weeks but for at least 24 hours preoperatively[78]
- bronchodilators, beta$_2$ agonists, theophylline derivatives, ipratropium bromide
- steroids
- antibiotics.

Renal disease

Chronic renal disease has been reported in many studies to be an important factor in postoperative morbidity and mortality[79]. Many studies have found a link factor between abnormal renal function and increased cardiac mortality in the perioperative period. Patients are often anaemic (with a compensatory chronic rise in cardiac output) and have hypertension, both of which will increase myocardial oxygen demand. One study showed a significant increase in postoperative dialysis dependence (0.0% vs 9%) and mortality (0.6% vs 8.0%) rates in patients with a creatinine clearance of < 45 ml/min undergoing vascular surgery when compared to those with normal renal function[80]. Patients with end-stage renal failure facing amputations have an especially high rate of in-hospital mortality. One centre quoted mortality rates of 43% for bilateral and 38% for unilateral above-knee amputations in this group of patients[81].

Cross-clamping of the aorta below the level of the renal artery is known to reduce renal blood flow by about 40%, and this persists long into the postoperative period[82]. It is important, therefore, that patients undergoing aortic surgery who have renal impairment preoperatively are optimally prepared. Preparation may include overnight saline intravenous hydration and theophylline before any intravenous contrast media are given. Radiographic contrast media can induce renal failure, and theophylline has been found to preserve glomerular filtration after angiography, perhaps due to its effect in antagonizing the vasoconstrictor effect of adenosine[83].

Problems associated with renal disease that must be considered in the perioperative period include:

- altered drug metabolism/excretion
- salt and water retention, causing hypertension and oedema
- hyperkalaemia
- acidosis; aim for pH > 7.25
- hypocalcaemia with hyperphosphataemia
- anaemia from decreased erythropoietin, bone marrow suppression, decreased erythrocyte lifespan
- ischaemic heart disease, accelerated atherosclerosis, uraemic cardiomyopathy
- prolonged bleeding time from reduced platelet function/adhesiveness
- high incidence of malnutrition

- delayed gastric emptying
- impaired immune system and increased likelihood of infections
- care needed with fistulas and shunts
- nephrotoxicity of angiographic contrast media.

Diabetes

Diabetic patients have a high incidence of peripheral vascular disease, coronary artery disease and renal failure. Blood sugar levels should usually be controlled perioperatively with one of the various insulin/sugar/potassium regimens that exist. Patients not usually requiring insulin and facing more minor surgery can have their oral medication stopped preoperatively and restarted soon after surgery without the need for insulin infusions. Postoperative infection and poor wound healing are common, and myocardial ischaemia is more likely to be silent. Hypoglycaemic episodes are more likely to be dangerous than slight hyperglycaemia, and any patient showing signs of sympathetic stimulation/sweating should have the blood sugar measured and corrected quickly if low.

Preoperatively, patients should be assessed for the presence of:

- cardiac disease
- renal disease
- insulin requirements
- neuropathy.

Diabetic neuropathy affects all nerves and can result in autonomic neuropathy. This can produce instability under anaesthesia, with a tendency to hypotension (especially with positive pressure ventilation). There is no reliable test of autonomic function, but a reduced tachycardic response to the valsalva manoeuvre and on standing up, especially if associated with postural hypotension, may indicate possible problems. Gastric stasis may also occur as a result of autonomic neuropathy and aspiration is possible even if the patient is starved.

Recommended further reading

Patterson D, Treasure T. *Disorders of the Cardiovascular System.* Edward Arnold, 1993.

References

1. Boyd AM. The natural course of arteriosclerosis of the lower extremities. *Angiol* 1960; **11**: 10–16.
2. Young JR, Hertzer NR, Bevan EG *et al.* Coronary artery disease in patients with aortic aneurysm; a classification 302 coronary angiograms and results of surgical management. *Ann Vasc Surg* 1986; **1**: 36–42.
3. Tarhan S, Moffitt EA, Taylor WF *et al.* Myocardial infarction after general anaesthesia. *JAMA* 1972; **220**: 1451–4.

 4. Goldman L, Caldera DL, Southwick FS *et al.* Cardiac risk factors and complications in non-cardiac surgery. *Medicine* 1978; **57**: 357–70.
 5. Glazier JJ, Chierchia S, Brown MJ *et al.* Importance of generalized defective perception of painful stimuli as a cause of silent myocardial ischaemia in chronic stable angina pectoris. *Am J Cardiol* 1986; **58**: 667–72.
 6. American College of Cardiologists/American Heart Association Task Force Report. Guidelines for perioperative cardiovascular evaluation for noncardiac surgery. *Circulation* 1996; **93**: 1278–1317.
 7. Steen PA, Tinker JH, Tarhan S. Myocardial reinfarction after anesthesia and surgery. *JAMA* 1978; **239**: 2566–70.
 8. Landesburg G, Luria MH, Cotev S *et al.* Importance of long-duration postoperative ST segment depression in cardiac morbidity after vascular surgery. *Lancet* 1993; **341**: 715–9.
 9. Dawood MM, Gupta DK, Southern J *et al.* Pathology of fatal perioperative myocardial infarction; implications regarding pathophysiology and prevention. *Int J Cardiol* 1996; **57**: 37–44.
10. Tuman KJ, McCarthy RJ, March RJ *et al.* Effects of epidural anesthesia and analgesia on coagulation and outcome after major vascular surgery. *Anesth Analg* 1991; **73**: 696–704.
11. Goldman L, Caldera DL, Nussbaum SR *et al.* Multifactorial index of cardiac risk in non-cardiac surgical procedures. *N Engl J Med* 1977; **297**: 845–50.
12. Jeffrey CC, Kunsman J, Cullen DJ *et al.* A prospective evaluation of cardiac risk index. *Anesthesiology* 1983; **58**: 462–4.
13. Domaingue CM, Davies MJ, Cronin KD. Cardiovascular risk factors in patients for vascular surgery. *Anaesth Intensive Care* 1982; **10**: 324–7.
14. Detsky AS, Abrams HB, McLaughlin JR *et al.* Predicting cardiac complications in patients undergoing non-cardiac surgery. *J Gen Intern Med* 1986; **1**: 211–9.
15. Payne SP, Galland RB. The use of a simple clinical cardiac risk index predictive of long-term outcome after infrarenal aortic reconstruction. *Eur J Vasc Endovas Surg* 1995; **9**: 138–42.
16. Eagle KA, Coley CM, Newell JB *et al.* Combining clinical and thallium data optimizes preoperative assessment of cardiac risk before major vascular surgery. *Ann Intern Med* 1989; **110**: 859–66.
17. Goldman L. Assessment of the patient with known or suspected ischaemic heart disease for non-cardiac surgery. *Br J Anaesth* 1988; **61**: 38–43.
18. Fisher JD. New York Heart Association Classification. *Arch Intern Med* 1972; **129**: 836.
19. O'Hara PJ, Hertzer NR, Krajewski LP *et al.* Ten-year experience with abdominal aortic aneurysm repair in octogenarians; early results and late outcome. *J Vasc Surg* 1995; **21**: 830–7.
20. Shah KB, Kleinman BS, Sami H *et al.* Re-evaluation of perioperative myocardial infarction in patients with prior myocardial infarction undergoing non-cardiac operations. *Anesth Analg* 1990; **71**: 231–5.
21. Rao TL, Jacobs KH, El-Etr AA. Reinfarction following anesthesia in patients with myocardial infarction. *Anesthesiology* 1983; **59**: 499–505.
22. Mangano DT, Browner WS, Hollenberg M *et al.* Association of perioperative myocardial ischaemia with cardiac morbidity and mortality in men undergoing non-cardiac surgery; The Study of Perioperative Ischaemia Research Group. *New Engl J Med* 1990; **323**: 1781–8.
23. Prys-Roberts C, Meloche R, Foex P. Studies of anaesthesia in relation to hypertension. I; cardiovascular responses of treated and untreated patients. *Br J Anaesth* 1971; **42**: 122–37.
24. Prys-Roberts C, Greene LT, Meloche R. Studies in relation to hypertension; II. Haemodynamic consequences of induction and endotracheal intubation. *Br J Anaesth* 1971; **43**: 531–47.
25. Assidao CB, Donegan JH, Whitesell RC *et al.* Factors associated with perioperative complications during carotid endarterectomy. *Anesth Analg* 1982; **61**: 631–7.

26. Goldman L, Caldera DL. Risks of general anesthesia and elective operation in the hypertensive patient. *Anesthesiology* 1979; **50**: 285–92.
27. Sever P, Beevers DG, Bulpitt C *et al*. Management guidelines in essential hypertension; report of the second working party of the British Hypertension Society. *BMJ* 1993; **306**: 983–7.
28. Wolfsthal SD. Is blood pressure control necessary before surgery? *Med Clin North Am* 1993; **77**: 349–63.
29. Howell SJ, Sear YM, Yeates D *et al*. Risk factors for cardiovascular death after elective surgery under general anaesthesia. *Br J Anaesth* 1998; **80**: 14–19.
30. Rose DK, Cohen MM, DeBoer DP. Cardiovascular events in the postanesthesia care unit; contribution of risk factors. *Anesthesiology* 1996; **84**: 772–81.
31. Allman KG, Muir A, Howell SJ *et al*. Resistant hypertension and preoperative silent myocardial ischaemia in surgical patients. *Br J Anaesth* 1994; **73**: 574–8.
32. Gill NP, Wright B, Reilly CS. Relationship between hypoxaemic and cardiac ischaemic events in the perioperative period. *Br J Anaesth* 1992; **68**: 471–3.
33. Burkart F, Pfisterer M, Kiowski W *et al*. Effect of anti-arrhythmic therapy on mortality in survivors of myocardial infarction with asymptomatic complex ventricular arrhythmias; Basel Anti-arrhythmic Study of Infarct Survival (BASIS). *J Am Coll Cardiol* 1990; **16**: 1711–18.
34. Ukani ZA, Ezekowitz MD. Contemporary management of atrial fibrillation. *Med Clin North Am* 1995; **79**: 1135–52.
35. Wong T, Detsky AS. Preoperative cardiac risk assessment for patients having peripheral vascular surgery. *Ann Intern Med* 1992; **116**: 743–53.
36. Schueppert MT, Kresowik TF, Corry DC *et al*. Selection of patients for cardiac evaluation before peripheral vascular operations. *J Vasc Surg* 1996; **23**: 802–8.
37. Poldermans D, Arnese M, Fioretti PM *et al*. Sustained prognostic value of dobutamine stress echocardiography for late cardiac events after major non-cardiac surgery. *Circulation* 1997; **95**: 53–8.
38. Kontos MC, Akosah KO, Brath LK *et al*. Cardiac complications in non-cardiac surgery; value of dobutamine stress echocardiography versus dipyridamole-thallium imaging. *J Cardiothorac Vasc Anesth* 1996; **10**: 329–35.
39. Mantha S, Roizen MF, Barnard J *et al*. Relative effectiveness of four preoperative tests for predicting adverse cardiac outcomes after vascular surgery; a meta-analysis. *Anesth Analg* 1994; **79**: 422–33.
40. Mayo Clinic Cardiovascular Working Group on Stress Testing. Cardiovascular stress testing; a description of the various types of stress tests and indications for their use. *Mayo Clin Proc* 1996; **71**: 43–52.
41. Robotham JL, Takata M, Berman M *et al*. Ejection fraction revisited. *Anesthesiology* 1991; **74**: 172–83.
42. Debusk RF, Blomqvist CG, Kouchoukos NT *et al*. Identification and treatment of low-risk patients after acute myocardial and coronary artery bypass graft surgery. *N Engl J Med* 1986; **314**: 161–6.
43. Pedersen T, Kelbaek H, Munck O. Cardiopulmonary complications in high-risk surgical patients; the value of preoperative radionuclide cardiography. *Acta Anaesthesiol Scand* 1990; **34**: 183–9.
44. Pasternak PF, Imparato AM, Bear G *et al*. The value of radionuclide angiography as a predictor of perioperative myocardial infarction in patients undergoing abdominal aortic aneurysm resection. *J Vasc Surg* 1984; **1**: 320–5.
45. McCann RL, Wolfe WG. Resection of abdominal aortic aneurysms in patients with low ejection fractions. *J Vasc Surg* 1989; **10**: 240–4.
46. Franco CD, Goldsmith J, Veith FJ *et al*. Resting gated pool ejection fraction; a poor predictor of perioperative myocardial infarction in patients undergoing vascular surgery for infrainguinal bypass grafting. *J Vasc Surg* 1989; **10**: 656–61.
47. Raby KE, Barry J, Creager MA *et al*. Detection and significance of intraoperative and postoperative myocardial ischaemia in peripheral vascular surgery. *JAMA* 1992; **268**:

222–7.

48. Raby KE, Goldman L, Creager MA *et al*. Correlation between preoperative ischaemia and major cardiac events after peripheral vascular surgery. *New Engl J Med* 1989; **321**: 1296–300.

49. Pasternak PF, Grossi EA, Baumann FG *et al*. The value of silent myocardial ischaemia monitoring in the prediction of perioperative myocardial infarction in patients undergoing peripheral vascular surgery. *J Vasc Surg* 1989; **10**: 617–25.

50. Edwards ND, Troy G, Yeo W *et al*. Early detection and treatment of myocardial ischaemia after operation using continual ambulatory arterial pressure monitoring and ECG ST segment analysis. *Br J Anaesth* 1995; **75**: 491–4.

51. Bodenheimer MM. Non-cardiac surgery in the cardiac patient; what is the question? *Ann Intern Med* 1996; **124**: 763–6.

52. Boucher CA, Brewster DC, Darling RC *et al*. Determination of cardiac risk by dipyridamole-thallium imaging before peripheral vascular surgery. *N Engl J Med* 1985; **312**: 389–94.

53. Emlein G, Villegas B, Dahlberg S *et al*. Left ventricular cavity size determined by preoperative dipyridamole-thallium scintigraphy as a predictor of late cardiac events in vascular surgery patients. *Am Heart J* 1996; **131**: 907–14.

54. Myers WO, Schaff HV, Gersh BJ *et al*. Improved survival of surgically treated patients with triple vessel coronary artery disease and severe angina pectoris. A report from the Coronary Artery Surgery Study (CASS) registry. *J Thorac Cardiovasc Surg* 1989; **97**: 487–95.

55. Foster ED, Davis KB, Carpenter JA *et al*. Risk of non-cardiac operation in patients with defined coronary disease; The Coronary Artery Surgery Study (CASS) Registry Experience. *Ann Thorac Surg* 1986; **41**: 42–50.

56. Rihal CS, Eagle KA, Mickel MC *et al*. Surgical therapy for coronary artery disease among patients with combined coronary artery and peripheral vascular disease. *Circulation* 1995; **91**: 46–53.

57. Hertzer NR, Young JR, Bevan EG *et al*. Late results of coronary bypass in patients with infrarenal aortic aneurysms. The Cleveland Clinic Study. *Ann Surg* 1987; **205**: 360–7.

58. Fleisher LA, Eagle KA. Screening for cardiac disease in patients having non-cardiac surgery. *Ann Intern Med* 1996; **124**: 767–72.

59. Krupski WC, Bensard DD. Preoperative cardiac risk management. *Surg Clin North Am* 1995; **75**: 647–63.

60. Cruchley PM, Kaplan JA, Hug CC Jr *et al*. Non-cardiac surgery in patients with prior myocardial revascularization. *Can Anaesth Soc J* 1983; **30**: 629–34.

61. Huber KC, Evans MA, Bresnahan JF *et al*. Outcome of non-cardiac operations in patients with severe coronary artery disease successfully treated preoperatively with coronary angioplasty. *Mayo Clin Proc* 1992; **67**: 15–21.

62. Elmore JR, Hallett JW Jr, Gibbons RJ *et al*. Myocardial revascularization before abdominal aortic aneurysmorrhaphy; effect of coronary angioplasty. *Mayo Clin Proc* 1993; **68**: 637–41.

63. RITA-2 trial participants. Coronary angioplasty versus medical therapy for angina; the second randomized intervention treatment of angina (RITA-2) trial. *Lancet* 1997; **350**: 461–8.

64. Hlatky MA, Boineau RE, Higginbotham MB *et al*. A brief self-administered questionnaire to determine functional capacity (the Duke Activity Status Index). *Am J Cardiol* 1989; **64**: 651–4.

65. Fleisher LA, Beattie C. Current practice in the preoperative evaluation of patients undergoing major vascular surgery; a survey of cardiovascular anesthesiologists. *J Cardiothorac Vasc Anesth* 1993; **7**: 650–4.

66. Michaels JA, Payne SP, Galland RB. A survey of methods used for cardiac risk assessment prior to major vascular surgery. *Eur J Vasc Endovasc Surg* 1996; **11**: 221–4.

67. Mangano DT. Preoperative assessment of the patient with cardiac disease. *Curr Opin Cardiol* 1995; **10**: 530–42.

68. Cohen MC, McKenna C, Lewis SM *et al.* Requirements for controlled clinical trials of preoperative cardiovascular risk reduction. *Control Clin Trials* 1995; **16**: 89–95.
69. Berlauk JF, Abrams JH, Gilmour IJ *et al.* Preoperative optimization of cardiovascular hemodynamics improves outcome in peripheral vascular surgery; a prospective, randomized clinical trial. *Ann Surg* 1991; **214**: 289–97.
70. Boyd O, Grounds RM, Bennett ED. A randomized clinical trial of the effect of deliberate perioperative increase of oxygen delivery on mortality in high-risk surgical patients. *JAMA* 1993; **270**: 2699–707.
71. Garrison RN, Wilson MA, Matheson PJ *et al.* Preoperative saline loading improves outcome after elective, noncardiac surgical procedures. *Am Surg* 1996; **62**: 223–31.
72. Mangano DT, Layug EL, Wallace A *et al.*, for the Multicenter Study of Perioperative Ischemia Research Group. Effect of atenolol on mortality and cardiovascular morbidity after non-cardiac surgery. *N Engl J Med* 1996; **335**: 1713–20.
73. Pasternak PF, Imparato AM, Baumann FG *et al.* The hemodynamics of beta blockade in patients undergoing abdominal aortic aneurysm repair. *Circulation* 1987; **76**: III1–III7.
74. Yeager RA, Moneta GL, Edwards JM *et al.* Reducing perioperative myocardial infarction following vascular surgery. The potential of beta blockade. *Arch Surg* 1995; **130**: 869–72.
75. Celli BR, Rodriguez K, Snider GL. A controlled trial of positive pressure breathing, incentive spirometry and deep breathing exercise in preventing pulmonary complications after abdominal surgery. *Am Rev Respir Dis* 1984; **130**: 12–15.
76. Pedersen T, Eliasen K, Henriksen E. A prospective study of risk factors and cardiopulmonary complications associated with anaesthesia and surgery; risk indicators of cardiopulmonary morbidity. *Acta Anaesthesiol Scand* 1990; **34**: 144–55.
77. Kroenke K, Lawrence VA, Theroux JF *et al.* Operative risk in patients with severe obstructive pulmonary disease. *Arch Int Med* 1992; **152**: 967–71.
78. Warner MA, Offord KP, Warner ME *et al.* Role of preoperative cessation of smoking and other factors in postoperative pulmonary complications; a blinded prospective study of coronary artery bypass patients. *Mayo Clin Proc* 1989; **64**: 609–16.
79. Pedersen T, Eliasen K, Henriksen E. A prospective study of mortality associated with anaesthesia and surgery; risk indicators of mortality in hospital. *Acta Anaesthesiol Scand* 1990; **34**: 176–82.
80. Powell RJ, Roddy SP, Meier GH *et al.* Effect of renal insufficiency on outcome following infrarenal aortic surgery. *Am J Surg* 1997; **174**: 126–30.
81. Dossa CD, Shepard AD, Amos AM *et al.* Results of lower extremity amputations in patients with end-stage renal disease. *J Vasc Surg* 1994; **20**: 14–19.
82. Gamulin Z, Forster A, Morel D *et al.* Effects of infrarenal aortic cross-clamping on renal hemodynamics in humans. *Anesthesiology* 1984; **61**: 394–9.
83. Osswald H, Gleiter C, Muhlbauer B. Therapeutic use of theophylline to antagonize renal effects of adenosine. *Clin Nephrol* 1995; **43**(suppl 1); S33–S37.

4

Monitoring during surgery

Statistical evidence that basic monitoring makes anaesthesia safer does not exist, and is unlikely ever to be produced because of ethical difficulties with a non-monitored control group. However, anaesthesia has become progressively safer over the last 30 years as minimal monitoring standards have been introduced, though there are clearly other factors contributing to this improved outcome[1]. Monitoring does not in itself prevent potential or actual damage to patients; it simply aims to provide an early warning of developing problems, and so allow extra time for the anaesthetist to identify and correct the abnormality. For this reason, recommendations on intraoperative monitoring invariably stress that the most important monitor is the presence of a competent and alert anaesthetist with the patient[2].

A complete discussion of intraoperative monitoring is beyond the scope of this book, and it is therefore assumed that basic monitoring is already in place. Similarly, detailed practical guidance on the insertion of invasive monitoring lines is not provided here as it is assumed that anaesthetists have acquired these basic skills before embarking upon major vascular surgical cases. This chapter describes the implications of vascular surgery on basic monitoring procedures, and introduces some of the more invasive and complex monitoring used for major vascular surgery.

Electrocardiography

It would be unusual nowadays to see any form of anaesthesia administered without using an electrocardiogram (ECG) for monitoring, and in most developed countries it is now recommended for use in all patients undergoing general anaesthesia[2,3,4]. In spite of this, in a study of 2000 critical incidents during anaesthesia only 7% were first detected with an ECG[5], most of which related to changes in heart rate which could have been detected with other monitors such as pulse oximeters. Over half the critical incidents were detected by the anaesthetist without the aid of any monitors, and it must be remembered that an ECG may be normal in a patient who is almost dead.

With the prevalence of coronary vascular disease amongst patients presenting for vascular surgery being so high (p. 85) it would, however, be most unwise not to utilize an ECG during anaesthesia. Because of its significance in vascular patients it is important to maximize the usefulness of the ECG, particularly with respect to detecting myocardial ischaemia by correct placement of electrodes and interpretation of the resulting ECG trace.

Positioning of ECG leads

Intraoperative ECG is most useful if the trace obtained can accurately reproduce one or more of the 12-lead ECG leads recorded preoperatively. This will allow comparison with the resting preoperative state and so provide useful information about any changes in rhythm or degree of ischaemia. Almost any lead will provide suitable information about rhythm changes, although standard lead II has been anecdotally described as the best for monitoring atrial arrhythmias[6]. For detection of ischaemia during anaesthesia, the precordial lead V_5 has been shown to have far greater sensitivity than any other lead (Figure 4.1)[7]. In an ideal world (and to maximize the sensitivity of ECG monitoring) all 12 leads should be recorded throughout the perioperative period, but this is clearly impractical, and several compromises have been developed.

Three lead configuration is the simplest, in which two electrodes act as the positive and negative recording electrodes for an ECG lead whilst the third acts as the neutral (ground) electrode. ECG monitors allow the use of different combinations of the three recording electrodes, such that with electrodes sited in the positions shown in Figure 4.2a the ECG trace

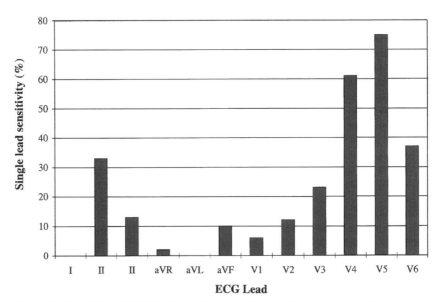

Figure 4.1 Sensitivity of ECG leads for detection of ischaemia during non-cardiac surgery. Sensitivity is the number of times ST depression is detected in a single lead, as a proportion of the number of occurrences of ST depression detected in any lead. The pattern of ST depression occurring in leads V_4–V_5 and lead II reflects the clinical pattern of ischaemia in the anterior and inferior regions of the left ventricle respectively. (After London *et al.*[7], with permission of the publishers of *Anesthesiology*.)

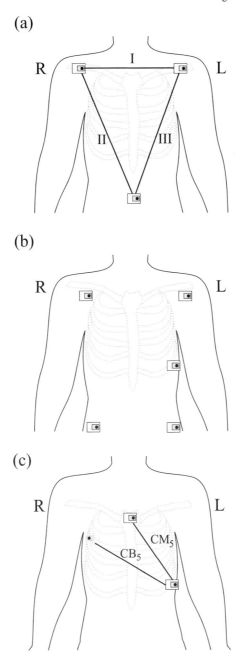

Figure 4.2 Siting of electrodes for ECG recording. (a) Three lead configuration. Lines show the lead recorded when the electrodes at each end are the active electrodes, the remaining electrode always being ground; (b) Five-lead configuration in which four electrodes correspond to the limb leads of a 12-lead ECG. The precordial electrode shown is at the V_5 position. Addition of only two more electrodes has allowed monitoring of seven different ECG leads; (c) CM_5 and CB_5 configuration. For CB_5, the right arm electrode is over the right scapula. The position of the 3rd (ground) electrode is irrelevant.

displayed can be switched between either of standard leads I, II or III. Although suitable for many anaesthetics, this combination of leads does not allow adequate monitoring of all regions of the heart that may develop ischaemia during surgery in patients with ischaemic heart disease.

Five lead configuration (Figure 4.2b) allows recording of all six standard ECG leads and one precordial lead, usually V_5 (see below). The addition of two further electrodes therefore allows monitoring of regions of myocardium broadly supplied by all three major branches of the coronary arteries:

- II, III, aVF–inferior left ventricle and conducting system, supplied by right coronary artery
- V_5–anterior left ventricle, supplied by left anterior descending artery
- aVL,V_5–lateral left ventricle, supplied by branches of circumflex artery.

CM$_5$ or CB$_5$ monitoring[8]. Monitoring of only standard limb leads excludes the anterior region of the left ventricle, so inclusion of a precordial lead is desirable. This may be achieved by using a five lead system, or, if not possible, by using the three lead configuration (monitor set to lead I) and placing the left arm electrode in the position of V_5 (5th intercostal space, anterior axillary line) and the right arm electrode either on the upper sternum (CM$_5$) or over the right scapula (CB$_5$) (Figure 4.2c). If only a single ECG lead is to be displayed during anaesthesia, then a CM$_5$ or CB$_5$ is useful because they:

- have a tall positive QRS which reduces the impact of interference (high signal:noise ratio)
- have a tall positive P wave which facilitates diagnosis of arrhythmias
- monitor the territory supplied by the left coronary artery, where ischaemia is common
- have a high sensitivity for detection of intraoperative ischaemia (Figure 4.1)
- can be compared with lead V_5 from preoperative ECGs (either resting, exercise or stress).

Based on all this information, for intraoperative monitoring of ECG:

- ideally, five leads (including V_5) should be used
- with two leads, II and V_5 are required, and over 80% of ischaemic events will be detected
- if only one lead is available, V_5 should be used.

ECG changes with myocardial ischaemia

Myocardial ischaemia during surgery may result in almost any ECG abnormality, including rhythm disturbances, conduction defects and T wave changes. However, these ECG changes exist preoperatively in many vascular surgery patients, and are not particularly specific to ischaemia. For this reason, ST segment analysis remains the best method of detecting the onset, or changes in severity, of myocardial ischaemia. Most of the research on ST

ECG patterns commonly associated with ischaemia

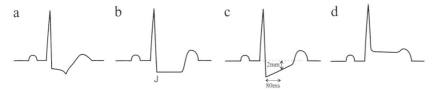

ECG patterns not usually associated with ischaemia

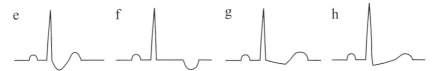

Figure 4.3 ST segment changes with myocardial ischaemia during exercise testing (see text for details). (After Goldschlager[9] with the permission of Dr Goldschlager and the publishers of *Annals of Internal Medicine*.)

segment changes is derived from studies of exercise testing in patients with angina, but in several respects (for instance changes in heart rate and blood pressure) this may be equated to the perioperative situation. When assessing the ST segment for ischaemia, care must be taken in interpretation (Figure 4.3)[9].

Minimum criteria for the diagnosis of ischaemia include either:

- 1 mm J point depression with horizontal or downsloping ST segment (Figure 4.3, a and b)
- 2 mm ST depression 80 msec after the J point with an upsloping ST segment (Figure 4.3, c), or
- 1 mm ST segment elevation (Figure 4.3, d).

Patterns of ST segment depression with exercise testing have been correlated with the severity of coronary artery disease[10]. Horizontal or up-sloping ST segment depression is the least severe; down-sloping ST segment usually indicates severe two or three vessel disease, and ST elevation represents transmural ischaemia associated with obstruction of the proximal coronary arteries.

Figure 4.3, e–h, show ECG patterns which are not normally associated with myocardial ischaemia during exercise testing. It can be seen that, in spite of abnormal ST segments, the J point is less than 1 mm from the baseline in all cases.

Many modern ECG machines now automatically measure the amount of ST segment depression on a real time basis[11]. This is usually done at 80 msec past the J point (ignoring the ST segment slope), and the value displayed in millimetres, corrected to the normal ECG vertical gain irrespective of the amplification of the displayed trace. The resulting figure must be interpreted with care, and with full knowledge of the electrode positions and lead being monitored, but does show reasonable agreement with changes found on monitoring multiple leads[12].

Arterial blood pressure

Frequent blood pressure measurement is now recommended for all patients having general anaesthesia[2,4]. It is primarily responsible for the detection of only 6.5% of critical incidents during anaesthesia, once again being greatly outnumbered by incidents detected by the anaesthetist without recourse to monitors (48%)[13].

Non-invasive measurement

Manual methods of blood pressure measurement involving brachial artery occlusion and either palpation or auscultation of the distal pulse have now become almost obsolete in the operating theatre setting, although they remain essential skills for the rare occasion when equipment failure occurs. Automated measurement of non-invasive blood pressure (NIBP) was introduced in the 1970s, and is based on the oscillometric method[14]. The artery is occluded by inflation of a cuff around the limb, and the cuff is then allowed to deflate in a stepwise fashion every 3–5 seconds. During each plateau the cuff pressure is measured and the rate of change (differential) of the pressure calculated, amplifying the pulsations transmitted to the cuff from the partially occluded artery beneath. The pulsations begin to increase at the systolic arterial pressure, reach a peak at the mean pressure, and level off at diastolic pressure (corresponding to phase 5 using Korotkoff sounds).

Values for blood pressure obtained by automated NIBP correlate well with blood pressure measured manually[15] or with arterial lines[14]. At normal values, the 95% confidence limits for NIBP readings of mean blood pressure compared with intra-arterial monitoring are ± 15 mmHg[14]. When compared with systolic and diastolic values, mean blood pressure measured by an oscillometric technique is more accurate as the maximal oscillations are the easiest to detect. As a result, at extremes of blood pressure NIBP machines may only display a mean result.

Sources of error from NIBP measurement include:

- inappropriate cuff size
- motion artefacts from the patient or staff
- kinking or obstruction of the cuff inflation or sensing tubes
- leaks from the cuff or tubes
- poor peripheral perfusion (may still read mean pressure)
- arrhythmias, particularly atrial fibrillation
- sudden changes in blood pressure during the NIBP inflation cycle, e.g. release of the aortic clamp.

The latter two problems cause changes to the pulsations in the cuff, which can disturb the algorithms within the NIBP machine microprocessor and result in extreme 'rogue' values. Blood pressure should therefore if possible be measured during periods of stability, and suspect values, including those which take longer than normal to determine, be repeated or confirmed by another method.

The convenience of repeated measurements with an automated technique can lead to over-enthusiastic NIBP recordings with almost continuous cuff inflation, which may lead to complications including ulnar nerve damage[16].

Direct arterial pressure measurement

An indwelling arterial cannula is now routine for all but the fittest of patients having major arterial surgery. An arterial line provides accurate beat-to-beat measurement of blood pressure, and facilitates blood sampling for assessment of pulmonary function and metabolic status. Arterial lines are not infallible in their ability to measure blood pressure, and attention to detail is required in their use.

Siting arterial cannulae in vascular patients. In the majority of vascular patients the radial artery is used because there is normally a good collateral supply to the hand from the ulnar artery, and in the wrist the radial artery is very superficial, allowing relatively easy insertion of an arterial cannula. In patients with shock, such as those with leaking aortic aneurysms, the radial artery may not be palpable and intense vasoconstriction may lead to inaccurate blood pressure measurement from peripheral arteries; the femoral or brachial artery should therefore be used. Patients presenting for arterial surgery may have significant disease of the subclavian arteries and, though uncommon in those having lower limb or aortic surgery, it is worth considering in patients presenting for carotid artery surgery before choosing the ideal site for an arterial cannula. Finally, lower limb revascularization may require the harvesting of arm veins, which will limit access to the cannula during surgery.

Arterial puncture in vascular surgery patients is often complicated by the presence of heavily calcified atheromatous arteries throughout the body, leading in particular to problems with threading the cannula along the lumen of the artery. This problem is usually overcome by using a Seldinger technique, in which a wire is thread through a needle into the artery lumen and then used to guide the cannula into the artery, a method associated with greater success than direct puncture[17]. Some examples of arterial cannulae are shown in Figure 4.4. For routine use with an easily palpable pulse, the cannula-over-needle system (Figure 4.4a) is normally sufficient; if unsuccessful it is usual to progress to the closed system Seldinger type arterial cannulae (Figure 4.4b). For particularly difficult arteries or patients with severely reduced cardiac output, an open Seldinger technique is required (Figure 4.4c), a method which results in too much blood spillage for routine use.

Measurement of blood pressure from arterial lines. This requires the arterial pressure waveform within the artery to be transmitted to a transducer, usually some distance away, which converts the pressure into an electrical signal for analysis by the monitoring system. Between the artery and transducer two problems can arise:

(a) Cannula over needle system

(b) Cannula over needle with built-in wire

(c) Separate needle, wire and cannula

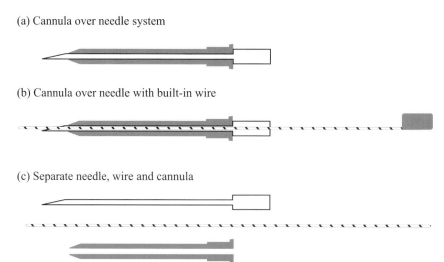

Figure 4.4 Types of arterial cannulae available. (a) Simple catheter over needle type; (b) Catheter over needle with built in wire for Seldinger technique; (c) Separate needle, wire and catheter set.

1 Damping. Energy contained in the arterial pressure wave is absorbed by elasticity of the tubing or compression of the fluid within, such that the peaks and troughs of the trace will be blunted with subsequent inaccuracy of the systolic and diastolic pressures (which will approach the mean pressure).
2 Resonance. Rigid tubing walls will result in pressure peaks 'bouncing' off the walls of the tube and resonating within the fluid column of the monitoring line. Individual frequency components of each arterial pulse may therefore become additive, and again cause inaccuracy of the systolic and diastolic pressures (which will diverge from the mean pressure).

Some degree of damping is therefore vital to prevent resonance, but not so much that the peaks and troughs are blunted. Thus in practice a compromise is needed, and arterial line monitoring systems are designed to provide 'critically' damped systems which result in accurate blood pressure readings at the transducer. This is achieved by having the correct length of tubing of the correct elasticity and diameter for the transducer concerned. Any modifications to the monitoring system, such as extensions to the tubing, will invalidate the systolic and diastolic readings. Air (which is very compressible) within the arterial line tubing is normally the cause of 'over-damping'. It is worth remembering that damping and resonance have no effect on the reading of mean blood pressure, which is therefore the most reliable and accurate parameter to observe, as in the case of NIBP above.

The blood pressure reading obtained from an arterial line is always relative to the transducer, and the height of the transducer is therefore vital. A technique in which the transducer is physically attached to the patient, level with the heart, is ideal, and it is particularly important to make sure that the transducer travels with the patient as the height of the operating table changes for the comfort of the surgeon. During carotid endarterectomy it is usual to place the patient in a head-up position, and the anaesthetist usually resides near the feet. In this case, the transducer must be positioned at the height of the patient's heart (or brain), and not at the feet.

Complications of arterial lines. These are numerous but rarely serious, and include:

● infection, localized or systemic
● pain in awake patients, particularly when flushing the cannula
● haemorrhage
● arterial trauma from dissection of the artery wall
● haematoma, potentially leading to pseudoaneurysm formation
● thrombosis
● embolism of thrombus or air (may be proximal to arterial line following rapid flushing or injection into small arteries)
● injection of drugs leading to distal arterial thrombosis.

Prevention of complications relies upon strict attention to detail, particularly with regard to asepsis and the equipment and technique of insertion used. Arterial lines should be left in place for as short a time as possible, and should only be used by adequately trained staff. Commercially available systems allow small volumes of heparinized saline to continually flush the cannula and so reduce thrombotic complications.

Central venous and pulmonary vascular pressures

Central venous pressure

In a similar fashion to arterial cannulae, the use of central venous pressure (CVP) lines for arterial surgery has increased over recent years. Fluctuations in vascular resistance and the potential for catastrophic blood loss make their use in patients having aortic surgery mandatory. They are useful during anaesthesia in any patient with significant heart disease having prolonged surgery, in order to monitor cardiac preload and provide suitable venous access for infusion of drugs. Other reasons for the popularity of CVP lines in vascular surgery include:

● frequent use of epidural analgesia with subsequent peripheral vasodilatation
● monitoring of insidious blood loss during prolonged lower limb revascularization
● venous access in patients whose arm veins are harvested for the surgery
● monitoring of fluid balance postoperatively, particularly when reperfusion injury is occurring.

Any patient in whom a CVP line is justified normally requires a multiple lumen line, usually a triple lumen catheter in which one lumen is used for monitoring, one for continuous drug infusions and one for giving drug boluses. The site and method of insertion is one of personal choice, but a

Seldinger technique using a guide wire is universal for the insertion of multilumen CVP lines. In cases that involve opening the chest cavity it is wise to site the CVP line on the side of surgery, to ensure the CVP line is uppermost when the patient is in the lateral position. Complications of CVP line insertion include:

- trauma to nearby structures, including arteries, nerves and other veins
- haematoma formation
- pneumothorax; more common during positive pressure ventilation
- air embolism
- arrhythmias, particularly when using a guide wire
- catheter damage and possible embolism
- perforation of vena cava or right atrium and haemothorax
- infection; either local or systemic.

Measurement of central venous pressure. Damping is less critical than for arterial lines, as only a mean pressure is required. However, the small magnitude of CVP means that positioning of the transducer at mid-heart level is important.

Pulmonary arterial catheterization

Use of a CVP line to measure cardiac filling pressure in the right atrium is many steps away from assessing the main determinant of cardiac output, the left ventricular end-diastolic volume (p. 5). This problem will be particularly pronounced in groups of patients who may be predicted to have different filling pressures on the right and left sides of the heart, including those with severe respiratory disease and consequent pulmonary hypertension or those with cardiac failure. In these cases, an indication of the filling pressure in the left atrium may be useful. A balloon-tipped pulmonary arterial catheter can provide this information by occluding a branch of the pulmonary artery, so allowing the pressure from the left atrium to be transmitted back through the pulmonary veins and capillaries and measured distal to the occlusion. This measurement is usually referred to as pulmonary capillary wedge pressure (PCWP).

The addition of a thermistor to the tip of a pulmonary artery catheter allows intermittent measurement of cardiac output by the thermal dilution technique, which is discussed in detail below.

Finally, a pulmonary artery (PA) catheter also allows measurement of mixed venous oxygen saturation, either by intermittent sampling or continuously with a fibre-optic oximeter. This, in conjunction with other easily obtained measures, may then be used to calculate oxygen delivery and consumption and the oxygen extraction ratio to provide an assessment of circulatory function.

For clinical use, the most commonly used device is a flow-directed balloon flotation catheter first described by Swan and Ganz, who developed the idea of using the blood flow through the heart to direct a balloon after watching boats sailing in Santa Monica Bay in 1967[18].

Insertion of a Swan–Ganz catheter. This is usually done via a large-diameter introducer catheter in either the internal jugular or subclavian vein,

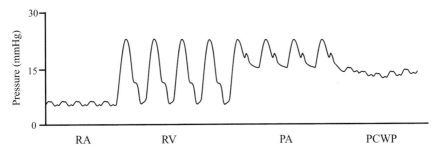

Figure 4.5 Pressure waveforms seen during insertion of a balloon flotation PA catheter. RA, right atrium; RV, right ventricle; PA, pulmonary artery; PCWP, pulmonary capillary wedge pressure.

but may also be done from the femoral vein. After inserting 15–20 cm of the catheter, to ensure the balloon is not within the introducer, the balloon is inflated and the catheter advanced slowly whilst continuously monitoring the pressure at the tip. The typical tracings for right atrial, right ventricular (RV) and pulmonary arterial pressure are observed (Figure 4.5), and pressures recorded if required. If it is intended to measure PCWP, the catheter is advanced until the balloon occludes a branch of the pulmonary artery and the PCWP trace is observed (Figure 4.5). The balloon is then deflated to check that a normal PA trace returns. Beyond the right ventricle there is little that the anaesthetist can do to influence where the catheter goes, particularly in low cardiac output states, but the following pitfalls should be avoided:

- check that the inflation syringe, balloon and tap all work before insertion
- Swan–Ganz catheters have a slight bend in the distal few centimetres, which should be aimed medially when in the right atrium to assist passage through the tricuspid valve into the RV
- coils of catheter in the RV may cause arrhythmias, and are likely if the PA is not entered when over 30 cm of catheter has been inserted
- arrhythmias are common on crossing the pulmonary valve, and the catheter should quickly be advanced further into the PA
- the balloon should always be fully deflated before pulling the catheter back, to prevent prolapse of the heart valves.

Complications relating to the insertion of Swan–Ganz catheters include all those associated with CVP line insertion; in addition, arrhythmias, knotting, cardiac perforation and valvular damage may occur, though fortunately the last two are very rare.

Measurement of PA pressures and PCWP. Pressure in the PA is measured in the same way as for systemic arterial pressure; the PA waveform is pulsatile and of low pressure, so it is important to ensure correct positioning and damping of the transducer system. Measurement of PCWP requires inflation of the balloon whilst observing the PA waveform and ensuring that the trace changes to a PCWP trace (Figure 4.5), identified by its similarity to the CVP trace and respiratory oscillations. Mean pressure is recorded, usually during expiration. Finally, the balloon must be deflated and the trace observed to ensure that it returns to a PA trace, otherwise the wedged balloon will cause pulmonary infarction.

Mixed venous oxygen saturation is measured by an oximeter, using optical fibres within the PA catheter which transmit infrared light and record the absorption by blood at the tip of the catheter. Mixed venous oxygen saturation (Svo_2) is normally around 75% compared with ≈100% in arterial blood, indicating an extraction ratio of 0.75. With rapidly changing cardiac output, tissue oxygen consumption tends to remain constant, so oxygen extraction must increase with a consequent fall in Svo_2. In this way, Svo_2 correlates with changes in cardiac output, particularly acute changes. However, changes in oxygen delivery or consumption also will affect Svo_2 and therefore confuse the relationship between Svo_2 and cardiac output. Acute changes in temperature and haemoglobin concentration seen during surgery therefore limit the use of Svo_2 monitoring in this setting.

Indications for perioperative use of a pulmonary arterial catheter. Measurement of PCWP and cardiac output is an empirically useful thing to do when managing patients with a compromised circulation. However, proof of benefit (in terms of improved outcome) when using PA catheters has been elusive, even in an intensive care setting where patients generally have more complex cardiovascular problems than in theatre. Perioperatively, patients having vascular surgery generally suffer from low cardiac output states related to myocardial ischaemia, hypovolaemia and aortic clamping, whilst the primary problem in many intensive care patients is sepsis with a picture of high cardiac output and low vascular resistance. Therefore, extending recommendations on PA catheter use from intensive care studies to surgical patients is unlikely to be valid.

Recently there has been renewed debate about the value of PA catheters, initiated by a large study of intensive care patients showing an increased mortality associated with their use[19,20]. This led to the establishment of a Pulmonary Artery Catheter Consensus Conference, held in 1996, specifically to address the benefits and risks of PA catheterization under many circumstances[21]. For peripheral vascular surgery, the consensus panel concluded that there was weak evidence that use of PA catheters reduced complications, but only if used correctly to optimize haemodynamics, and that their contribution to reducing mortality was uncertain. For abdominal aortic aneurysm surgery, there was good evidence of no benefit from using PA catheters in low-risk patients, but weak evidence of benefit when used in high-risk patients.

It is therefore left to the individual anaesthetist to decide in which patients a PA catheter may be useful. In most centres, PA catheters are used only for major vascular surgery in high-risk patients such as those with clinical evidence of heart failure, poor left ventricular function, pulmonary hypertension or severe ischaemic heart disease, though the threshold for their use is generally lower in the USA than in Europe.

Cardiac output and left ventricular function

Assessment of left or right heart filling pressures is adequate for most patients undergoing vascular surgery, but for high-risk procedures cardiovascular measurement needs to be taken a step further, and cardiac output (CO) determined as well. This then completes the analysis of cardiovascular function by enabling the assessment of myocardial contractility (relationship between preload and cardiac output) and systemic vascular resistance (relationship between blood pressure and cardiac output) as described in Chapter 1.

Over the years many techniques have been described for measuring CO, but only those that have become popular in clinical use are described here.

Measurement of cardiac output by thermodilution[22]

Indicator dilution is a method used in physiology for measuring blood flow through any system. An indicator is injected into the circulation at one point, and its concentration further along the circulation measured continuously to produce a concentration–time curve. Provided the indicator is not removed from the circulation by absorption or metabolism between the points of injection and measurement, the resulting indicator concentration curve can be used to calculate the blood flow between the two points selected. To assess CO, blood flow through the lungs is usually measured as these are the only organs through which all the CO flows (with the exception of a small amount of anatomical shunt blood flowing through the bronchial arteries and Thebesian veins of the left ventricle). Indocyanine green is the indicator generally used because it is non-toxic and easily measured in arterial blood. However, the necessity for continuous sampling of arterial blood and the accumulation of indicator dye with repeated measurement has led to the replacement of this technique with thermodilution.

Swan–Ganz catheter for CO measurement[23]. The principle of thermodilution is identical to that of indicator dilution, but relatively cool saline is used as the indicator, and a change in temperature distal to the injection point may then be equated to the indicator concentration. When using a Swan–Ganz catheter, 10 ml of cool saline (of known temperature) is injected into the RA through a proximal lumen, and the temperature measured in the PA by a thermistor built into the tip of the catheter. With this information a computer can then calculate CO, and although recirculation of the cool bolus is very occasionally detected, the indicator cannot accumulate with repeated measurements. Reproducibility of a single measurement may be poor, so three injections are usually performed a few minutes apart and the mean result correlates very well with blood flows measured either *in vitro* or *in vivo* using other methods.

Many technical factors will affect the CO reading obtained, including the injectate used (saline or dextrose), initial injectate temperature (near freezing or room temperature), injectate volume (3, 5 or 10 ml) and dead space for the injectate within the catheter (usually as much as 0.86 ml). Commercially available CO computers will automatically correct the result for all of these factors, but only if the correct information is provided concerning the type of catheter, injectate solution and volume being used. In general, larger injectate volumes provide more accurate results but increase the fluid load administered to the patient, and cooler injectate temperatures theoretically give more accurate results, although this is not borne out in practice because of greater variation in the injectate temperature when it reaches the circulation.

Patient factors that may lead to inaccurate readings are numerous, and include:

- rapidly changing CO of whatever cause
- patient movement
- intrapulmonary shunting
- valvular heart disease
- hypothermia (inadequate temperature difference between patient and injectate)
- respiration.

Respiration affects CO measurement in two ways. First, respiration causes cyclical changes in venous return and therefore CO; second, it is believed that inspiration may transiently cool the RV and pulmonary vessels by a direct effect from the gases in the lung tissue. These effects will be exaggerated during positive pressure ventilation and/or PEEP, when the effects on CO may be dramatic. Herein lies another reason for always undertaking measurements in triplicate and, in patients with controlled ventilation, performing each one at the same point in the respiratory cycle.

Continuous thermodilution technique. Injection of cool saline bolus remains the standard clinical method of measuring CO, but results will always be limited to intermittent recordings and by potentially large volumes of fluid administration. An ingenious modification of the thermodilution technique has been devised in which a small heating element built into the proximal part of a Swan–Ganz catheter intermittently produces a warm bolus of blood, the temperature change further along the circulation is measured, and CO is again calculated from the temperature curve obtained. The temperature change achieved is much less, and its measurement is therefore more difficult because of the natural variations in PA temperature described above[23]. Electronic processing of the temperature signal has managed to overcome these difficulties, and CO can be displayed every 30 seconds with no necessity for fluid injections. Under ideal conditions, the results obtained by this technique have an average error of only ± 3.6% when compared with intermittent cool bolus[24].

Oesophageal Doppler[25]

This technique requires the insertion of a small (6 mm diameter) flexible probe into the patient's oesophagus during anaesthesia. The probe tip contains a Doppler-based device that measures the velocity of blood passing along the descending aorta, which is displayed against time. Using a nomogram, the patient's height and weight are used to derive an estimate of aortic cross-sectional area, which is then used in conjunction with aortic flow velocity to estimate cardiac output. Cardiac output is displayed continuously and, although average figures compare favourably with other measures of CO, it is advisable only to regard the displayed figure as an estimate on which observation of trends in CO may be made. As may be predicted, aortic cross-clamping in the abdomen does reduce the accuracy of oesophageal Doppler,

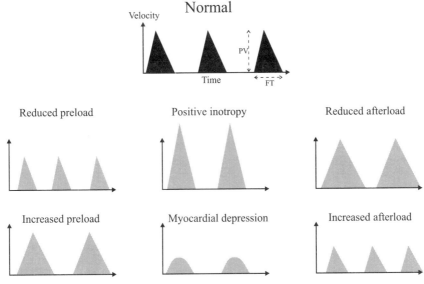

Figure 4.6 Schematic representation of normal and abnormal oesophageal Doppler traces. PV, peak velocity; FT, flow time, which must be corrected for heart rate. (After Singer[25], with permission from Dr M Singer and the publishers of *International Anesthesiology Clinics*.)

but trends in CO again mirror the actual CO measured by thermodilution[26].

The value of oesophageal Doppler lies not only in the continuous estimate of CO but also in wider interpretation of the trace obtained. Trace height (peak velocity) represents the contractility of the myocardium, and the width of the trace (flow time corrected for heart rate, FTc) is a function of the preload and afterload of the heart. Representative traces for many common cardiovascular disturbances are shown in Figure 4.6.

Using an oesophageal Doppler monitor, cardiac preload assessed by FTc can be actively manipulated by fluid loading during surgery, even in the absence of CVP monitoring. In cardiac and orthopaedic surgery this technique has been shown to improve some measures of patient well-being, and in the case of the latter even to reduce hospital stay, although no studies have been performed for vascular surgery[27,28,29].

Transoesophageal echocardiography

Transoesophageal echocardiography (TOE) involves technology that has been available for some years but has only recently been adopted by anaesthetists. A flexible ultrasound probe is inserted into the oesophagus facing anteriorly, where it can be brought into close proximity to the heart, allowing the production of clear images of most cardiac structures.

Techniques

Use of TOE is contraindicated in patients with oesophageal pathology such as tumour, varices and stenosis. Complications of insertion (generally trauma to the pharynx or oesophagus) are rare, occurring in less than 1% of cases, and fatalities related to the technique are approximately 1 in 7000–10 000[30,31]. Current standard technology includes a biplane probe, which rapidly rotates backwards and forwards through a 90° arc to produce a quarter circle view. Many different anatomical views of the heart can be obtained by advancing the probe to different positions along the oesophagus, tilting the tip in specific directions and scanning in specific planes, but for intraoperative use there are four standard views[31]:

- *three chamber view*, showing both ventricles, the left atrium and the left ventricular outflow tract
- *aortic views*, which are obtained at the same time as three chamber views by rotating the probe within the oesophagus to obtain views of the ascending aorta and aortic valve or the descending aorta to the side of the oesophagus
- *four chamber view*, showing a longitudinal section of all four cardiac chambers and the mitral and tricuspid valves
- *ventricular short axis view*, obtained by scanning the heart from within the stomach, which provides a cross-sectional view of both ventricles.

Some of these views are illustrated in Figure 4.7.

Assessment of valvular function

Standard TOE images clearly display aortic, mitral and tricuspid valves. TOE evidence of valvular dysfunction may include abnormalities of heart chamber dimensions, such as an enlarged left atrium in mitral valve disease, valve dimensions when open (stenosis) or closed (regurgitation), valve leaflet movements (prolapse), or flow abnormalities. The last of these is assessed by superimposing colour flow Doppler pictures on the TOE image to show the direction and flow rate of blood within the heart. Either valvular stenosis or regurgitation then results in a dramatically coloured 'jet' of blood within the heart chambers, the size of which provides an accurate method of quantifying the functional severity of a valvular lesion.

Assessment of ventricular function

The ventricular short axis view allows several aspects of ventricular function to be assessed.

Systolic function depends on a combination of preload, contractility and afterload (p. 5). Preload is best measured as left ventricular end-diastolic volume, which will be closely related to the end-diastolic cross-sectional area seen with TOE. Similarly, end-systolic volume, or cross-sectional area, equates to afterload. Contractility is assessed mainly by direct observation of ventricular wall motion, but may be quantified by comparing end-systolic

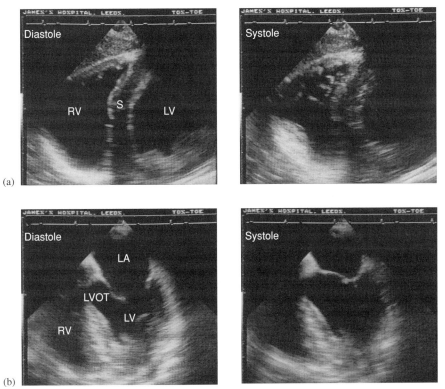

Figure 4.7 Standard images obtained using transoesophageal echocardiography in a normal subject. (a) Ventricular short axis view. (b) Three chamber view. RV, right ventricle; LV, left ventricle; S, ventricular septum; LA, left atrium; LVOT, left ventricular outflow tract.

and end-diastolic cross-sectional areas, the ratio of which approximates to ejection fraction measured by other techniques. The problem with all these observations is their dependence on each other and on the compliance of the ventricular wall, which will be influenced in turn by many other factors including diastolic function.

Diastolic function resulting in impaired ventricular filling dynamics is difficult to assess even with TOE, and has only recently been identified as an important component of ventricular dysfunction during heart failure, myocardial ischaemia and anaesthesia[32]. Flow velocity across the mitral valve during diastole, again measured with colour flow Doppler, gives a reasonable assessment of ventricular filling rate[31].

Ischaemia and infarction are detected with TOE by segmental wall motion abnormalities (SWMA). Following the onset of ischaemia, abnormalities of ventricular wall motion occur in a few seconds, well before ECG changes or clinical symptoms. A SWMA may involve hypokinesia (reduced movement in the correct direction), akinesia (no movement) or dyskinesia (movement in the wrong direction). Ventricular scarring from previous infarction will be evident at the outset, but new SWMAs developing during surgery are

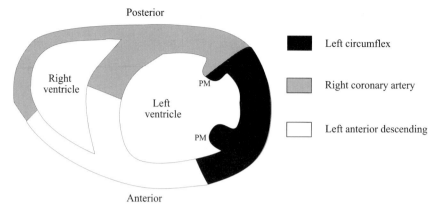

Figure 4.8 Schematic drawing of ventricular short axis view obtained with TOE (Figure 4.7a), showing the usual areas supplied by each coronary artery branch. Segmental wall motion abnormalities in these areas therefore provide detailed identification of the arterial abnormality. PM, papillary muscle.

excellent indicators of ischaemia, and form the basis of the preoperative investigation of stress echocardiography. A ventricular short axis image at the level of the origins of the papillary muscle allows the territory of each major branch of the coronary artery to be assessed (Figure 4.8).

TOE use in vascular surgery

TOE is now an accepted technique in cardiac surgery, particularly in valvular reconstruction surgery (where Doppler flows allow immediate assessment of the surgical outcome) and in high-risk coronary artery bypass surgery (when the development of SWMA post-bypass indicates technical problems with the graft to that area of myocardium). However, routine use of TOE for monitoring in vascular surgery remains controversial[33]. New valvular abnormalities will be uncommon, and although TOE is undoubtedly a good method of detecting the onset of ischaemia, the therapeutic interventions available when a SWMA occurs during non-cardiac surgery are less beneficial than those following coronary revascularization surgery, when the arterial lesion can be rectified directly and quickly. In addition, TOE is an expensive technology, both in terms of the initial expenditure on equipment and on the time required to train anaesthetists in its use. In the USA, where TOE is used much more widely than in Europe, specific guidelines now exist on training anaesthetic personnel in its use[34]. However, as technology advances TOE will become progressively less expensive and more user-friendly, and its use will undoubtedly become more widespread in the future.

Renal function[35]

In keeping with the generalized nature of vascular disease, patients presenting for arterial surgery commonly have impaired renal function before surgery due either to hypertensive renal disease or renal artery disease. Prolonged anaesthesia and surgery, accompanied by significant reperfusion injury and surgical stress response, lead to alterations in renal physiology. Aortic clamping, whether above or below the renal arteries, has profound effects on renal blood flow (p. 177). Postoperative renal failure remains a significant part of the morbidity and mortality associated with vascular surgery, and monitoring of renal function is therefore important in any patient having major arterial surgery.

Measurement of urine output. Catheterization of the bladder and recording of urinary flow rates is in most institutions the sole method for assessing renal function. A minimum urine production of 0.5 ml/kg per hr is generally accepted as adequate, and a patient who fails to maintain this during surgery should be treated aggressively with appropriate fluid monitoring and therapy, and diuretics if necessary. With this fundamental approach, postoperative renal failure seems to be less common than 20 years ago. However, many studies have failed to show a relationship between intraoperative oliguria and postoperative renal failure[35], the latter being better predicted by the age, preoperative serum creatinine level and cardiac function of the patient.

Other tests of renal function depend on biochemical approaches to measuring either glomerular filtration rate (GFR) or tubular function and include:

- urine to plasma (U/P) ratios for urea; U/P creatinine ratio or urinary sodium excretion require laboratory analysis of the samples and provide an indication of whether existing renal failure is prerenal or intrinsic in origin
- creatinine clearance measures GFR, but requires at least 2 hours of urine sampling and is known to have significant diurnal variations with lower values in the morning. Interpretation of a single measurement is therefore very difficult
- renal blood flow determination by para-aminohippurate clearance or isotope methods is useful but impractical in the perioperative setting
- tubular function can be assessed by measurement of urinary β_2-microglobulin (βMG) excretion. This small plasma protein passes easily through the glomerulus and is normally totally reabsorbed by the renal tubules, so its presence in urine indicates tubular damage. Unfortunately, βMG is unstable at room temperature and requires a complex laboratory analysis, and the relationship between βMG, evidence of tubular damage and clinically significant renal failure is unclear.

Urine output, in spite of its lack of predictive value, therefore currently remains the only practical method for monitoring renal function during surgery.

Temperature[36]

Induction of general anaesthesia immediately disturbs temperature regulation, causing a reduction in body temperature of approximately 1°C in the first half hour due to redistribution of body heat causing an equalization of the body core and the normally relatively cool periphery. Without intervention, continued anaesthesia results in a gradual decline in temperature to approximately 34°C before it stabilizes. The situation in vascular surgery is complicated by periods of ischaemia, when exposed non-perfused tissues such as the legs cool even further and add to body hypothermia when reperfused. Following ischaemia tissues may show profound compensatory vasodilatation, which increases heat loss, and this often continues long into the postoperative period before normal local thermoregulatory mechanisms return.

Significance of temperature measurement. Hypothermia may be beneficial in many circumstances in vascular surgery by reducing tissue metabolism and therefore oxygen consumption, anaerobic metabolism and cellular damage during ischaemia. The magnitude of the effect is significant, with a 7% decrease in oxygen consumption for each °C reduction in temperature. This effect is most commonly utilized for neurological tissue protection by allowing some degree of hypothermia during carotid surgery (p. 187) or suprarenal aortic surgery, when the brain and spinal cord respectively are at risk of ischaemic damage.

Conversely, for many body systems moderate hypothermia (32–35°C) is detrimental:

- heart–reduced contractility, irritability of the myocardium and more arrhythmias
- blood vessels–vasoconstriction resulting in hypertension and therefore increased afterload, with detrimental effects on myocardial oxygen supply and demand
- central nervous system–confusion, irritability or drowsiness
- respiration–reduced CO_2 production and depressed respiration; reduced ventilatory responses to hypercapnia or hypoxia with associated increased risk postoperatively
- haematology–increased blood viscosity, so poor perfusion to at-risk tissues (important following vascular surgery) and impaired haemostasis
- musculoskeletal–shivering occurs normally at 36.5°C, so is common in recovering patients and results in a large increase in oxygen consumption and possibly hypoxia.

Sites for temperature measurement. Many sites are used for temperature measurement during anaesthesia, and these are shown in Table 4.1 along with their principal advantages and problems. The preferred site depends on which organ system is most at risk from hypothermia. For example, in cardiac surgery myocardial temperature is vital so blood or oesophageal sites are used, whilst in most other instances (including vascular surgery) brain temperature is important for adequate emergence from anaesthesia so nasopharyngeal or aural sites are appropriate. The problem of heparin-induced bleeding from positioning temperature probes is minimized by siting the probe as early as possible before heparin administration, and when epistaxis or aural bleeding occurs it is usually of little significance compared with the potential complications of hypothermia.

Table 4.1 Sites for intraoperative temperature measurement showing their advantages and problems

Probe site	Advantages	Problems
Nasopharynx	Close to core (brain)	Epistaxis with heparin, easily displaced
PA catheter	Central blood temperature	Invasive solely as temperature monitor
Oesophagus	Close to cardiac temperature	Pharyngeal trauma, inaccurate if chest or pericardium open
Rectal	Convenient, few complications	May not reflect core temperature due to faeces, or mesenteric ischaemia
Skin	Convenient, few complications	Variable relationship to core temperature. Easily displaced, skin temperature very variable, poor when using convective heaters
Tympanic membrane	Close to core (brain)	Small risk of perforation or bleeding

Haemostasis

Normal haemostasis has three components, namely blood vessel constriction, activation of the plasma clotting factors and platelet activation, all of which are closely dependent on each other. Our ability to monitor these systems separately is hindered by the interdependence of each system. For example, activated platelets are involved in causing both blood vessel constriction and amplifying the intrinsic and extrinsic clotting cascades, whilst the endothelial lining of a traumatized blood vessel attracts the platelets and also activates clotting factors. When considering haemostasis it is also important not to overlook the fibrinolytic system, which once again is very closely linked with these factors. Thus in a normal subject there is a very delicate balance between all these biological systems, and any assessment of a single aspect of haemostasis or fibrinolysis is unlikely to give a true picture of the whole system.

Assessment of blood vessel constriction is extremely difficult, although fortunately abnormalities of this aspect of haemostasis are rare. Platelet *numbers* can be measured with ease in the haematology laboratory, but assessment of platelet *function* is more complex and requires either the performance of a bleeding time or the addition of several platelet activators to whole blood or platelet-rich plasma before measuring platelet aggregation[37]. Assessment of coagulation factor activity is relatively easy, with many laboratory and bedside tests available.

Whichever test is used, there are three factors which must be considered when performing coagulation tests during surgery:

1 *Temperature* has a profound effect on the rate at which clotting factor cascades proceed and the ability of platelets to be activated. Thus in a cold

patient, tests of haemostasis (usually performed at 37°C) may overestimate *in vivo* haemostatic activity.

2 *Haemodilution* with rapid infusion of crystalloid or colloid solutions will dilute the clotting factors and platelets and reduce their activity.

3 *Accidental heparinization.* Blood samples for tests of haemostasis during surgery are commonly taken from indwelling cannulae. It is particularly important in these cases to ensure there is no contamination of the sample with heparin from the flushing system used with the arterial or CVP line. Although present in quite dilute solution, heparin will have a profound effect on the often very small volumes of blood analysed. With meticulous technique, there is no difference in coagulation results between samples obtained from arterial lines with a 4.5 ml discard volume and those obtained using peripheral venepuncture[38].

Reasons for haemostasis monitoring in vascular patients

Patients arriving in the vascular operating theatre will rarely have normal haemostasis, even at the start of surgery. They are typically hypercoagulable, with high plasma fibrinogen levels as a result of both smoking and widespread arterial disease. In addition, patients are now commonly taking low-dose aspirin preoperatively to limit the progression of their vascular disease, and may have recently received low-dose heparin for the prophylaxis of deep vein thrombosis. Patients having surgery acutely for embolic or thrombotic arterial occlusion may be receiving intravenous heparin or have already received thrombolytic agents.

During surgery, there are two situations where monitoring of haemostasis is vital. First, control of heparin dosage is critical to prevent clots forming in distal arteries during clamping whilst allowing adequate haemostasis of often complex anastomoses once revascularization is complete. Second, in situations where blood loss is rapid or large, clotting factors and platelets will become depleted, resulting in a severe abnormality of haemostasis which requires correction.

Finally, following arterial reconstruction it is preferable to maintain a small degree of anticoagulation to reduce the incidence of early graft thrombosis or embolism, whilst once again allowing adequate haemostasis.

Assessment of coagulation factors and heparin activity

Laboratory tests of clotting activity most commonly involve measurement of the prothrombin time (PT), thrombin time (TT), activated partial thromboplastin time (aPTT) and fibrinogen levels. The aPTT test is the most useful as it mainly tests the intrinsic pathway which is inhibited by heparin, though at high doses of heparin the aPTT loses its linearity and therefore its ability to contribute to the clinical picture. The test requires technical expertise, involving the initial anticoagulation of the blood, separation of the plasma, reactivation of coagulation, careful monitoring of the progress of clot formation and adequate control samples. This test is therefore of limited use in the operating theatre context, but is a valuable part of the range of coagulation assays required to guide therapy following major haemorrhage.

Activated clotting time (ACT)[39] was first described over 30 years ago, as an attempt to bring laboratory coagulation tests closer to the patient. It involves the addition of blood to a warmed test chamber containing diatomaceous earth to activate factor XII and initiate clotting, and a mechanism for detecting clot formation. The ACT is simply the time in seconds between activation and clot formation, and is normally between 70–110 seconds. Commercially available ACT monitors are now available which are almost 'pocket sized', and provide reproducible and accurate results when operated by staff with only minimal training. ACT is prolonged by heparin administration in a linear fashion up to approximately 600 seconds, though a target of 200 seconds is more usual for vascular surgery and 400 seconds for cardiopulmonary bypass. At low plasma heparin concentrations ACT is less sensitive for detecting residual heparinization than the aPTT or thromboelastograph (see below), but as a rapid bedside test it remains useful[40]. Inter- and intraindividual variations in the metabolism of heparin are large, and the ACT should ideally be measured before heparin administration, a few minutes after intravenous heparin, and at regular intervals throughout surgery.

A prolonged ACT may result from a relative overdose of heparin or from other causes such as dilution of clotting factors by fluid administration or other anticoagulants, for example in transfused blood. For this reason, some systems are now available which perform the ACT in duplicate, with one test also containing heparinase which immediately inactivates any heparin present in the sample. Thus any difference between the two results can be ascribed to the presence of heparin in the sample, and methods are available to use this difference to derive the required dose of protamine. A similar technique employs multiple ACT tests preloaded with known doses of protamine[39,40].

Thromboelastography[41]

Thromboelastography (TEG) is a viscoelastic measurement of clot formation in whole blood, so it represents an overall picture of coagulation, platelet activity and the interaction between the two. A warmed cuvette containing 0.35 ml of blood has a slowly rotating piston lowered into it, and the torque between the piston and cuvette is measured. As a clot forms the torque increases and is plotted against time, resulting in a characteristic tracing (Figure 4.9a).

Four measurements are normally made from the tracing to quantify the results (Figure 4.9):

- R time, from starting the test to clot beginning to form, equates to coagulation times
- α angle, the rate at which clot forms once begun, dependent on clotting factors and platelet activity
- MA (maximum amplitude), the maximum width of the trace equating to final clot strength, also dependent on both clotting factors and platelets
- A60 (amplitude after 60 minutes), which as a ratio with MA quantifies thrombolysis.

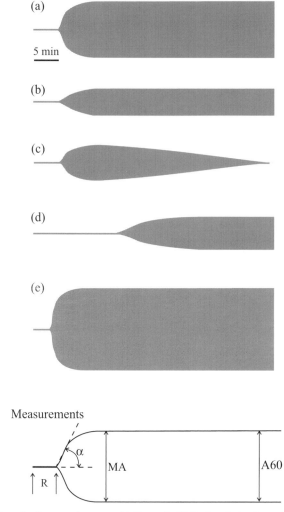

Figure 4.9 Thromboelastograph traces. (a) Normal; (b) Reduced platelet activity (e.g. aspirin or thrombocytopenia); (c) Thrombolysis; (d) Reduced coagulation factors (e.g. haemodilution, haemophilia); (e) Hypercoagulable state (e.g. postoperative aortic aneurysm surgery).

TEG may easily be performed in the operating theatre environment but, as can be seen from Figure 4.9, still requires nearly 30 minutes before any useful information is obtained and even longer to assess thrombolysis. Although slow to perform, the TEG is now widely used perioperatively because it provides a better 'snapshot' of the *in vivo* situation than any other single test. As shown in Figure 4.9, it is capable of demonstrating a wide variety of abnormalities including the hypercoagulable state associated with vascular surgery[42].

References

1. Lagasse RS. Monitoring and analysis of outcome studies. *Int Anesthesiol Clin* 1996; **34**: 263–78.
2. *Recommendations for Standards of Monitoring during Anaesthesia and Recovery.* Association of Anaesthetists of Great Britain and Ireland, 1994.
3. American Society of Anesthesiologists. Standards for basic intraoperative monitoring. *Anesthesia Patient Safety Foundation Newsletter* 1990; **54**: 17–19.
4. International Task Force on Anesthesia Safety. International standards for a safe practice of anaesthesia. *Eur J Anaesthesiol Suppl* 1993; **10**(7): 12–15.
5. Ludbrook GL, Russell WJ, Webb RK *et al.* The electrocardiograph: applications and limitations–an analysis of 2000 incident reports. *Anaesth Intensive Care* 1993; **21**: 558–64.
6. Kistner JR, Miller ED, Epstein RM. More than V_5 needed (letter). *Anesthesiology* 1977; **47**: 75–6.
7. London MJ, Hollenberg M, Wong MG *et al.* Intraoperative myocardial ischaemia: localization by continuous 12-lead electrocardiography. *Anesthesiology* 1988; **69**: 232–41.
8. Bazaral MG, Norfleet EA. Comparison of CB_5 and V_5 leads for intraoperative electrocardiographic monitoring. *Anesth Analg* 1982; **60**: 849–53.
9. Goldschlager N. Use of the treadmill test in the diagnosis of coronary artery disease in patients with chest pain. *Ann Intern Med* 1982; **97**: 383–8.
10. Goldschlager N, Selzer A, Cohn K. Treadmill stress tests as an indicator of presence and severity of coronary artery disease. *Ann Intern Med* 1976; **85**: 277–86.
11. Muller JG, Barash PG. Automated S–T segment monitoring. *Int Anesthesiol Clin* 1993; **31**: 45–55.
12. Ellis JE, Shah MN, Briller JE *et al.* A comparison of methods for the detection of myocardial ischaemia during non-cardiac surgery: automated S–T segment analysis systems, electrocardiography, and transoesphageal echocardiography. *Anesth Analg* 1992; **75**: 764–72.
13. Cockings JGL, Webb RK, Klepper ID *et al.* Blood pressure monitoring–applications and limitations: an analysis of 2000 incident reports. *Anesth Intensive Care* 1993; **21**: 565–9.
14. Hutton P, Dye J, Prys-Roberts C. An assessment of the Dinamap 845. *Anaesthesia* 1984; **39**: 261–7.
15. Silas JH, Barker AT, Ramsay LE. Clinical evaluation of Dinamap 845 automated blood pressure recorder. *Br Heart J* 1980; **43**: 202–5.
16. Sy WP. Ulnar nerve palsy possibly related to use of automatically cycled blood pressure cuff. *Anesth Analg* 1981; **60**: 687–8.
17. Mangar D, Thrush DN, Connell GR *et al.* Direct or modified Seldinger guide wire-directed technique for arterial catheter insertion. *Anesth Analg* 1993; **76**: 714–17.
18. Swan HJC, Ganz W. Hemodynamic monitoring: a personal and historical perspective. *Can Med Assoc J* 1979; **121**: 868–71.
19. Connors A, Speroff T, Dawson N *et al.* The effectiveness of right heart catheterization in the initial care of critically ill patients. *JAMA* 1996; **276**: 889–97.
20. Soni N. Swan song for the Swan–Ganz catheter. *BMJ* 1996; **313**: 763–4.
21. Pulmonary Artery Catheter Consensus Conference Participants. Pulmonary Artery Catheter Consensus Conference: Consensus Statement. *Crit Care Med* 1997; **25**: 910–25.
22. Jansen JRC. The thermodilution method for the clinical assessment of cardiac output. *Intensive Care Med* 1995; **21**: 691–7.
23. Mantin R, Ramsay JG. Cardiac output technologies. *Int Anesthesiol Clin* 1996; **34**: 79–108.
24. Boldt J, Menges T, Wollbruck M *et al.* Is continuous cardiac output measurement using thermodilution reliable in the critically ill patient? *Crit Care Med* 1994; **22**: 1913–18.

25. Singer M. Esophageal Doppler monitoring of aortic blood flow: Beat-by-beat cardiac output monitoring. *Int Anesthesiol Clin* 1993; **31**: 99–125.
26. Klotz KF, Klingsiek S, Singer M *et al*. Continuous measurement of cardiac output during aortic cross clamping by the oesophageal Doppler monitor ODM-1. *Br J Anaesth* 1995; **74**: 655–60.
27. Gan TJ, Arrowsmith JE. The oesophageal Doppler monitor. *BMJ* 1997; **315**: 893–4.
28. Sinclair S, James M, Singer M. Intraoperative intravascular volume optimization and length of hospital stay after repair of proximal femoral fracture: randomized control trial. *BMJ* 1997; **315**: 909–12.
29. Mythen M, Webb AR. Intraoperative gut mucosal hypoperfusion is associated with increased postoperative complications and cost. *Intensive Care Med* 1994; **20**: 99–104.
30. Townend JN, Hutton P. Transoesophageal echocardiography in anaesthesia and intensive care. *Br J Anaesth* 1996; **77**: 137–9.
31. Oxorn D, Edelist G, Smith MS. An introduction to transoesophageal echocardiography: II Clinical applications. *Can J Anaesth* 1996; **43**: 278–94.
32. Marsch SCU, Dalmas S, Philbin DM *et al*. Post-ischemic diastolic dysfunction. *J Cardiothorac Vasc Anaesth* 1994; **8**: 611–17.
33. George SJ. Transoesophageal echocardiography in anaesthesia and intensive care. *Br J Anaesth* 1996; **77**: 700.
34. Practice Guidelines for Perioperative Transoesophageal Echocardiography. A Report by the American Society of Anesthesiologists and Society of Cardiovascular Anesthesiologists Task Force on Transoesophageal Echocardiography. *Anesthesiology* 1996; **84**: 985–1006.
35. Garwood S, Hines RL. Renal function monitoring. *Int Anesthesiol Clin* 1996; **34**: 175–91.
36. Young CC, Sladen RN. Temperature monitoring. *Int Anesthesiol Clin* 1996; **34**: 149–74.
37. George JN, Shattil SJ. The clinical importance of acquired abnormalities of platelet function. *N Engl J Med* 1991; **324**: 27–39.
38. Heap MJ, Ridley SA, Hodson K *et al*. Are coagulation studies on blood sampled from arterial lines valid? *Anaesthesia* 1997; **52**: 640–5.
39. Stanley TE, Reves JG. Cardiovascular monitoring. In: Miller RD ed. *Anesthesia*, 4th edn. Churchill Livingstone, 1994.
40. Murray DJ, Brosnahan WJ, Pennell B *et al*. Heparin detection by the activated coagulation time: a comparison of the sensitivity of coagulation tests and heparin assays. *J Cardiothorac Vasc Anesth* 1997; **11**: 24–8.
41. Mallett SV, Cox DJA. Thrombelastography. *Br J Anaesth* 1992; **69**: 307–13.
42. Gibbs NM, Crawford GPM, Michalopoulos N. Thromboelastographic patterns following abdominal aortic surgery. *Anaesth Intensive Care* 1994; **22**: 534–8.

5

Carotid endarterectomy

Carotid endarterectomy is a prophylactic operation, and involves removal of an atheromatous lesion of the carotid artery that is likely to lead to a future stroke if left alone. However, patients who might benefit from carotid endarterectomy also have high levels of coronary artery disease, and the operation carries a significant morbidity and mortality from stroke and myocardial infarction. Risk–benefit analysis is therefore of the utmost importance in the treatment of these patients, to enable selection of those patients likely to benefit from surgery.

Patient selection has been an area of controversy for many years, but has recently been clarified with the publication of large multicentre trials into the efficacy of carotid endarterectomy in patients with both symptomatic and asymptomatic carotid artery disease.

Controversy still exists in the selection of the optimal method of anaesthesia and in the merits of the various methods of detecting peroperative cerebral ischaemia.

Cerebrovascular disease

Stroke

A stroke is defined as a rapidly developing, irreversible neurological deficit caused by a vascular lesion. A reversible ischaemic neurological deficit (RIND) is defined as one that lasts longer than 24 hours but has completely resolved at 3 weeks. A transient ischaemia attack (TIA) is a neurological event that lasts less than 24 hours (usually less than 1 hour) but then resolves completely. The annual incidence is about 2 per 1000 of the population per year, and the average GP with a practice of 2500 will see about five new stroke patients a year. The mortality is about 30%.

Aetiology

Strokes are mainly caused by infarction or haemorrhage. Infarction is more common, causing about 80% of strokes, compared to about 10% caused by intracerebral haemorrhage and about 10% by subarachnoid haemorrhage[1].

The Oxfordshire Community Stroke Project[2] looked at 244 cases of first stroke caused by cerebral infarction, proven by CT scan or at post mortem. Of these patients:

- 52% had hypertension
- 38% had ischaemic heart disease
- 25% had peripheral vascular disease
- 20% had a cardiac source of embolism
- 14% had TIAs
- 14% had a cervical arterial bruit.

This study shows that most patients presenting with cerebral infarction have hypertension or clinical evidence of atheromatous disease, and this emphasizes the potentially large public health benefits of effective treatment of high blood pressure. It also shows the large number of patients in this group with angina or previous myocardial infarction. The presence of pre-stroke TIAs or asymptomatic carotid bruits was a significant but much less common factor than the presence of hypertension. The problem is whether or not prophylactic carotid endarterectomy in these patients will produce a net reduction in the future stroke rate.

Prevention

Various treatment options are known to reduce the incidence of stroke:

- treatment of hypertension
- stopping smoking
- anti-platelet treatment, (in patients with TIAs)
- carotid endarterectomy (in suitable patients)
- warfarin (in patients with non-valvular atrial fibrillation).

Transient ischaemic attacks

Transient ischaemic attacks (TIAs) are mainly due to emboli from the heart or extracranial vessels, especially from unstable atheromatous lesions at the junction of the internal and external carotid artery. They are characterized by a sudden onset of neurological deficit that gradually recovers over 5–30 minutes[3]. Motor symptoms are more common than sensory symptoms, although transient monocular blindness (amaurosis fugax) can occur from emboli in the ophthalmic artery. Bilateral symptoms, vertigo, or diplopia may be due to vertebrobasilar TIAs. Drops in blood pressure and cardiac output can also cause TIAs. Interestingly, the patient who underwent the first reported carotid endarterectomy in 1954 suffered TIAs during episodes of palpitations[4]. Presumably the lower blood pressure or cardiac output during these attacks was enough to cause cerebral ischaemia. The TIAs resolved with excision of her tight carotid stenosis, but the palpitations continued.

Only about 14% of strokes are preceded by a TIA, and TIAs with severe carotid stenosis will progress to stroke in about 12–13% of patients at 1 year and 30–35% of patients in the next 5 years.

Medical treatment of TIAs includes aspirin 300 mg/day or ticlopidine 250 mg twice a day in patients intolerant of aspirin or who develop neurological deficits while on aspirin. Both treatments significantly reduce the risk of a stroke and of death[5]. Surgical treatment has been recently clarified with the publication of trials looking at the efficacy of carotid endarterectomy in patients with TIAs.

Asymptomatic carotid artery disease

Cervical bruits due to lesions of the carotid artery are heard high up in the neck under the angle of the mandible. Bruits heard lower down may be due to transmitted sounds from the aortic valve, the subclavian artery or a vertebral artery, stenosed at its origin. The sound of a carotid artery bruit is due to turbulent flow from an atheromatous lesion, and implies a stenosis of greater than 25%. However, high grades of stenosis may cause such a reduction in flow that no bruit is audible; an occluded artery will have no flow or bruit. In one study looking at the natural history of 500 patients with asymptomatic cervical bruits followed up for up to 4 years (mean 23 months), a risk of stroke of 1.7% at 1 year was noted. This was not as high as the risk of a cardiac ischaemic event in the same patients[6] (7%). Another study looking at asymptomatic patients measured carotid and vertebral artery stenosis with continuous-wave Doppler[7]. During follow-up of 11 months to 3 years, 23/122 patients died, 10 from a cardiac cause and only 3 from a cerebrovascular accident. Both these stroke rates are less than that following carotid endarterectomy.

Asymptomatic carotid and vertebral artery disease therefore seems to have a low likelihood of progressing to stroke, and appears to be more predictive of fatal coronary events. There seems to be, on average, an annual stroke rate of 1–2% and an annual cardiac death rate of 2–4% in patients with asymptomatic cervical bruits[8]. The complications of carotid endarterectomy in these patients are likely to outweigh any benefit, unless the complication rate is kept very low.

Although the degree of stenosis of the internal carotid artery is the most important factor in the subsequent risk of stroke from an atheromatous plaque, other factors play a part. Echolucent or heterogeneous plaques (on ultrasound) embolize more frequently, and are 4–6 times more likely to be associated with cerebral infarction than echogenic plaques[9]. This is presumably due to the high lipid or blood content of these plaques, which makes them unstable. Ulcerated lesions have a higher risk of causing a stroke, and the rate of progression of the stenosis is also important as this can vary widely, with some lesions even regressing.

Surgical considerations in carotid endarterectomy

Asymptomatic Carotid Atherosclerosis Study

The position on carotid endarterectomy in asymptomatic patients with a high degree of stenosis has been recently clarified with the publication of the Asymptomatic Carotid Atherosclerosis Study (ACAS)[10]. In this study, patients with an asymptomatic stenosis of 60% or more were allocated either to optimal medical treatment (including aspirin and risk-factor management) or optimal medical treatment plus carotid endarterectomy. The study was stopped when the 721 patients in the carotid endarterectomy group showed a statistically significantly better outcome. This was a reduction in risk of ipsilateral stroke of 5.8% at 5 years. The combined rate of surgical and arteriographic mortality and stroke rate was 2.3%. This is, however, only a small decrease in stroke rate, and no advantage was seen for women. This advantage would be lost if the overall operative surgical risk of morbidity and serious mortality in a centre operating on these patients were to rise above 3%, and it is therefore only really applicable to low-risk patients.

Carotid endarterectomy in patients with TIAs

The North American Symptomatic Carotid Endarterectomy Trial (NAS-CET)[11] randomized 659 patients with a history of TIA or non-disabling stroke in the previous 120 days and a 70–99% stenosis of the appropriate carotid artery, either to optimum medical therapy or carotid endarterectomy (CE). The overall risk for major or fatal strokes was 2.6% in the CE group, compared to 13.1% in the medically treated group, $P < 0.001$. This benefit was maintained at 3 years, and the survival curves showed no signs of converging. Early perioperative strokes and death produced an initial detriment to those undergoing CE, but the curves crossed at about 1 month and from then on outcome was better in the surgical group.

The MRC European Carotid Surgery Trial (ECST)[12] randomized 778 patients with a similar pathology to the above study, into either medical or surgical treatment. They found a risk of death or severe stroke to be 6% in the surgical group and 11% in the medical group, $P < 0.05$. This trial also looked at patients with 0–29% stenosis and TIAs or stroke, but found that the overall risk of stroke over 3 years in those patients treated medically was small and the early morbidity and mortality of surgery produced no overall benefit. The results of the intermediate group, 30–69% stenosis, were inconclusive, and recruitment continues.

Conclusions. Patients with 70–99% stenosis of the ipsilateral carotid artery and TIAs or non-disabling stroke do significantly better with carotid endarterectomy compared to optimal medical treatment.

- In patients with 0–29% stenosis of the ipsilateral carotid artery and TIAs or non-disabling stroke, there is no overall benefit from carotid endarterectomy.

Overall guidelines or indications for carotid endarterectomy

In 1995, the American Heart Association published the findings of a multidisciplinary committee into the performance of carotid endarterectomy[13]. The committee looked at 96 possible indications for this operation, and classified the results into four groups. These results are applicable only to a centre or surgeon with a less than 6% morbidity and mortality.

- *Group 1.* This indication was classed as proven, from the results of properly randomized prospective trials.

- *Group 2.* Acceptable but not proven. Supported by data, but not absolutely certain.
- *Group 3.* Uncertain. Insufficient data available to define the risk–benefit ratio clearly.
- *Group 4.* Proven inappropriate. The risk of surgery outweighs benefit for the patients in this group.

For symptomatic patients

Group 1. TIAs/mild stroke in the previous 6 months and a carotid stenosis >70%.

Group 2. TIAs/mild/moderate stroke in the previous 6 months and a carotid stenosis of 50–69%.

Carotid endarterectomy ipsilateral to the TIAs combined with coronary artery bypass grafting.

For asymptomatic patients

Group 1. None.

Group 2. Patients with carotid stenosis >60% diameter reduction (with the publication of the ACAS trial, this indication is now considered proven and moves to Group 1).

Measurement of carotid stenosis

Angiography. Cerebral angiography was the gold standard measurement of carotid artery disease, but is invasive and associated with a 1% mortality from stroke[14]. It is also inaccurate in predicting the state of the vessel wall, as it only outlines the lumen. Its role as the main imaging modality has been taken over by Duplex sonography and magnetic resonance angiography.

Duplex scanning. This is combined B-mode ultrasound and range-gated pulsed Doppler flow. It is non-invasive, accurate and acceptable for determining the extent of the stenosis and estimating flow reduction, although there is a small risk of falsely diagnosing a high-grade stenosis as an occlusion. It is also useful in the diagnosis of postoperative carotid thrombosis.

MR scanning. Magnetic resonance angiography is a non-invasive alternative to conventional angiography. Regions of tight stenosis are often 'seen' as a gap in the flow pattern when the signal is lost (Figure 5.1). When compared to conventional angiography this implies a stenosis of at least 70%, with a sensitivity and specificity similar to carotid duplex ultrasonography[15].

Surgical procedure[16]

Operative technique is very important to ensure minimal cerebral emboli and ischaemia, and a low operative morbidity and mortality. The patient is positioned slightly head-up, with the face pointed away from the surgeon, shoulders slightly raised and head supported on a ring. The incision is on the

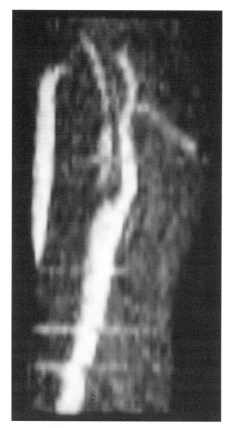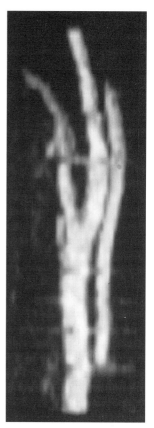

Figure 5.1 Magnetic resonance angiography (2D, time of flight) of carotid arteries. (a) Left side showing diseased artery. The flow gap at the origin of the internal carotid implies a stenosis of over 70%. (b) Right side showing the normal arterial layout. The other structure seen in each illustration is the vertebral artery.

side of the neck along the anterior border of the sternocleidomastoid, from just below the ear to just above the sternal notch. The common carotid and its bifurcation into the external and internal carotid are then fully exposed. Care must be taken to avoid damage to the hypoglossal nerve at the superior end of the wound and the vagus nerve running in the carotid sheath. The mandibular branch of the facial nerve and the recurrent laryngeal nerve can also be damaged during dissection. Heparin is given at this point, usually 5000 i.u., and after waiting 3 minutes to allow the heparin to circulate, the arteries can be clamped. The area of stenosis is carefully identified and the common carotid and the external carotid artery are clamped. At this time the stump pressure can be measured by direct arterial puncture with a needle attached to an invasive pressure measuring set and inserted into the internal carotid on the cerebral side of the atheromatous lesion above the arterial clamp. If the pressure is low, the surgeon may want to insert a shunt. The shunt is inserted into the distal end of the internal carotid first, and allowed to bleed back. It is then inserted into the proximal end of the common carotid artery, taking care to avoid air bubbles or particulate embolism. Once shunted, the endarterectomy continues with a blunt-ended dissection instrument in the correct plane for dissection of the thickened intimal layer. This may involve following the atheromatous lesion around the bifurcation of the common carotid artery and up into the external carotid. The distal end of the endarterectomy should be allowed to 'feather out' into very thin strands of intima. Sometimes small stitches are needed to tack down flaps of distal intima onto the arterial wall, to prevent them being lifted off in the postoperative period and causing an arterial dissection and occlusion. The artery is closed with a running stitch, or a patch may be sewn in if the artery is very small to avoid postoperative stenosis. Just before closing the arteriotomy, any shunt is removed and the lumen fully washed out ensuring there are no air bubbles. After closure of the artery, flow is restored to the external carotid first, as embolic phenomenon are less dangerous in this artery, and then the internal carotid. The wound is closed in two layers and a drain left in, which is usually removed at 24 hours.

Insertion of a shunt

Intuitively, it may seem a good idea to place a shunt during performance of the endarterectomy, to preserve distal blood flow and avoid strokes due to low flow ischaemia. However, shunt placement is not without complications and the number of patients in which shunts are needed may be small. Shunt placement can cause embolization and make the surgery more difficult by interfering with performance of the endarterectomy and identification of the end of the plaque. Intimal dissection may be precipitated, and the shunt can kink or thrombose peroperatively. Studies looking at results from centres that routinely insert shunts into all patients do not consistently show significant reductions in stroke rate when compared to those centres that rarely place shunts or which only insert shunt in selected patients. One study looking at 359 patients undergoing carotid endarterectomy under local anaesthesia found that only 4% of patients exhibited neurological symptoms on cross-clamping of the internal carotid artery and needed shunting[17]. Under general anaesthesia this percentage may well be less as cerebral metabolic rate and oxygen requirements are reduced, as is, presumably, the critical blood flow needed to avoid cerebral hypoxia. Under general anaesthesia clinical signs of cerebral ischaemia are not available, and as yet there is no perfect monitor to predict the need for shunt placement. Even patients who exhibit abnormal EEGs on cross-clamping may not develop neurological deficits if shunts are not inserted[18].

Good results have been reported without the use of a shunt at all. In one study involving 304 carotid endarterectomies using general anaesthesia without a shunt, only 2.6% of patients woke with a new neurological deficit. Another 2.6% developed deficits later, but overall only 0.6% died and 1.6% had a permanent neurological deficit[19]. Another study of 280 consecutive operations performed without a shunt reported no patients waking with a new neurological deficit and an overall stroke rate of 1.1%. All operations in this series were done under general anaesthetic, with hypertension during the performance of the endarterectomy, and total carotid occlusion time averaged only 10 minutes[20], representing extremely quick surgery.

Generally, most centres seem to use cerebral monitoring and insert shunts into those patients in whom the cerebral monitoring indicates potential cerebral ischaemia during cross-clamping. Patients with severe contralateral internal carotid artery disease or a recent cerebral infarction seem to be at high risk of ischaemia if shunts are not placed, and should probably have a shunt inserted.

Carotid angioplasty

Recently, interest has increased in the use of angioplasty for carotid artery stenosis[21]. Initially it may seen to be a very risky procedure, with a large chance of embolization and stroke. Using transcranial Doppler, many emboli can be detected during the angioplasty but the majority seem to be asymptomatic. Angioplasty can be combined with the use of stenting, and good results have been reported[22]. The exact place of this treatment remains to be decided, and is the focus of ongoing trials.

Anaesthesia for carotid endarterectomy

Preoperative assessment

Ischaemic heart disease. Carotid endarterectomy is followed by fatal myocardial infarction in about 1–2% of cases, forming about 60% of the total death rate. As well as all the normal risk factors for coronary artery disease, there is a close association between degree of carotid artery stenosis and subsequent myocardial ischaemia[6]. Unfortunately, this means that the patients more likely to benefit from surgery are also those more likely to be at risk of myocardial infarction. The reverse is also true, in that patients with coronary artery disease have a much greater cerebrovascular morbidity than patients without.

Pre-existing cardiac disease is a highly significant independent risk factor for perioperative mortality[23]. The guidelines for management of the patient with cardiovascular disease are dealt with in Chapter 3. Controversy surrounds the correct management of patients with coexistent severe coronary and carotid artery disease. Should carotid surgery precede coronary surgery, or the other way around, or should both be performed together? Meta-analysis published by the American Heart Association showed mixed results (Table 5.1).

These are high-risk patients, however, and overall the combined operation fared quite well, although the value of combined operations cannot be considered definitely proven. Overall, though, many studies have reported showing beneficial results of combined carotid and coronary surgery in patients with angina requiring carotid artery surgery[24–26], and this now appears to be the approach favoured in many centres.

Cerebrovascular disease. Increasing severity of preoperative neurological symptoms leads to increasing risk of postoperative stroke. Asymptomatic patients are at low risk. Patients with very frequent or 'crescendo TIAs' develop neurological deficits more often than those with infrequent TIAs, and patients with a stroke in evolution are at the highest risk. On angiography, patients with an occlusion of the contralateral internal carotid

Table 5.1 Risk of adverse events in patients requiring CEA and CABG

Operative order	Risk of adverse postoperative events		
	CVA	MI	Death
Simultaneous CABG + CEA	6.2%	4.7%	5.6%
CEA then CABG later	5.3%	11.5%	9.4%
CABG then CEA later	10%	2.7%	3.6%

CVA, cerebrovascular accident; MI, myocardial infarction; CEA, carotid endarterectomy; CABG, coronary artery bypass grafting. (After The American Heart Association[13].)

artery have increased peroperative risks[27]. If the presenting symptom is an ocular TIA (amaurosis fugax or retinal artery occlusion), then there is less operative risk than if the TIA is in cerebral artery territory[27].

There is a high morbidity for carotid endarterectomy in patients with a recent stroke. A wait of 5 weeks has been advocated[28], but operating early will avoid the risk of a further stroke in the intervening period and good results have been reported with earlier operation[29]. Pritz[30] reports good results within days of a stroke if the patient is fully conscious, the infarction was small and if there is no mass effect on CT scanning.

Age. Old age is associated with an increased risk of stroke and death after carotid endarterectomy[27]. However, this operation can be performed on the elderly (those over the age of 75 years) with good short- and long-term results[31,32], and old age in itself should not be a contraindication to surgery.

Hypertension. Hypertension occurs in 50–70% of patients presenting for carotid endarterectomy. Systolic blood pressure greater than 180 mmHg is a risk factor for postoperative stroke or death[27]. It is not clear whether preoperative treatment of this hypertension would reduce the subsequent risks. A few measurements of the patient's normal blood pressure should be taken on the ward preoperatively. A mean figure 10–20% higher than the mean of this reading can be used as a target for induced hypertension during performance of the endarterectomy. Hypertensive patients may have right shift of the cerebral autoregulation curve, and may need higher blood pressures generally to ensure adequate cerebral blood flow. Blood pressure should be measured in both arms, as there is occasionally also subclavian artery disease, which will give a falsely low impression of blood pressure.

Diabetes. Diabetes predisposes the patient to an increased incidence of cardiac pathology. However, using logistic regression analysis, diabetes in itself is not an independent risk factor in the development of a postoperative cardiac event[33], stroke or death[27].

Renal failure. Chronic renal failure is a significant risk factor for operative mortality and operative stroke[23].

Sex. Females seem to have an increased risk of stroke or death compared to males[27]. The reasons for this are not clear, but may be due to problems resulting from the smaller size of their internal carotid arteries.

Peripheral vascular disease. The presence of coincidental peripheral vascular disease is a strong predictor of subsequent peroperative stroke or death[27].

General anaesthesia

The aims of anaesthetic management are to provide adequate cerebral blood flow, especially during the period of carotid cross-clamping, and to avoid cardiac ischaemia in patients likely to be affected by significant coronary arterial disease. These two goals are somewhat contradictory, as maximizing cerebral blood flow involves inducing hypertension during cross-clamping. The overall result must be a balance between the two, and if high blood pressure is causing cardiac ischaemia it should be lowered.

Generally a 'light' general anaesthetic with muscle relaxation, intubation and ventilation is preferred, to avoid the cardiovascular depression of deep anaesthesia and allow rapid awakening at the end. As with most types of anaesthesia, results depend not so much on which drugs are used as on how carefully they are used to produce their desired effect.

Premedication

Long-acting premedication is not recommended, as the patient should be awake quickly after the operation to enable detection of new neurological deficits and immediate return for further surgery if indicated. If a premed is needed at all, 10–20 mg of temazepam given 2 hours prior to surgery should suffice.

Drugs

Induction agents. All the commonly used intravenous induction agents are acceptable, as long as the induction dose used does not cause undue hypotension. Propofol reduces blood pressure more than thiopentone, but the patient will awake more clear-headed. Ketamine increases intracranial pressure and is associated with unpleasant emergence phenomena, and is best avoided.

It may be appropriate to blunt the hypertensive response to laryngoscopy and intubation with alfentanil 1 mg, lignocaine 1.5 mg/kg or esmolol 1 mg/kg, particularly in the hypertensive patient.

Volatile agents. Nitrous oxide is avoided by some anaesthetists as there is a risk that any air emboli will increase in size. However, it is commonly used to prevent awareness and for its analgesic effect, and no significant increase in stroke rate has been reported with its use. Isoflurane at 0.5–1.0% MAC is the volatile agent of choice, as there is evidence that lower cerebral blood flows can be tolerated without cerebral ischaemia than with other volatile agents[34].

Muscle relaxants. General anaesthesia usually involves a muscle relaxant, intubation and a positive pressure ventilation technique. This avoids cardiovascular depression caused by high concentrations of volatile agent, and so allows a higher blood pressure to be maintained and decreases the use of vasopressors. Pancuronium is favoured by some anaesthetists for its hypertensive effect, but it can cause tachycardia as well and other anaesthetists prefer to used more cardio-stable relaxants such as atracurium or vecuronium and to induce hypertension by other means.

Opioids. Carotid endarterectomy is not associated with a large amount of postoperative pain, and this combined with the desire for a rapid return to full consciousness means that small doses of opioids are usually used. Fentanyl 1–2 µg/kg is usually sufficient. There may be a place for the use of the ultra short-acting opioid remifentanil in allowing rapid assessment of neurological state postoperatively. Postoperatively, intramuscular opioids and oral analgesics usually suffice for analgesia.

Vasopressors. Ephedrine in 6 mg increments is useful, especially if there is an accompanying bradycardia. Phenylephrine in 100 µg increments is a potent vasopressor but only lasts for 5–10 minutes, so has to be repeated often or given by infusion. Methoxamine in 4–6 mg boluses can also be used, and noradrenaline 5 mg in 50 ml of dextrose given at 2–6 ml/hr can produce stable cardiovascular conditions. In one study of 683 endarterectomies, however, the use of vasopressors in patients with known heart disease was associated with a significant increase in the postoperative myocardial infarction rate from 2.0 to 8.1%[35].

Monitoring

All the standard monitoring is routinely used, with the addition of an arterial line (see p. 123). As well as detecting beat-to-beat variations in arterial blood pressure, an arterial line also allows easy measurement of the stump pressure as an extra monitoring line and needle can be attached to the same transducer via a three-way tap.

Central venous pressure lines and pulmonary artery catheters are not routinely inserted, as the operation rarely involves large blood loss or fluid shifts. They may be needed if the patient has severe cardiac disease. The internal jugular on the same side as the operation is obviously an unsuitable site. The contralateral internal jugular site runs the risk of puncturing and damaging the contralateral carotid artery, which is essential for cerebral flow during cross-clamping, and the neck is therefore best left alone. The subclavian approach has a 1–2% risk of pneumothorax, but is otherwise suitable. Long lines placed in the antecubital fossa may also be used for the infusion of vasoactive drugs that are occasionally needed perioperatively. The more medial basilic vein is the best choice, as the lateral cephalic vein may be kinked at the clavipectoral fascia and insertion may fail. This is relatively complication-free, and can be used for per- and postoperative infusion of potent vasoactive drugs.

Cerebral monitoring

The best method of cerebral monitoring is to have the patient awake. If there are no new neurological signs during a test carotid clamping of 1 minute, it is generally safe to assume cerebral blood flow is adequate and that a shunt will not be needed. Under general anaesthesia there is as yet no perfect monitor for detection of low flow cerebral ischaemia occurring on cross-clamping.

Stump pressure. Measuring the pressure in the internal carotid artery distal to the occluding clamp is commonly used as an estimate of adequate collateral flow through the circle of Willis. It is unusual to observe strokes in patients with stump pressures greater than 50 mmHg, and it is easy to measure stump pressure once invasive arterial monitoring is in place.

However, pressure does not equal flow, and flow may be low in the presence of a high stump pressure if the resistance in the arterial tree is high due to widespread atheromatous change, especially in the presence of significant disease of the middle cerebral artery. Conversely, flow may be adequate even with low stump pressures, which may lead to the insertion of unnecessary shunts. There also seems to be little relationship between stump pressure and ischaemic changes on the EEG. In one study, 11 out of 17 patients with EEG changes suggestive of ischaemia had stump pressures greater than 59 mmHg. This is a level that would normally imply that a shunt is not needed[36]. Another problem with stump pressure is that it is a 'one off' measurement, while EEG monitoring is a continuous monitor of cerebral function for the whole duration of carotid cross-clamping.

Electroencephalogram (EEG). The EEG continuously detects electrical activity in the brain, mainly from the more superficial areas of the brain (the cortical neurones). It involves the placement of multiple electrodes around the head, and requires expensive equipment and a dedicated trained technician to interpret changes.

Factors affecting the EEG include:

- anaesthetics, volatile agents, depth of anaesthesia
- hypertension and hypotension
- temperature, hypothermia
- hypocarbia, hypoxia
- low cerebral blood flow.

Anaesthetic conditions should therefore be stable at the time of cross-clamping. EEG changes purely from low cerebral blood flow are then more clearly seen, and are not complicated by changing anaesthetic conditions. EEG changes due to low blood flow include an ipsilateral slowing of the waveform frequency and a decrease in amplitude of the EEG occurring a few seconds after clamping. This occurs at a higher blood flow than that which will cause neuronal ischaemia and death–flattening of the EEG occurs at flows of about 15 ml/min per 100 g, and neuronal death at flows below 10 ml/min per 100 g. This may be seen as a safety feature, but could also lead to the insertion of a shunt when one is not strictly needed.

The EEG is less reliable in patients with areas of neuronal death following previous strokes, who presumably have areas of pre-existing abnormal electrical activity. One study advocated the routine use of a shunt in such patients as EEG monitoring (and stump pressure) were found to be unreliable in predicting the need for a shunt[37].

Proponents of the EEG as a cerebral monitor maintain that maintenance of a normal EEG during carotid endarterectomy ensures that the patient has not had a stroke due to low blood flow. However, one centre reports EEG changes in only 6 patients out of 12 who woke with a neurological deficit, giving a sensitivity of only 50%[38]. As the EEG detects mainly cortical waveforms, ischaemia deeper in the brain may not be detected. Other centres have reported low stroke rates when using EEG monitoring to predict the need for shunts[39].

A normal EEG during cross-clamping of the artery is reassuring and allows the use of vasopressors to raise blood pressure to be avoided, thereby minimizing cardiac stress. A change in EEG after successful insertion of a shunt may imply a problem with the shunt, and could lead to the detection of a problem and avoidance of a stroke.

Processed EEG. The raw EEG data can be processed and analysed to extract the data required to make a judgement on cerebral ischaemia while simplifying the display. Spectral edge frequency, cerebral function monitors and processed EEGs have all been used, but may not be as accurate as the full 16 channel EEG[40].

Somatosensory evoked potentials (SSEP). Measuring the cerebral potentials 'evoked' by stimulation of the peripheral nervous system is one method of looking at the integrity and viability of neural pathways and testing for ischaemia in deeper layers of the brain not accessed by the EEG. A peripheral nerve is stimulated, and after a latent period the cortical electrical responses are monitored. It seems likely that SSEP monitoring gives the same information as EEG monitoring, and reliable results have been reported[41,42]. A reduction in amplitude of the primary cortical wave by 50% and prolongation of conduction time by 1 ms have been given as criteria for shunting[43].

Cerebral oximetry, niroscopy. Passing light at the near-infrared wavelength through the skin, scalp, skull, and brain and looking at the changes in the absorption spectra of the reflected light can allow estimates of changes in concentration of oxyhaemoglobin and deoxyhaemoglobin and the reduction–oxidation state of the cytochrome oxidase enzymes in the brain. Measurement of these parameters gives an indication of ischaemia and hypoxia occurring in the brain during the operation[44]. Measured changes will have a contribution from skin and scalp blood flow, and only areas of the brain directly below the optode will be examined. Exactly what the results mean in clinical terms is as yet unknown; however, it may compare well to other presently used methods of detecting cerebral hypoxia on cross-clamping[45]. The place of this monitor in clinical practice is still under evaluation.

Transcranial Doppler (TCD). By placing Doppler probes at various 'windows' in the skull (areas of relatively thin bone that allow passage of sound waves), intracerebral arteries can be insonated with sound waves, the reflected signal analysed and the velocity of the blood flow in that vessel calculated. This is the basis of TCD, and gives a real time read out of cerebral blood flow velocity. The usual parameter that is measured is the mean blood flow velocity. Drops in middle cerebral artery blood flow velocity do correlate well with EEG changes on clamping of the internal carotid artery[46]; however, this is not the same as flow because changes in vessel wall diameter are not known. There is a poor overall correlation between stump pressure and blood flow velocity in the middle cerebral artery, but patients with low stump pressures do tend to a low blood flow velocity[47]. The critical changes in blood flow velocity and the 'cut-off' level for shunting have not as yet been accurately defined.

Emboli are readily detected, and are heard as 'blips' in the normal whooshing sound of the trace. One possible advantage of detecting them is that surgeons may be able to modify their technique during the operation to minimize production of emboli. TCD may also be of use in the detection of cerebral hyperperfusion after carotid endarterectomy, when very high blood flow velocities may predict patients at risk of cerebral haemorrhage[48].

One disadvantage of TCD monitoring is that the probe can sometimes become displaced during the procedure, and it may be difficult to replace peroperatively. Also, a number of patients are unsuitable because of technical problems of getting a signal at the beginning.

Jugular venous oxygen saturation. The saturation of the blood in the internal jugular vein depends on the balance between cerebral blood flow and cerebral uptake of oxygen. If the brain is extracting a normal amount of oxygen, a drop in cerebral blood flow will lead to a drop in jugular vein oxygen saturation (SjO_2). A low SjO_2 is therefore assumed to be indicative of global cerebral ischaemia. Catheters can be placed into the jugular vein and directed up towards the skull base by the surgeon after exposure of the vessels during surgery.

Conduct of anaesthesia

The principle of anaesthesia is to maintain adequate cerebral oxygenation by avoiding hypoxia and hypotension. Cardiac ischaemia must be watched for and, if ST segment depression occurs, appropriate steps taken to relieve it, including blood pressure reduction. An arterial line and a large-bore intravenous cannula with extension line are usually inserted. An antecubital or subclavian central venous pressure line can be inserted if considered necessary.

Hypotension should be avoided post-induction and during the period of carotid cross-clamping, when the mean blood pressure should be increased to 10–20% more than the patient's normal mean blood pressure to help ensure adequate collateral cerebral blood flow. This is less important if a shunt has been inserted. Dissection and exposure of the artery may cause pressure on the carotid sinus and stimulate the baroreceptors. This results in a reflex bradycardia and hypotension. The surgeon will often warn that the sinus is being approached, but extreme vigilance is always required, as sudden severe drops in heart rate and blood pressure are possible. If this occurs, a vagolytic such as glycopyrolate 0.2 mg may be given and the surgeon told to stop operating until conditions return to normal. Occasionally the surgeon will anaesthetize the sinus with lignocaine or leave an epidural catheter *in situ* for injections of local anaesthetic in the post-operative period if necessary.

Ventilation to normocarbia is the general rule. Hypoventilation raises $Paco_2$, causes cerebral vasodilatation and raises intracranial pressure. The resulting vasodilatation of normal blood vessels may cause a 'steal' of blood away from ischaemic areas that are already maximally vasodilated. Hyperventilation will vasoconstrict intracerebral blood vessels except those in ischaemic areas, which will remain maximally vasodilated. This will potentially increase blood flow to ischaemic areas, but there is no convincing evidence of a significantly beneficial effect of this technique.

In one study hypocarbia was shown to be associated with fewer neurological complications than hypercarbic anaesthesia, although this difference failed to reach statistical significance. There was, however, a statistically significant increase in the incidence of arrhythmias in the hypercarbic group[49].

Some centres give a large dose of thiopentone (10–20 mg/kg) for cerebral protection just before cross-clamping of the internal carotid artery. This enables them to avoid the use of a shunt, and good results with a low incidence of major neurological events are reported[50]. Blood pressure is supported with vasopressors as necessary.

Large amounts of intravenous fluid are not needed, and 1 l of normal saline is all that is usually required. Glucose-containing solutions should be avoided, as there is evidence that patients with cerebral injury have worse neurological outcomes if their blood sugar is high at the time of injury.

Heparin 5000 i.u. is given before clamping the carotid artery and measuring stump pressure. It is usually not necessary to reverse the heparin with protamine, and there have been some reports of increased stroke rate if protamine is used[51]. If generalized bleeding is a big problem it may be due to aspirin therapy, and platelet transfusion could be indicated.

In the United Kingdom the operation takes about 2 hours (± 1 hour), and after extubation the patient is assessed neurologically and taken to the recovery room. Intra-arterial monitoring should be continued for at least 6 hours. Most patients can be managed on a high dependency unit (HDU), as only a few require intensive care. If no HDU facilities are available, the patient should be kept in the recovery area for as long as possible with invasive monitoring of blood pressure until a stable cardiovascular state is achieved. Any change in neurological condition must be immediately reported to the surgeons, as re-exploration may be necessary.

Carotid endarterectomy under local anaesthesia

There is no overwhelming evidence that carotid endarterectomy performed under local anaesthesia produces better results than when it is performed under general anaesthesia. There is a hint that a slight reduction in myocardial infarction rate is possible[52,53], but this cannot be considered to be proven. Many studies have presented large series of patients with good outcomes under local anaesthesia[54], including a reduction in cardiac and respiratory morbidity and a shorter hospital stay[55].

Overall, regional anaesthesia does not produce the same cerebral protection as general anaesthesia, as there is no fall in cerebral metabolic rate. However, autoregulation seems to be better preserved than in patients having general anaesthesia[56].

Advantages include:

- reliable cerebral monitoring
- good postoperative recovery
- less blood pressure fluctuation?
- less myocardial infarction?
- less need for vasoactive infusions peroperatively?

Disadvantages include:

- the requirement for patient and surgeon co-operation
- discomfort
- the need to pass urine
- boredom if the procedure is lengthy
- the tendency for a higher blood pressure peroperatively
- possible loss of control during cerebral ischaemia.

Conduct of regional anaesthesia

Sensory block of the C2–C4 dermatomes is required, as the C1 nerve root carries no sensory nerve fibres. This entails blocking the greater auricular, lesser occipital, supraclavicular and transverse cervical nerves, which are branches of the cervical plexus. This can be achieved in a number of ways:

- deep cervical plexus block
- superficial cervical plexus block
- local infiltration
- combination of the above
- cervical epidural.

In practice, deep cervical plexus block is usually combined with superficial cervical plexus block and with local infiltration by the surgeon as necessary.

Deep cervical plexus block. Care should be taken to handle the neck as little as possible to avoid dislodging emboli from the carotid plaques. With the head turned slightly to the side and the neck extended, the tubercle of the transverse process of C2 is gently palpated inferior to the mastoid process. A line drawn from the mastoid process to the tubercle of Chassaignac (the easily palpable transverse tubercle of C6) will indicate the approximate positions of the C3 and C4 tubercles, as they lie along this line at about 2 cm intervals down from C2. With the three needles in position on the transverse tubercles, 5–8 ml of local anaesthetic can be injected into each needle. Alternatively, a single injection technique can be used[57]. Phrenic nerve block often occurs but is seldom serious. Inadvertent vertebral artery injection is possible from a needle that passes too deep, and careful aspiration should be undertaken before injection to avoid this.

Superficial cervical plexus block. This is used to block the nerves as they emerge from around the posterior border of the sternocleidomastoid. With the neck in the same position as above, the posterior border of the sternomastoid is identified at the point at which the external jugular vein crosses. A single puncture point is used to inject local anaesthetic in front of, behind, and up and down the edge of the muscle from this point.

Local infiltration by the surgeon is a useful adjunct to cervical plexus block, and during performance of a carotid endarterectomy under local anaesthesia the surgeon should have a supply ready for use if the patient feels pain.

Cervical epidural. Epidural anaesthesia has been used successfully for the performance of carotid endarterectomy. The danger here is of cervical cord damage, epidural haematoma and bilateral phrenic nerve block, but good results have been reported[58].

Postoperative management

The main problems after carotid endarterectomy are:

- neurological deficit
- blood pressure control
- wound haematomata
- airway problems
- nerve damage
- ICU or HDU?

Neurological deficit

Postoperative neurological deficit is a major cause of morbidity and mortality after carotid endarterectomy surgery, and occurs in about 3–5% of cases. About 60–70% of strokes occur peroperatively, of which about 20% are due to low blood flow[59]. Information on the timing of neurological events has come from studies of patients undergoing carotid endarterectomy under local anaesthesia. During surgery, deficits may develop during dissection of the carotid bifurcation or occlusion of the artery, on release of the clamp, and in the postoperative period. Most peroperative deficits are embolic in nature, and only a few are attributable to low cerebral blood flow during carotid cross-clamp[17].

Meticulous surgical technique is of the utmost importance to minimize embolic events. Cerebral monitoring is used to identify patients in need of a temporary shunt, and may prevent strokes by identifying patients who don't need a shunt, thereby avoiding the insertion of a device that may cause an embolus. No technique of cerebral monitoring has been shown to be superior to any other.

Postoperatively, thrombosis of the internal carotid artery is possible, as the newly endarterectomized site is highly thrombogenic. Some centres use dextran to help prevent platelet aggregation, and the patients are usually on aspirin anyway. New symptoms (especially hemiplegia) developing a few hours after a 'successful' carotid endarterectomy are highly suggestive of an arterial thrombosis or dissection. If suspected, immediate Duplex scanning (and re-exploration if appropriate) should be undertaken for best results[60].

Postoperative blood pressure control is of paramount importance to ensure adequate cerebral perfusion by avoiding hyper- or hypotension.

Causes of neurological deficit following carotid endarterectomy include:

- intraoperative embolic phenomenona
- intraoperative hypoperfusion
- postoperative hypotension
- postoperative hypertension and hyperperfusion

- carotid artery thrombosis
- intracerebral haemorrhage
- cranial nerve injuries.

Blood pressure control

After carotid endarterectomy, blood pressure instability is common for the first 12–24 hours. Both hypertension and hypotension can occur, and lead to neurological deficit through hypoperfusion or cerebral bleeding.

Hypotension. Postoperatively, the carotid sinus may be exposed to the full force of the arterial blood pressure without the damping effect of the atheromatous plaque that was previously present. This overstimulation may lead to a reflex hypotension and bradycardia, which if severe can place the patient at risk of cerebral hypoperfusion. The usual course of this hypotension is however benign and transient. If necessary, blood pressure can be maintained by infusions of dopamine 1–10 µg/kg per min via a central line, or by anaesthetizing the carotid sinus with lignocaine through a pre-inserted epidural catheter. If the patient is asymptomatic, over-zealous attempts to raise the blood pressure may be inappropriate, but it would seem wise to aim for a systolic pressure of within 30% of preoperative levels. Hypovolaemia should be excluded. Hypotension usually resolves in the first 24 hours as the baroreceptors slowly 'reset' themselves.

Hypertension. The reason for postoperative hypertension is less clear. The patient may have been hypertensive preoperatively, and returns to this state postoperatively. Pain may be a factor, and should be considered and treated. Various other possible causes have been put forward for unexplained hypertension, including cerebral renin release[61], cerebral oedema, cerebral ischaemia during cross-clamping[62] and cerebral noradrenaline release[63].

Hypertension occurs more often in patients who have received intra-operative blocking of the carotid sinus with local anaesthetics. The brain may misinterpret this lack of baroreceptor input as a low blood pressure and act to raise systemic pressure. This may possibly also occur if the carotid sinus nerve has been damaged during surgery.

Hypertension is dangerous as it can cause bleeding from the wound site, which may compromise the airway, or bleeding from fragile vessels in the brain, leading to intracerebral haemorrhage. It also causes increased myocardial oxygen demands on a heart likely to have significant coronary heart disease. Blood pressures higher than the patient's norm should be avoided, and it is probably wise to aim for a pressure slightly lower than this to avoid excess strain on the arteriotomy suture line. Treatment can include nitrate or labetolol infusions. Hydralazine has also been used effectively as a hypotensive agent in the postoperative period[64]. Care must be taken to ensure that the patient is not over-treated, becoming hypotensive.

Hyperperfusion syndrome

A small number of patients develop hyperperfusion of the brain through the newly endarterectomized artery[65]. This can lead to severe unilateral fronto-temporal headaches, eye and face pain, seizures, confusion, cerebral oedema and even cerebral haemorrhage. This usually occurs 5–7 days postoperatively, and changes on post mortem resemble the changes seen with malignant hypertension[66]. Patients at risk of this complication seem to be those requiring endarterectomy of a very high degree of stenosis who have had a prolonged period of cerebral hypoperfusion. This leads to progressive intracerebral arteriolar vasodilatation and loss of autoregulation in order to maintain cerebral blood flow. Hypertension is usually (although not invariably) present, and treatment should be aimed at reducing the blood pressure, even in normotensive patients, in order to prevent cerebral haemorrhage. If cerebral oedema is present, mannitol and dexamethasone may be indicated. Transcranial Doppler has been used to document the high intracerebral blood velocities in this condition, and been found useful in the diagnosis[67]. Defective autoregulation due to chronic cerebral ischaemia has been implicated, as the cerebral blood flow velocities in these patients vary with blood pressure[68]. Cerebral autoregulation seems to 'reset' itself after 5–7 days, and the symptoms subside[68].

Cranial nerve damage

Transient damage to the adjacent cranial nerves is relatively common, but permanent damage is rare. Most injuries are neuropraxias, probably related to retraction or oedema, and patients recover within a year[69].

- The hypoglossal nerve lies at the rostral end of the incision, and passes anterior to the external carotid artery to enter the base of the tongue. Damage causes paralysis of the muscles of the tongue. and the tongue deviates to the side of the lesion on protrusion.
- The superior laryngeal nerve is a branch of the vagus, and splits into the internal and external laryngeal nerves supplying the larynx. Symptoms of damage are mild and are not usually noticed, but include a difficulty with high-pitched sounds.
- The marginal mandibular branch of the facial nerve is sometimes damaged and causes a drooping of the corner of the mouth.
- Recurrent laryngeal nerve injury or vagal nerve injury will produce paralysis of the vocal cord on that side, and hoarseness of the voice postoperatively. The patient may also be unable to cough effectively and, if damage is bilateral, may develop airway obstruction.
- The spinal accessory nerve is sometimes damaged, and can lead to weakness or aching of the shoulder.

Bleeding and wound haematomata

Preoperative aspirin, peroperative heparin and hypertension can combine in some patients to cause generalized ooze from the operation site. This is the case in about 80% of cases of wound haematomata. In about 20% of cases, bleeding from the artery is the cause[70]. Small haematomata can be left, larger ones need evacuation, and the rare, quickly expanding arterial bleed needs urgent decompression to avoid life-threatening airway obstruction. Some centres recommend local anaesthesia for evacuation of haematomata, as this avoids the dangers of general anaesthesia in the potentially compromised airway.

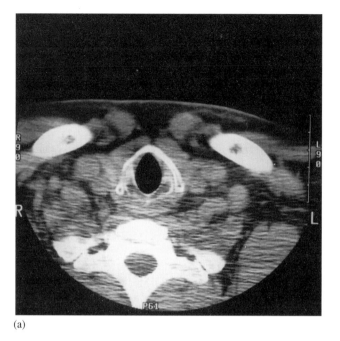

(a)

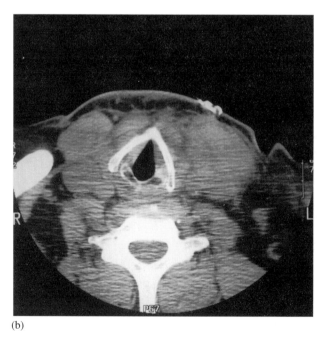

(b)

Figure 5.2 Computed tomography scans of the neck at cricoid level before surgery and the following morning. (a) Preoperative scan; (b) postoperative scan in the same patient showing moderate airway oedema;

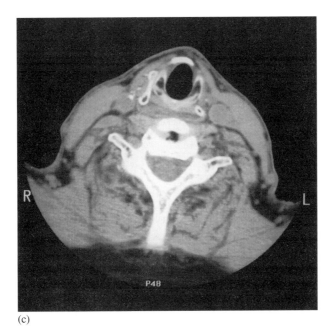

(c)

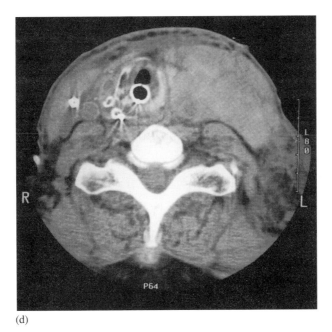

(d)

Figure 5.2 (*continued*) (c) preoperative scan; (d) postoperative scan in the same patient showing severe airway swelling requiring intubation, with large left-sided haematoma displacing the airway. We are grateful to Dr G McGuire of the Toronto Hospital for kindly providing the scans.

Airway problems

The airway can become compromised by direct damage during intubation, external compression from an expanding haematoma or from venous obstruction leading to engorgement and oedema of the airway (Figure 5.2)[71,72]. In extreme circumstances, airway obstruction can develop very quickly and intubation can obviously be very hazardous, if not impossible. Early recognition of wound haematomata and prompt evacuation, possibly under local anaesthesia, can hopefully avoid serious problems. In practice, when faced with a swollen neck and a compromised airway, local anaesthesia has its drawbacks. It will be very difficult to get good anaesthesia with such abnormal anatomy, and often removing the clot does not relieve the obstruction because this is commonly due to oedema of the upper airway and not to direct compression from the haematoma. An emergency tracheostomy using oxygen and a volatile agent in a spontaneous breathing technique is often the best option. Intubation under local anaesthesia using a fibreoptic technique is possible, if there is time.

High dependency unit or intensive care unit?

Patients with severe neurological damage, vocal cord paralysis with airway compromise or haemodynamic instability requiring large doses of vasoactive drugs should be admitted to intensive care. In practice, this is rarely required. The vast majority of patients can return to the ward or high dependency unit, if one is available. Postoperatively, all patients should have arterial monitoring for 4–6 hours until stable, or longer if haemodynamic instability persists. In units with no high dependency beds this can mean a prolonged stay in the post-anaesthetic care unit. After this, the majority of patients can return to the ward[73].

Problems following bilateral carotid endarterectomy

Bilateral carotid endarterectomy, either performed during the same operation or separated by a period of time, can cause damage to both carotid bodies. This can lead to:

● a significantly impaired ventilatory response to hypoxia
● extreme sensitivity to respiratory depressants
● long-term hypoventilation with a chronically raised Pa_{CO_2}[74,75].

These patients will obviously need close observation in the recovery period to ensure adequate ventilation. These factors, added to the increased risk of airway obstruction following bilateral surgery, makes bilateral carotid endarterectomy an unwise procedure at one sitting. If bilateral carotid endarterectomy is necessary, a staged procedure is recommended.

References

1. McLeod JG, Lance JW, Davies L. Cerebral vascular disease. In: *Introductory Neurology*. Blackwell Science, 1993.

2. Sandercock PAG, Warlow CP, Jones LN *et al.* Predisposing factors for cerebral infarction: the Oxfordshire community stroke project. *BMJ* 1989; **298**: 75–80.

3. Nadeau SE. Transient ischemic attacks: diagnosis, and medical and surgical management. *J Fam Pract* 1994; **38**: 495–504.

4. Eastcott HHG, Pickering GW, Rob CG. Reconstruction of internal carotid artery in a patient with intermittent attacks of hemiplegia. *Lancet* 1954; **2**: 994–6.

5. Barnett HJ, Eliasziw M, Meldrum HE. Drugs and surgery in the prevention of ischemic stroke. *N Engl J Med* 1995; **332**: 238–48.

6. Chambers BR, Norris JW. Outcome in patients with asymptomatic neck bruits. *N Engl J Med* 1986; **315**: 860–865.

7. Hennerici M, Rautenberg W, Mohr S. Stroke risk from symptomless extracranial disease. *Lancet* 1982; **2(8309)**: 1180–3.

8. Chambers BR, Norris JW. The case against surgery for asymptomatic carotid stenosis. *Stroke* 1984; **15**: 964–7.

9. Sterpetti AV, Schultz RD, Feldhaus RJ *et al.* Ultrasonographic features of carotid plaque and the risk of subsequent neurologic effects. *Surgery* 1988; **104**: 652–60.

10. Young B, Moore WS, Robertson JT *et al.* An analysis of perioperative surgical mortality and morbidity in the asymptomatic carotid atherosclerosis study. ACAS Investigators. Asymptomatic Carotid Atherosclerosis Study. *Stroke* 1996; **27**: 2216–24.

11. North American Symptomatic Carotid Endarterectomy Trial Collaborators. Beneficial effect of carotid endarterectomy in symptomatic patients with high-grade carotid stenosis. *N Engl J Med* 1991; **325**: 445–53.

12. European Carotid Surgery Trialists Collaborative Group. MRC European Carotid Surgery Trial: interim results for symptomatic patients with severe (70–99%) or with mild (0–29%) carotid stenosis. *Lancet* 1991; **337**: 1235–43.

13. A Multidisciplinary Consensus Statement from the ad hoc Committee, American Heart Association. Guidelines for Carotid Endarterectomy. *Stroke* 1995; **26**: 188–201.

14. Davies KN, Humphrey PR. Complications of cerebral angiography in patients with symptomatic carotid territory ischaemia screened by carotid ultrasound. *J Neurol Neurosurg Psych* 1993; **56**: 967–72.

15. Heiserman JE, Zabramski JM, Drayer BP *et al.* Clinical significance of the flow gap in carotid magnetic resonance angiography. *J Neurosurg* 1996; **85**: 384–87.

16. Thompson JE. Carotid endarterectomy. In: Greenhalgh RM ed. *Vascular and Endovascular Surgical Techniques.* WB Saunders, 1994.

17. Steed DL, Peitzman AB, Grundy BL *et al.* Causes of stroke in carotid endarterectomy. *Surgery* 1982; **92**: 634–41.

18. Evans WE, Hayes JP, Waltke EA *et al.* Optimal cerebral monitoring during carotid endarterectomy: neurologic response under local anaesthesia. *J Vasc Surg* 1985; **2**: 775–7.

19. Baker WH, Dorner DB, Barnes RW. Carotid endarterectomy: is an indwelling shunt necessary? *Surgery* 1977; **82**: 321–6.

20. Bland JE, Lazar ML. Carotid endarterectomy without a shunt. *Neurosurgery* 1981; **8**: 153–7.

21. Brown MM. Balloon angioplasty for cerebrovascular disease. *Neurol Res* 1992; **14**: 159–63.

22. Roubin GS, Yadav S, Iyer SS *et al.* Carotid stent-supported angioplasty: a neurovascular intervention to prevent stroke. *Am J Cardiol* 1996; **78**: 8–12.

23. Plecha EJ, King TA, Pitluk HC *et al.* Risk assessment in patients undergoing carotid endarterectomy. *Cardiovasc Surg* 1993; **1**: 30–2.

24. Ennix CL, Lawrie GM, Morris GC Jr *et al.* Improved results of carotid endarterectomy in patients with symptomatic coronary disease: an analysis of 1546 consecutive carotid operations. *Stroke* 1979; **10**: 122–5.

25. Chang BB, Darling RC III, Shah DM *et al.* Carotid endarterectomy can be safely performed with acceptable mortality and morbidity in patients requiring coronary artery

bypass grafts. *Am J Surg* 1994; **168**: 94–6.

26. Akins CW, Moncure AC, Daggett WM *et al*. Safety and efficacy of concomitant carotid and coronary artery operations. *Ann Thorac Surg* 995; **60**: 311–17.

27. Rothwell PM, Slattery J, Warlow CP. Clinical and angiographic predictors of stroke and death from carotid endarterectomy: a systematic review. *BMJ* 1997; **315**: 1571–7.

28. Giordano JM, Trout HH, Kozloff L *et al*. Timing of carotid artery endarterectomy after stroke. *J Vasc Surg* 1985; **2**: 250–5.

29. Gasecki AP, Ferguson GG, Eliasziw M *et al*. Early endarterectomy for severe carotid artery stenosis after a nondisabling stroke: results from the North American Symptomatic Carotid Endarterectomy Trial. *J Vasc Surg* 1994; **20**: 288–95.

30. Pritz MB. Carotid endarterectomy after recent stroke: preliminary observations in patients undergoing early operation. *Neurosurgery* 1986; **19**: 604–9.

31. Perler BA, Williams GM. Carotid endarterectomy in the very elderly: is it worthwhile? *Surgery* 1994; **116**: 479–83.

32. Coyle KA, Smith RB III, Salam AA *et al*. Carotid endarterectomy in the octogenarian. *Ann Vasc Surg* 1994; **8**: 417–20.

33. Akbari CM, Pomposelli FB Jr, Gibbons GW *et al*. Diabetes mellitus: a risk factor for carotid endarterectomy? *J Vasc Surg* 1997; **25**: 1070–5.

34. Messick JM Jr, Casement B, Sharbrough FW *et al*. Correlation of regional cerebral blood flow (rCBF) with EEG changes during isoflurane anaesthesia for carotid endarterectomy. *Anesthesiology* 1987; **66**: 344–9.

35. Riles TS, Kopelman I, Imparato AM. Myocardial infarction following carotid endarterectomy: a review of 683 operations. *Surgery* 1979; **85**: 249–52.

36. Brewster DC, O'Hara PJ, Darling RC *et al*. Relationship of intraoperative EEG monitoring and stump pressure measurements during carotid endarterectomy. *Circulation* 1980; **62**: 14–17.

37. Rosenthal D, Stanton PE Jr, Lamis PA. Carotid endarterectomy. The unreliability of intraoperative monitoring in patients having had stroke or reversible ischemic neurologic deficit. *Arch Surg* 1981; **116**: 1569–75.

38. McCarthy WJ, Park AE, Koushanpour E *et al*. Carotid endarterectomy. Lessons from intraoperative monitoring–a decade of experience. *Ann Surg* 1996; **224**: 297–305.

39. Whittmore AD, Kauffman JL, Kohler TR *et al*. Routine electroencephalographic (EEG) monitoring during carotid endarterectomy. *Ann Surg* 1983; **197**: 707–13.

40. Kearse LA Jr, Martin D, Mcpeck K *et al*. Computer-derived density spectral array in detection of mild analog electroencephalographic ischemic pattern changes during carotid endarterectomy. *J Neurosurg* 1993; **78**: 884–90.

41. Russ W, Fraedrich G, Hehrlein FW *et al*. Intraoperative somatosensory evoked potentials as a prognostic factor of neurologic state after carotid endarterectomy. *Thorac Cardiovasc Surg* 1985; **33**: 392–6.

42. Schwartz ML, Panetta TF, Kaplan BJ *et al*. Somatosensory evoked potential monitoring during carotid surgery. *Cardiovasc Surg* 1996; **4**: 77–80.

43. Gigli GL, Caramia M, Marciani MG *et al*. Monitoring of subcortical and cortical SSEPs during carotid endarterectomy: comparison with stump pressure levels. *Electroenceph Clin Neurophysiol* 1987; **68**: 424–32.

44. Kirkpatrick PJ, Smielewski P, Whitfield PC *et al*. An observational study of near-infrared spectroscopy during carotid endarterectomy. *J Neurosurg* 1995; **82**: 756–63.

45. Kuroda S, Houkin K, Abe H *et al*. Near infra-red monitoring of cerebral oxygenation state during carotid endarterectomy. *Surg Neurol* 1996; **45**: 450–8.

46. Arnold M, Sturzenegger M, Schaffler L *et al*. Continuous intraoperative monitoring of middle cerebral artery blood flow velocities and electroencephalography during carotid endarterectomy. A comparison of the two methods to detect cerebral ischemia. *Stroke* 1997; **28**: 1345–50.

47. Kalra M, al-Khaffaf H, Farrell A *et al*. Comparison of measurement of stump pressure and transcranial measurement of flow velocity in the middle cerebral artery in carotid

surgery. *Ann Vasc Surg* 1994; **8**: 225–31.

48. Jansen C, Sprengers AM, Moll FL *et al.* Prediction of intracerebral haemorrhage after carotid endarterectomy by clinical criteria and intraoperative transcranial Doppler monitoring. *Eur J Vasc Surg* 1994; **8**: 303–8.

49. Baker WH, Rodman JA, Barnes RW *et al.* An evaluation of hypocarbia and hypercarbia during carotid endarterectomy. *Stroke* 1976; **7**: 451–4.

50. Frawley JE, Hicks RG, Gray LJ *et al.* Carotid endarterectomy without a shunt for symptomatic lesions associated with contralateral severe stenosis or occlusion. *J Vasc Surg* 1996; **23**: 421–7.

51. Mauney MC, Buchanan SA, Lawrence WA *et al.* Stroke rate is markedly reduced after carotid endarterectomy by avoidance of protamine. *J Vasc Surg* 1995; **22**: 264–9.

52. Youngberg JA, Gold MD. Carotid artery surgery: perioperative anesthetic considerations. In: Kaplan JA ed. *Vascular Anesthesia*. Churchill Livingstone, 1991.

53. Prough DS, Scuderi PE, Stullken E *et al.* Myocardial infarction following regional anaesthesia for carotid endarterectomy. *Can Anaesth Soc J* 1984; **31**: 192–6.

54. Shah DM, Darling RC III, Chang BB *et al.* Carotid endarterectomy in awake patients: its safety, acceptability and outcome. *J Vasc Surg* 1994; **19**: 1015–9.

55. Young-Beyer P, Frisella P, Sicard GA. The influence of anaesthetic technique on perioperative complications. *J Vasc Surg* 1994; **19**: 834–42.

56. McCleary AJ, Dearden NM, Dickson DH *et al.* The differing effects of regional and general anaesthesia on cerebral metabolism during carotid endarterectomy. *Eur J Vasc Endovasc Surg* 1996; **12**: 173–81.

57. Winnie AP, Ramamurthy S, Durrani Z *et al.* Interscalene cervical plexus block: a single-injection technique. *Anesth Analg* 1975; **54**: 370–5.

58. Bonnet F, Derosier JP, Pluskwa F *et al.* Cervical epidural anaesthesia for carotid artery surgery. *Can J Anaesth* 1990; **37**: 353–8.

59. Krul JMJ, van Gijn J, Ackerstaff RGA *et al.* Site and pathogenesis of cerebral infarction associated with carotid endarterectomy. *Stroke* 1989; **20**: 324–8.

60. Takolander R, Bergentz S-E, Bergqvist D *et al.* Management of early neurologic deficits after carotid thromboendarterectomy. *Eur J Vasc Surg* 1987; **1**: 67–71.

61. Smith BL. Hypertension following carotid endarterectomy: the role of cerebral renin production. *J Vasc Surg* 1984; **1**: 623–7.

62. Archie JP Jr. The relationship of early hypertension following carotid endarterectomy to intraoperative cerebral ischaemia. *Ann Vasc Surg* 1988; **2**: 108–13.

63. Ahn SS, Marcus DR, Moore WS. Post-carotid endarterectomy hypertension: association with elevated cranial norepinephrine. *J Vasc Surg* 1989; **9**: 351–60.

64. Davies MJ, Cronin KD. Post-carotid endarterectomy hypertension. *Anaesth Intensive Care* 1980; **8**: 190–4.

65. Naylor AR, Ruckley CV. The post-carotid endarterectomy hyperperfusion syndrome. *Eur J Vasc Endovasc Surg* 1995; **9**: 365–7.

66. Bernstein M, Fleming JF, Deck JH. Cerebral hyperperfusion after carotid endarterectomy: a cause of cerebral haemorrhage. *Neurosurgery* 1984; **15**: 50–6.

67. Magee TR, Davies AH, Horrocks M. Transcranial Doppler evaluation of cerebral hyperperfusion syndrome after carotid endarterectomy. *Eur J Vasc Surg* 1994; **8**: 104–6.

68. Jorgensen LG, Schroeder TV. Defective cerebrovascular autoregulation after carotid endarterectomy. *Eur J Vasc Surg* 1993; **7**: 370–9.

69. Hertzer NR, Feldman BJ, Beven EG *et al.* A prospective study of the incidence of injury to the cranial nerves during carotid endarterectomy. *Surg Gynaecol Obstet* 1980; **151**: 781–4.

70. Kunkel JM, Gomez ER, Spebar MJ *et al.* Wound hematomas after carotid endarterectomy. *Am J Surg* 1984; **148**: 844–7.

71. Munro FJ, Makin AP, Reid J. Airway problems after carotid endarterectomy. *Br J Anaesth* 1996; **76**: 156–9.

72. Carmichael FJ, McGuire P, Wong DT *et al.* Computed tomographic analysis of airway dimensions after carotid endarterectomy. *Anesth Analg* 1996; **83**: 12–17.
73. McGrath JC, Wagner WH, Shabot MM. When is ICU care warranted after carotid endarterectomy? A three-year retrospective analysis. *Am Surg* 1996; **62**: 811–14.
74. Wade JG, Larson CP Jr, Hickey RF *et al.* Effect of carotid endarterectomy on carotid chemoreceptor and baroreceptor function in man. *N Engl J Med* 1970; **282**: 823–9.
75. Lee JK, Hanowell S, Kim YD *et al.* Morphine-induced respiratory depression following bilateral carotid endarterectomy. *Anesth Analg* 1981; **60**: 64–5.

6

Abdominal aortic surgery

Abdominal aortic surgery may be required for atherosclerotic occlusive disease or aneurysmal dilation. These processes involve the aorta and its major branches, leading to ischaemia, rupture and bleeding. Atherosclerotic disease is rarely limited to one part of the arterial tree. The manifestations of atherosclerosis–coronary artery disease, aortic aneurysm formation, aorto-iliac and peripheral vascular occlusion and cerebrovascular disease–indicate the same disease process occurring throughout the arterial tree at varying times and rates of progress[1].

Higher morbidity and mortality rates in patients undergoing aortic surgery, largely related to the prevalence of ischaemic heart disease in this population, presents a challenge to those providing anaesthesia and perioperative care. Patients are usually elderly, surgery may be prolonged and involve major fluid shifts and/or blood loss and, may be emergent. Therefore, according to published guidelines for preoperative evaluation, most aortic surgery should be considered high risk for postoperative cardiac complications[2]. Additional problems contributing to morbidity and mortality including coexisting respiratory disease, diabetes and renal dysfunction, and these must also be considered in the perioperative management.

This chapter will focus on anaesthetic management of patients requiring surgery for obstructive or aneurysmal atherosclerotic lesions of the abdominal aorta.

Prevalence

Abdominal aortic aneurysms greater than 5 cm in diameter are present in 1.5% of patients over 50 years, and 95% of these occur below the renal arteries[3,4]. The aetiology of aortic aneurysm is atherosclerotic in 90% of cases, with a smaller number arising due to mycotic infection, medial degeneration (Marfan's syndrome or Takayasu's disease) or trauma[5].

Presentation

Most abdominal aortic aneurysms are asymptomatic; however, aneurysms greater than 5 cm in diameter often cause low back or lumbar pain. Aortic aneurysms may be a source of lower extremity embolism; larger aneurysms may present as a pulsatile abdominal mass, or may compress the duodenum causing partial small bowel obstruction. The diagnosis is confirmed by ultrasonography, computerized tomography scan or angiography. Renal arteries are involved in approximately 10% of cases.

Mortality and factors reducing mortality

The annual risk of rupture of an expanding 5 cm aneurysm is 4–10%, and 40% per year for aneurysms larger than 7 cm[6]. The operative mortality for elective aneurysm resection is less than 2%, while the overall mortality for aneurysm rupture is greater than 70%[7,8].

Factors contributing to declining mortality rates for elective surgery include improved surgical techniques, earlier surgical intervention, better preoperative management (including recognition and amelioration of risk factors), greater understanding of the underlying vascular pathophysiology, advances in haemodynamic monitoring, improved anaesthetic agents and techniques and intensive postoperative care.

Indications for surgery

Asymptomatic aneurysms gradually increase in size over time. Patients with aneurysms greater than 5 cm in diameter have improved prognosis if surgical resection is performed electively, particularly if the aneurysm is expanding.

Acute unstable aneurysmal expansion manifested by new abdominal or back pain in a patient with a previously asymptomatic aneurysm and confirmed by ultrasonographic measurement requires urgent surgery[9]. Often coexisting disease has not been adequately evaluated and optimized, and operative mortality is somewhat higher (1–6%) than for elective surgery[10,11].

Abdominal aortic aneurysm rupture causing rapid exsanguination is invariably fatal without rapid surgical intervention[12]. Mortality rates of up to 70% in shocked patients have remained almost unchanged over the past 25 years. The classic triad of abdominal pain, pulsatile mass and signs of hypovolaemic shock (systolic blood pressure <80 mmHg and tachycardia >100 per min) is present in 75% of patients. Temporary tamponade of the bleeding site by a retroperitoneal space haematoma allows initial survival of the rupture in some patients; however, once free rupture into the peritoneal cavity occurs, mortality approaches 100%[13]. Following diagnosis, patients with a ruptured aneurysm should immediately be taken to the operating theatre, where resuscitation and preparation for surgery are achieved simultaneously and laparotomy is performed as soon as possible.

Screening

Screening of patients at high risk of aortic aneurysm–men over 55 years with other signs of peripheral vascular disease and first-degree relatives of aneurysm patients–may be cost-effective[14].

Surgical approach

Aortic surgery is usually performed by a transperitoneal approach through a vertical midline incision. Alternatively, a retroperitoneal approach through a transverse flank incision is used, and may be associated with decreased evaporative fluid loss and decreased blood loss, intraoperative temperature stability, less bowel manipulation and shorter postoperative ileus and less postoperative respiratory problems[15]. Improved access to the suprarenal aorta is facilitated by this approach.

Aorto-iliac occlusive disease

Progressive occlusion of the aorto-iliac/femoral arterial tree results in vascular insufficiency of the lower extremities and produces gastrocnemius claudication.

Patients with aorto-iliac occlusive disease require aortic reconstruction, employing either aorto-iliac thrombo-endarterectomy, bypass or excision and graft placement. Operative mortality ranges from 2–4%[16,17].

As in aortic aneurysm resection, placement of a bifurcated aortofemoral graft for aortic reconstruction requires cross-clamping of the aorta and a period of lower extremity ischaemia. This well-established surgical procedure has good reported postoperative outcome in terms of lower limb blood flow, relief of ischaemic symptoms and improved life expectancy[18].

Preoperative evaluation

The perioperative mortality for aortic surgery (2–4%) remains higher than that reported for all patients undergoing a variety of surgical procedures (0.2–0.4%)[19,20]. This is in part due to the high incidence of perioperative myocardial infarction and left ventricular failure in the vascular surgery population[21]. Myocardial infarction alone is responsible for up to 70% of mortality associated with aortic surgery. However, improved survival for patients with electively resected aortic aneurysms and aorto-iliac reconstruction when compared with non-surgical patients indicates that aortic surgery effectively controls the disease and improves life expectancy, and may be offered to almost all patients[22].

Coexisting disease and perioperative risk

The prevalence of coexisting disease, particularly angina (20%), congestive heart failure (15%), previous myocardial infarction (50%), silent myocardial ischaemia (60%), hypertension (60%), chronic obstructive pulmonary disease (50%), renal dysfunction (25%) and diabetes mellitus (12%) is well documented[23–28], and can be used to effectively guide the preoperative evaluation of these patients.

Pre-existing conditions that have been shown by multivariate analysis to be associated with adverse outcome include angina[29,30], congestive heart failure[29], diabetes mellitus[30], ventricular ectopics or arrhythmia[26], abnormal ECG[29] and previous cerebrovascular accident[26].

Evaluation of cardiac risk using the cardiac risk index[31–33] underestimates the overall level of risk associated with aortic surgery, which may be two to three times as great[34,35]. This may be due to intraoperative haemodynamic deviations conferring specific risk[36]. Reduction or elimination of some risk factors is possible in the preoperative period[2], and this will contribute to a decrease in the risk of aortic surgery.

Specific clinical, laboratory and perioperative risk factors for aortic surgery are summarized in Table 6.1[25,26,29,30,34,35,37]. These can be used as a basis for the preoperative evaluation, which should aim to identify or exclude important coexisting disease in patients undergoing aortic surgery, including those who do not exhibit clinical manifestations. Conditions that are therefore particularly pertinent to preoperative evaluation and preparation of these patients include ischaemic heart disease, hypertension, congestive heart failure, renal function, electrolyte abnormalities, diabetes mellitus and respiratory disease.

Table 6.1 Aortic surgery–risk factors

Previous myocardial infarction
Angina
Heart failure
Dysrhythmias
Preoperative hypertension
Aortic valvular stenosis
Age > 70 years
Operative procedure
Coexisting disease; COAD, renal insufficiency

Plus
Abnormal ECG
Impaired thallium stress test
Intraoperative hypotension
Perioperative myocardial ischaemia
Intra- or postoperative renal failure

Data compiled from Diehl *et al.* 1983[25], Cooperman *et al.* 1978[26], Yeager *et al.* 1986[29], Eagle *et al.* 1989[30], Jeffrey *et al.* 1983[34], Domaingue *et al.* 1982[35], Slogoff and Keats 1989[37].

The specifics of preoperative evaluation, including indications for invasive and non-invasive investigations and risk stratification in vascular surgery patients, are detailed in Chapter 3.

Preoperative surgical considerations

Preoperative renal ultrasound may be helpful to detect ureteral obstruction caused by an aortic aneurysm. Selective angiography of the mesenteric vessels to detect occlusive processes in the superior or inferior mesenteric arteries may be appropriate in patients at risk of postoperative ischaemic colitis[38,39].

Pathophysiology of aortic cross-clamping and unclamping

Abdominal aortic surgery requires a period of aortic cross-clamping; either infrarenal aortic cross-clamping for abdominal aortic surgery or a more proximal site for abdominal lesions extending above the renal arteries. Aortic cross-clamping and unclamping are associated with severe homeostatic disturbances in almost all organ systems. Major physiological problems that result include acute left ventricular strain, ischaemia or hypoperfusion of the kidneys, spinal cord and abdominal viscera, and accumulation of metabolites in ischaemic tissues below the clamp. In addition, release of many mediators (described below) may reduce or aggravate the harmful effects of cross-clamping and unclamping. Injury to the kidney, lung, spinal cord and abdominal viscera is caused mainly by ischaemia and reperfusion, or by release of mediators from ischaemic and reperfused tissues.

Haemodynamic changes

The haemodynamic responses[40–43] to cross-clamping of the aorta comprise:

- increased arterial pressure
- increased systemic vascular resistance (up to 40%)
- no significant change in heart rate
- decreased cardiac output
- filling pressure changes are inconsistent, i.e. decrease, no change or increase.

Factors influencing the extent of response include:

- the preoperative coronary circulation and myocardial function
- the site of the cross-clamp
- the intravascular volume status at the time
- blood volume redistribution
- the anaesthetic technique and agents employed
- the surgical pathology.

Filling pressures and blood volume redistribution

Arterial hypertension results from an increase in impedence to left ventricular ejection producing increased after load, manifested as increased left ventricular end-systolic wall stress. During supracoeliac aortic cross-clamping, unchanged or increased filling pressures (central venous pressure, pulmonary occlusion wedge pressure or left-ventricular end-diastolic pressure) may result from blood flow redistribution from the splanchnic area (as splanchnic venous pressure decreases) to the area proximal to the area of occlusion, or may represent an afterload increase as the end-systolic volume progressively increases[43]. In contrast, infracoeliac aortic cross-clamping may be associated with a decrease in venous return[44] as blood volume pools in the splanchnic reservoir.

Oxygen consumption

Oxygen consumption in the tissues distal to the site of aortic cross-clamping decreases and, paradoxically, so does oxygen uptake in tissues above the occlusion. This may be due to an increase in sympathoadrenal discharge and arteriovenous shunting through the upper body during aortic cross-clamping, and/or accumulation of adenosine from ischaemic tissues below the aortic occlusion[43]. This may explain the improvement in cardiac output associated with vasodilator therapy (sodium nitroprusside, nifedepine, nitroglycerin) during aortic cross-clamping, i.e. altering blood flow distribution as well as decreasing afterload.

The combination of decreased oxygen consumption and increased mixed venous oxygen saturation and content is thought to reflect a decrease in the perfused mass of tissues, i.e. 'cross-clamp adapted oxygen consumption', and may indirectly be responsible for the decrease in cardiac output[43]. Since maximum arterial vasodilation is present in hypoxic tissue below the aortic cross-clamp, vasodilator therapy (including nitroglycerin) probably could not improve tissue oxygenation.

Myocardial function and coronary blood flow

Increased preload and afterload associated with aortic cross-clamping lead to an increase in myocardial oxygen demand. In patients without coronary artery disease, the myocardial oxygen supply is usually adequately increased by increased coronary blood flow and preservation of myocardial autoregulation and endocardial–epicardial flow ratios, thereby avoiding severe myocardial ischaemia and maintaining myocardial contractility ('the Anrep effect'). These patients, after an initial increase in left ventricular end-diastolic volume and pressure, demonstrate a decrease in pulmonary artery occlusion pressure and central venous pressure in response to aortic cross-clamping. This decrease in preload is consistent with a longer pre-ejection period and shorter ejection time in the normal left ventricle, seen on transoesophageal echocardiography[45].

However, in patients with atherosclerotic coronary artery disease, both left- and right-sided filling pressures increase[44], the decrease in cardiac index is exaggerated[46] and ECG evidence of myocardial ischaemia may be demonstrated[47] following aortic cross-clamping, indicating an inability to increase subendocardial blood flow in response to an increase in intraventricular pressure.

Echocardiography and ventriculography findings in post-myocardial infarction patients after aortic cross-clamping, include a longer pre-ejection period and a longer ejection time[45], impaired myocardial performance (the relation between cardiac index and end-diastolic index), and impaired systolic function (systolic blood pressure in relation to systolic volume index)[48]. These changes indicate that patients with pre-existing impaired myocardial contractility or increased left ventricular end-diastolic volumes cannot further mobilize the Frank–Starling mechanism, develop a decrease in the velocity and contraction of myocardial fibres[40] and proceed to develop left ventricular failure in response to myocardial ischaemia and release of myocardial depressant factor from ischaemic tissue. These changes may be somewhat attenuated by increased catecholamine release and by increased levels of adenosine and inosine in myocardial tissue, which improve myocardial blood flow and contractility.

Strategies for myocardial preservation during aortic cross-clamping therefore comprise decreasing afterload and normalizing preload, coronary blood flow and contractility.

Level of occlusion

Supracoeliac placement of the aortic cross-clamp is associated with significantly more dramatic increases in mean arterial pressure ($>50\%$), filling pressures (40%) and end-systolic area (70%), and decrease in ejection fraction (40%), compared to infrarenal cross clamping[49] (Table 6.2). In addition, the number of wall motion abnormalities increase significantly when the aortic clamp is placed more proximally[50].

Table 6.2 Effects of aortic cross-clamping: influence of site of cross-clamp

	Infrarenal	*Above coeliac artery*
Increased left ventricular end diastolic area	2%	54%
Decreased ventricular ejection fraction	8%	38%
Increased mean arterial pressure	2%	54%
Increased pulmonary artery occlusion pressure	0%	38%
Increase in number of left ventricular regional wall motion abnormalities	0%	92%

Data from Roizen *et al.* 1984[50].

Duration of clamping

With increasing duration of cross-clamping, systemic vascular resistance increases and cardiac output decreases. This may result from interstitial fluid shifts and decrease in blood volume and release of vasoactive substances.

Aortic cross-clamping and aortic occlusive disease

The haemodynamic[51] and metabolic[52] responses to aortic cross-clamping in patients with aortic occlusive disease are less dramatic and fluid requirements are lower compared to those in patients undergoing aortic aneurysm resection (minimal or unchanged cardiac index, stroke volume and systemic vascular resistance). This is probably related to the extent of chronic collateral circulation, which allows continuous perfusion of the pelvis and lower extremities during the clamp period. The magnitude of the response can therefore be predicted from the preoperative aortograms[52].

Haemodynamic responses distal to the aortic cross-clamp

Aortic pressure below the cross-clamp is decreased, and is directly dependent on proximal aortic pressure. Distal blood flow through collaterals, which depends on the distal aortic pressure, decreases significantly and is unaffected by fluid infusion or by increases in cardiac output. This implies that proximal and distal aortic pressures should be maintained as high as the heart can withstand, particularly when the clamp is placed more proximally on the aorta.

Aortic unclamping

During the period of aortic cross-clamping, ischaemic vasodilation and vasomotor paralysis develop in the lower extremities and pelvis[40,41]. Immediately following unclamping (10 seconds), systemic vascular resistance, carotid blood flow, venous return and left ventricular end-diastolic pressure decrease, and myocardial blood flow increases. Reactive hyperaemia is an important component of the later response to unclamping (15 minutes), i.e. increased blood flow to previously ischaemic areas caused by smooth muscle relaxation in the arterial tree due to hypoxia or passive dilation and/or accumulated lactic acid and products of anaerobic metabolism. This contributes to hypotension, myocardial dysfunction and renal vasoconstriction. However, changes in cardiac output depend critically on the intravascular volume status at the time of cross-clamp release.

Measures to prevent unclamping hypotension include a short aortic cross-clamping time, adequate fluid therapy, careful titration of vasoactive drugs and gradual release of the aortic clamp (to slow down the washout of vasoactive and cardiodepressant substances from ischaemic tissues).

Aortic unclamping and occlusive arterial disease

Following aortic cross-clamp release, well-hydrated patients with aorto-occlusive disease may increase their cardiac output[52]. In addition, reactive hyperaemia of the lower extremities may not be evident immediately, but occurs gradually over several hours.

Metabolic changes associated with aortic cross-clamping

During aortic cross-clamping, metabolic changes occur which also influence the haemodynamic alterations[43]. These include:

- metabolic acidosis and increased lactate concentration
- increased renin activity
- increased concentrations of adrenaline and noradrenaline
- hypophosphataemia (which persists into the postoperative period), due to haemodilution, tubular injury and increased excretion or resynthesis of high-energy phosphate compounds after reperfusion

- release of plasma adenosine, xanthine, inosine, hypoxanthine and oxygen free-radicals[53], which may increase vascular permeability and contribute to unclamping hypotension
- decreased lymphocyte count and increased neutrophil count after unclamping
- secretion of prostaglandin E[54], which reduces systemic vascular resistance and increases cardiac output
- increased levels of thromboxane A_2[55] and of its stable metabolite thromboxane B_2[56] during and after cross-clamping, as well as reduced Ca^{++}ATPase and Mg^{++}ATPase activity in the myocardial sarcoplasmic reticulum[57], contribute to depression of cardiac performance
- increased levels of anaphylotoxins C3a and C5a (which may be related to insertion of the prosthesis), causing smooth muscle contraction, increase in pulmonary vascular resistance and vascular permeability, release of histamine and activation of leukocytes and platelets. C3a also impairs AV conduction, and may cause coronary vasoconstriction
- release of myocardial depressant factor from ischaemic pancreatic tissue[58]
- release of endotoxin and tumour necrosis factor from ischaemic bowel, which may contribute to lung injury
- release of interleukin-1, interleukin-6 and endothelin-1.

The clinical significance of different mediators is difficult to establish, since their effects are often opposing and are sometimes overridden by physiologic variables (preload, afterload and contractility). Future therapeutic interventions will include use of specific and short-acting antagonists of humoral factors and mediators released during and after aortic cross-clamping.

Renal circulation and function

Renal failure occurs in 0.2–3% of elective aortic surgical patients, with associated mortality rates of 25%[59]. Contributing factors include pre-existing renal artery atherosclerosis, preoperative renal dysfunction[59], age[60], inadequate hydration following angiography, bowel preparation and preoperative starvation[61], as well as intravenous contrast material[62]. Suprarenal aortic cross-clamping is associated with higher rates of renal complications (17–51%)[63]. Perioperative factors include hypotension, renal artery embolism, large blood transfusion and intravascular myoglobin.

Ischaemia-reperfusion insult to the kidney plays a central role in the pathogenesis of renal failure associated with aortic surgery. Aortic cross-clamping affects both renal perfusion and blood flow distribution. Acute tubular necrosis[64], a 30% decrease in cortical blood flow[65] and increased renal vascular resistance[66,67] due to renin–angiotensin effects and sympathetic nervous system activation, microcirculation changes and micro-embolization have all been experimentally demonstrated. Other factors contributing to the intrarenal maldistribution of blood flow include endothelin release, inhibition of nitric oxide formation by myoglobin, and renal release of prostaglandins.

Renal haemodynamic changes persist after unclamping, and result in a prolonged decrease in glomerular filtration rate. In general, although experimental evidence strongly suggests a protective effect of diuretic agents (e.g. mannitol, frusemide) against ischaemic insult to the kidney, there is a lack of clinical evidence for this.

The changes in renal blood flow are significantly attenuated if adequate intravascular volume and cardiac output are maintained[68].

Spinal cord

Approximately 75% of the spinal cord is supplied by the anterior spinal artery, arising from multiple medullary branches of the aorta. Sacral supply to the distal cord arises from branches of the iliac arteries. Interruption of blood supply from the anterior spinal artery by mechanical means and/or hypotension may result in anoxia to the lower cord. The overall incidence of spinal cord damage associated with aortic aneurysm surgery is 0.25%, with greater prevalence in ruptured aneurysms and virtually none reported following surgery for aorto-occlusive disease[69]. The most common deficit is flaccid paraplegia with dissociated sensory loss.

Contributing factors[70–72] include:

- decreased perfusion pressure (the difference between distal aortic pressure/anterior spinal artery pressure and cerebrospinal fluid pressure/venous pressure), due to arterial hypertension above the clamp and increased intracranial blood volume during clamping
- hypotension
- higher site of cross-clamp
- longer clamp period (> 30 minutes for thoracic clamping)
- damage to lower intercostal and lumbar arteries, in particular the artery of Adamkiewicz
- sodium nitroprusside infusion, which decreases spinal cord perfusion pressure and also causes cerebral vasodilation.

Intestine

During aortic cross-clamping small bowel ischaemia may develop (up to 10% incidence), particularly in aorto-occlusive disease, due to further compromise of atheromatous coeliac and superior mesenteric vessels[73].

Contributing factors include:

- autoregulatory vasoconstriction[74]
- hypovolaemia
- inadequate cardiac output
- microembolism
- exacerbation of colonic ischaemia by nitroglycerin administration[75].

Lungs

The pathogenesis of respiratory complications following aortic surgery (8–26%)[63,76] may be due to:

- an increase in pulmonary vascular resistance during cross-clamping in response to increases in left ventricular end-diastolic pressure and

volume, and after cross-clamping, perhaps as a result of pulmonary microembolism and release of vasoconstrictive mediators from lung tissue
- thromboxane A_2 and B_2 generation, which increases pulmonary arterial pressure, induces neutrophil entrapment in the lungs and increases pulmonary microvascular permeability and pulmonary oedema
- intrapulmonary shunt of $> 10\%$
- oxygen free-radical generation and protease release from neutrophils
- increased pulmonary infection rate due to immune suppression (C3a and C5a increase).

Theoretically, therapeutic interventions directed towards attenuation of these effects include prostaglandin E_1 infusion, allopurinol and superoxide dismutase administration and heparin therapy[43]. Conventional pulmonary protection consists of careful fluid titration and pretreatment with mannitol 0.2 g/kg.

Anaesthetic considerations for aortic surgery

Optimum anaesthetic management includes smooth induction and provision of surgical anaesthesia and muscle relaxation; adequate tissue oxygenation, intravascular volume and urine output; maintenance of cardiovascular stability and metabolic homeostasis (which includes attenuating the haemodynamic consequences of aortic cross-clamping and unclamping and protection of vulnerable organs from ischaemic injury); and provision of intraoperative and postoperative analgesia.

Premedication

Generally all cardiac medications are continued up until surgery. However, some (e.g. diuretics for hypertension, digitalis for cardiac failure and long-acting beta blockers) may be discontinued at the anaesthetist's discretion, although sudden withdrawal of beta blockers may increase the risk of angina, arrhythmias and myocardial infarction. If digoxin is continued, potassium levels must be monitored perioperatively. Bronchodilators are continued until surgery. If the patient is receiving intravenous heparin, the infusion should be discontinued 4 hours before surgery.

Anxiety and pain release catecholamines, causing tachycardia and hypertension, which may result in myocardial ischaemia. A short-acting oral benzodiazepine may be required in some patients to produce anxiolysis without cardiopulmonary depression, with the added advantage of producing anterograde amnesia. Anticholinergics are sometimes used with premedication. Scopolamine has sedative, antisialogue, antiemetic and amnesic effects but may produce restlessness or agitation, particularly in the elderly. Glycopyrrolate does not cross the blood–brain barrier and is a good antisialogue, causing less tachycardia than atropine. Preoperative clonidine or atenolol (Chapter 2) may prevent hyperdynamic responses in the perioperative period.

Monitoring

The aim of all monitoring systems employed should be to reflect preservation of organ function. This includes myocardial, renal and pulmonary function as well as intravascular volume status and central nervous system function.

Basic monitoring includes electrocardiograph, non-invasive blood pressure determinations, pulse oximeter, capnograph and temperature. Additions required for aortic surgery include urine output measurement and arterial, central venous and often pulmonary artery catheters (Tables 6.3 and 6.4).

The electrocardiograph detects changes in rate and rhythm and myocardial ischaemia. Lead II demonstrates electrical changes over the long axis of the heart, and is useful to view P wave abnormalities as well as rhythm disturbances. Lead V_5 is useful for detecting intraoperative ischaemia, as is ST wave segment trending.

Table 6.3 Abdominal aortic surgery–standard monitoring

Basic
Electrocardiogram
– lead II dysrhythmia
– CM_5 ischaemia
Non-invasive blood pressure
Oximetry
Oesophageal stethescope
Temperature
Capnograph
Neuromuscular function

Organ function
Urine output
Direct intra-arterial pressure
Central venous pressure ± pulmonary artery pressure

Table 6.4 Abdominal aortic surgery–supplementary monitoring

Pulmonary artery catheter: measured and derived indices
– left ventricular function: left ventricular stroke work index
– cardiac output; thermodilution/continuous
– tissue oxygenation: mixed venous oximetry
– afterload: systemic vascular resistance

Two-dimensional transoesophageal echocardiography
– left ventricular preload
– ischaemia: wall motion abnormalities
– cardiac output: left ventricular ejection fraction
– afterload: left ventricular end-systolic wall stress

ST segment analysis

Somatosensory-evoked potentials

Direct intra-arterial pressure monitoring is indicated during aortic surgery due to the potential for rapid changes in arterial pressure, as well as the requirement for arterial blood sampling.

Pulmonary artery catheterization

A pulmonary artery catheter is indicated in the majority of patients presenting for aortic surgery[77] to detect changes in preload (pulmonary artery occlusion pressure) and cardiac output, to optimize intravenous fluid administration, and to detect ischaemic changes and adverse haemodynamic changes associated with aortic cross-clamping and release.

In patients with normal ventricular function ($> 50\%$ ejection fraction), central venous pressure correlates with pulmonary artery occlusion pressure during surgery[78] and following aortic cross-clamp and release[79]. However, in patients with significant coronary artery disease and/or ventricular dysfunction, changes in central venous pressure do not always accurately predict the magnitude and direction of pulmonary artery occlusion pressure changes. In addition, reduced cardiac and renal morbidity and mortality have been associated with pulmonary artery pressure monitoring and therapy based on the data recorded[61].

Central venous pressure monitoring may adequately reflect the balance between intravascular volume and left ventricular function in patients with aorto-iliac occlusive disease and no significant coronary artery disease or ventricular dysfunction because less marked haemodynamic changes follow aortic cross-clamp and release during this surgery, due to collateral circulation.

Pulmonary artery catheterization also faciliates derivation of indices, including stroke volume, cardiac index, left ventricular stroke work index, systemic vascular resistance (afterload) and pulmonary vascular resistance and intrapulmonary shunt. Myocardial ischaemia is often indicated by the appearance of V waves on the pulmonary artery occlusion pressure trace before ST segment changes occur[80]. Mixed venous oxygen saturation indicates tissue oxygenation, and may be used to monitor changes in cardiac output and responses to pharmacological management[81].

Transoesophageal echocardiography

Two-dimensional transoesophageal echocardiography estimates left ventricular dimensions and detects wall motion abnormalities. Left ventricular

Table 6.5 Indications for PA catheter monitoring

History of myocardial infarction
Angina
Cardiac failure
Decreased left ventricular ejection fraction
Abnormal ventricular wall motion
Redistribution on dipyridamole thallium imaging

end-diastolic volume and end-diastolic area measurements define preload more precisely than central venous and pulmonary artery occlusion pressure measurement[82]. Accurate monitoring of changes in left ventricular ejection fraction[83] and cardiac output, indicating alterations in function associated with induction of anaesthesia and critical events during surgery, facilitates rapid treatment.

Transoesophageal echocardiography may be a more sensitive monitor of intraoperative myocardial ischaemia than electrocardiographic changes or pulmonary artery catheter filling pressures and derived indices. Ischaemic changes are demonstrated as regional wall motion abnormalities. Hypokinesia of the endocardium occurs before coronary blood flow is sufficiently reduced to produce ST changes from epicardial leads[84].

Neurological monitoring

Somatosensory cortical evoked potential monitoring assesses dorsal column function. However, spinal cord ischaemia during aortic cross-clamping may be associated with motor loss and preservation of somatosensory cortical evoked potentials. Therefore, monitoring somatosensory cortical evoked potentials is usually reserved for thoracic aortic aneurysm surgery[85,86].

Monitoring motor evoked potentials by stimulation over the spinal tracts or over the motor cortex requires muscle activity, and may produce increases in heart rate and arterial pressure[87-89].

Anaesthetic techniques

No single agent or technique is ideal for all patients undergoing aortic surgery; no particular intravenous, epidural or volatile anaesthetic agent is specifically indicated or contraindicated. However, the anaesthesia management plan should consider the type and location of aortic pathology, the presence of coexisting disease and the physiologic condition of the individual patient, as well as the operation required[38,39].

The choices include opioid-based anaesthesia supplemented with volatile agent ± nitrous oxide[90], nitrous oxide–oxygen with incremental volatile agent, opioid–oxygen anaesthesia[91-94], oxygen with incremental volatile agent ± opioid supplementation[95] or combinations of epidural and general anaesthesia[96-102].

The goal of all anaesthetic techniques should be to produce low pressure and low myocardial demand, thereby preserving myocardial oxygenation.

Unsupplemented opioid–oxygen techniques (e.g. fentanyl 100 µg/kg) provide stable haemodynamics, i.e. preserve myocardial contractility in patients with ischaemic heart disease[103], suppress humoral and metabolic responses (catecholamine, cortisol and antidiuretic hormone release) to anaesthesia and surgery[104], and provide prolonged postoperative analgesia. This is particularly advantageous in patients undergoing aortic surgery who have high preoperative circulating levels of catecholamines. However, disadvantages include hyperdynamic responses to surgical stimuli and to aortic cross-clamping and release[91,105], and prolonged postoperative respiratory depression[92].

Anaesthetic techniques using nitrous oxide (nitrous oxide–oxygen–volatile agent and nitrous oxide–oxygen–opioid) have been associated with depressed left ventricular performance and myocardial ischaemia[106,107].

Volatile agents with oxygen moderately depress myocardial contractility and oxygen demand, which is beneficial in patients with ischaemic heart disease and good ventricular function. However, side-effects of these agents, including excessive depression of myocardial contractility in patients with heart failure, decreased aortic diastolic pressure and coronary perfusion pressure and early postoperative hypertension, must be considered[108,109].

Isoflurane may be the volatile agent of choice for aortic vascular surgery despite the cited disadvantages[90,110,111]. Coronary artery vasodilation producing coronary steal is not observed when inspired concentrations are less than 0.75%[23]. Cardiac output, hepatic artery, renal and cerebral blood flow are improved compared to earlier agents[112,113], and low concentrations may actually protect against myocardial ischaemia[114].

A combination technique, i.e. opioid–oxygen with low concentrations of volatile agent ± nitrous oxide titrated to prevent autonomic responses, is probably ideal, as it maintains reduced myocardial contractility and unchanged systemic vascular resistance and preserves myocardial oxygenation[108,109,115]. Supplementation with beta-adrenergic blockade and/or vasodilators may be appropriate.

Regional anaesthesia/analgesia

Combined general and epidural anaesthesia (with the epidural usually placed at approximately the T8 level) reduces volatile and opioid requirements during surgery, facilitates early extubation, improves graft flow and provides good postoperative analgesia and improved postoperative diaphragmatic function. The incidence of postoperative complications (including myocardial infarction, congestive heart failure and major infection) is reduced, as is postoperative mortality[99].

In addition, the haemodynamic responses to aortic cross-clamping and release are attenuated with combined general and epidural anaesthesia[98,111], and coronary blood flow may be redistributed to favour the endocardium thus improving left ventricular function during stress-induced myocardial ischaemia[116].

This technique may, however, be associated with increased intravascular volume requirements and reduced left ventricular function[117]. Although controversy surrounding the safety of anticoagulation following epidural catheter placement has been virtually dispelled by reports on large patient numbers[118], the technique has not been universally accepted[119]. However, in view of the advantages of continuous epidural anaesthesia and postoperative epidural analgesia, the combination with general anaesthesia should be considered as a beneficial approach for patients undergoing aortic surgery.

The epidural catheter is placed and a test dose (lignocaine 2%) administered prior to induction. A continuous infusion of, for example, dilute bupivacaine (0.1%) and fentanyl 10 µg/ml may be commenced early in the anaesthetic. Alternatively, the epidural may be placed preoperatively and used solely for postoperative analgesia.

Induction

The aim is to induce general anaesthesia without sympathetic or para-sympathetic stimulation or depression, titrating drugs to minimal haemodynamic changes and anaesthetic end-points. Critical events such as laryngoscopy and intubation may cause release of catecholamines, hypertension, tachycardia and possibly myocardial ischaemia. Induction agents are chosen to provide minimal myocardial depression, especially for patients with impaired left ventricular function. Etomidate and opioids are associated with least haemodynamic derangement, and are often selected as induction agents for this reason. Supplementation with esmolol 0.3–1.5 mg/kg or nitroglycerin 0.5–1.5 µg/kg per min may be useful in achieving haemodynamic control. Volatile agents are usually subsequently employed (1.3 MAC) in patients with good ventricular function.

Cardiovascular stability

Intraoperative myocardial ischaemia is common, and is associated with increased incidence of postoperative myocardial infarction[120,121]. Immediate recognition and treatment of haemodynamic changes (including arterial pressure changes, tachycardia and altered left ventricular filling pressures), which predispose to ischaemia, are important in improving postoperative outcome.

The major determinants of myocardial oxygen supply are coronary artery patency, coronary perfusion pressure and arterial oxygen content. Coronary artherosclerosis prevents dilatation. Therefore, in many aortic surgery candidates only the latter factors are amenable to intervention.

Determinants of myocardial oxygen demand include myocardial wall tension, contractility and heart rate. Myocardial wall tension increases with hypertension, increased afterload and left ventricular failure. Tachycardia increases cardiac work and decreases diastolic perfusion time, impairing myocardial perfusion.

Heat conservation

Cutaneous, visceral and respiratory evaporative losses as well as intravenous fluid administration and conductive losses contribute to heat loss during aortic surgery. This may lead to myocardial irritability and depression, renal dysfunction, coagulation abnormalities and postoperative shivering with increased oxygen consumption, and has been associated with increased postoperative morbidity and adverse outcome[122]. Preventative measures include a warm operating theatre (22–23°C), heated and humidifying inspired gases, warm intravenous fluids and blood and forced-air warming devices on arms and chest.

Bowel manipulation

Bowel manipulation is usually necessary to gain access to the aorta, and may be associated with hypotension due to a decrease in systemic vascular resistance exaggerated by coexisting sympathetic blockade. These changes are caused by release of vasodilators (including prostaglandins) from the bowel, and last for approximately 20 minutes. Treatment comprises additional intravenous fluids, reduction of anaesthetic depth and administration of vasoactive agents such as phenylephrine.

Fluid management and blood transfusion

Intravascular volume is depleted by haemorrhage, 'third space' losses into the bowel wall and peritoneal cavity, extensive retroperitoneal space oedema specifically associated with aortic surgery, and insensible losses associated with the large abdominal incision. The primary aim of intraoperative intravenous fluid administration is the restoration of normal intravascular and interstitial fluid volumes. In addition, fluid management includes preservation of adequate urine output, prevention of acid–base and electrolyte imbalance and maintenance of adequate haematocrit, oxygen carrying capacity and normal coagulation status.

Colloid administration may benefit patients with severe pulmonary disease in preventing postoperative respiratory problems associated with large volume crystalloid infusion. Patients with renal disease seem to progress better with crystalloids[123].

A combination of crystalloid and colloid is usually used, and administration is guided by central venous and pulmonary artery occlusion pressure monitoring or transoesophageal echocardiography, urine output and serial haematocrit measurements.

Initial fluid replacement is usually with crystalloid, and therapy is altered depending on plasma electrolyte, glucose and haematocrit measurements at hourly intervals. Pulmonary artery occlusion pressure is maintained within the normal range with crystalloid/colloid, and increased 3–6 mmHg above this just prior to release of the aortic cross-clamp.

Blood loss

Blood loss during aortic surgery occurs after the aneurysm has been opened and the lumbar arteries back-bleed, at the proximal and distal anastomoses, and following graft flushing. Contributory factors include heparinization, pre-existing bleeding diathesis and loss of clotting factors.

Transfusion should commence when blood loss exceeds 15% of estimated blood volume. Continued blood loss below a haematocrit of 30 (considered to improve myocardial tolerance of ischaemia) may reduce oxygen-carrying capacity sufficiently to impair ventricular function and precipitate myocardial ischaemia in patients with ischaemic heart disease. Generally, one unit of red cell concentrate will increase haemoglobin by 1 g/dl and the haematocrit by 3.

Large volume transfusion due to uncontrolled haemorrhage results in altered coagulation status, depleted platelets, shift of the oxyhaemoglobin curve to the left and impaired tissue oxygen delivery.

Techniques available to minimize homologous transfusion include autologous donation[124], storage and retransfusion during surgery, phlebotomy immediately preoperatively, haemodilution[125] and autologous transfusion, and intraoperative blood salvage and reinfusion[126,127].

Autotransfusion during surgery avoids up to 80% of homologous blood transfusion, without haemolysis or coagulapathy[128], has optimal 2–3 DPG content and prevents adverse cardiovascular effects associated with large volume homologous blood therapy. Autotransfused blood consists of washed red blood cells without platelets or clotting factors. Therefore, fresh frozen plasma and platelet transfusion may be necessary, guided by laboratory studies.

Management of aortic cross-clamping

Cardiovascular changes

Signs of left ventricular failure and/or myocardial ischaemia that develop following aortic cross-clamping require rapid treatment to avoid myocardial injury and further deterioration in ventricular function. Treatment includes decreasing left ventricular end-diastolic pressure (pulmonary artery occlusion pressure) and wall stress and restoring myocardial perfusion, and therefore improving contractility.

Nitroglycerin (1–2 μg/kg per min)[43,129] administration during aortic cross-clamping prevents increases in systemic vascular resistance and myocardial oxygen demand, favours coronary blood flow to the endocardium, maintains cardiac contractility and cardiac index[130] and preserves peripheral tissue blood flow. However, high doses may decrease intestinal blood flow during aortic cross-clamping[75].

Afterload reduction with sodium nitroprusside maintains normal renal blood flow distribution and splanchnic blood flow during cross-clamping[131]. However, if mean arterial pressure is reduced to less than 80 mmHg, myocardial ischaemia may develop due to decreased coronary perfusion pressure or coronary vasodilatory steal effect[131,132].

If stroke volume and cardiac output remain depressed after pulmonary artery occlusion has normalized, inotropic support[133] (e.g. amrinone, dobutamine infusion or calcium chloride) is appropriate.

Renal preservation

The incidence of acute renal failure is reduced when adequate hydration and urine flow are maintained. Intravenous fluids should be infused to maintain a pulmonary artery occlusion pressure of 10–15 mmHg and to ensure a urine output of at least 1 ml/kg per hour during the cross-clamp period.

If urine output is unsatisfactory despite adequate preload, diuretic therapy with mannitol 0.25 g/kg ± frusemide should be administered prior to cross-clamp application. Many anaesthetists routinely administer mannitol prior to cross-clamping. Mannitol improves renal cortical blood flow, reduces renal cell swelling following ischaemia and prevents sludging of cellular debris in the renal tubules[134,135]. Loop diuretics increase free water and sodium excretion and increase renal blood flow by stimulating release of intrarenal prostaglandin E[136]. Low-dose dopamine 1–3 μg/kg per min increases renal blood flow, glomerular filtration rate, urine output and sodium excretion, but has not been definitely associated with improved outcome[137].

If diuresis is inadequate during the cross-clamp period, additional mannitol, frusemide or dopamine may be given. However, clinical benefit from these interventions compared to intravascular volume expansion alone has not been demonstrated[138]. Minimal duration of ischaemia to the renal circulation and avoidance of dislodging material into the renal arteries during operative manipulation and clamping are also important in postoperative renal outcome.

Spinal cord preservation

In addition to surgical manoeuvres[139], prevention of anterior spinal artery syndrome is dependent on avoidance of hypotension and hyperglycaemia. Cerebrospinal fluid drainage has been advocated to increase spinal cord perfusion pressure during cross-clamping of the aorta. However, this has not been universally accepted due to conflicting reports regarding outcome[140].

Moderate hypothermia of the cord using local cooling of the distal aorta or the epidural space has been shown to be protective. The safe ischaemic time is prolonged by decreasing the metabolic rate and oxygen requirements[141].

Alternative measures include barbiturate (e.g. thiopentone) administration (which decreases cerebral blood flow and oxygen requirements and has membrane-stabilizing and free-radical scavenging effects), intrathecal papaverine, combination of hypothermia and thiopentone, cerebrospinal fluid drainage and steroid administration (although this is associated with a risk of hyperglycaemia), the use of shunts and bypasses, calcium channel antagonists or specific oxygen free-radical scavengers (e.g. allopurinol or superoxide dismutase)[43]. However, the definitive evidence for improved outcome following these therapeutic interventions is, to date, inconclusive.

Intestinal ischaemia

Postoperative ischaemic colitis due to inferior mesenteric artery ligation, trauma, hypotension and low cardiac output states, inadequate hypogastric flow and absence of collaterals between mesenteric and systemic vessels occurs in up to 2% of patients undergoing aortic surgery.

Prevention includes ligation of the inferior mesenteric artery close to the aorta to preserve collateral circulation, or reconstruction of the artery, maintenance of stable haemodynamics and avoidance of high-dose nitroglycerin infusion during cross-clamping. In addition, stress ulceration prophylaxsis should be routinely employed[142].

Aortic unclamping

Release of the aortic cross-clamp is associated with hypotension due to sudden loss of afterload. However, stroke volume and cardiac output may increase or decrease following cross-clamp release, depending on left ventricular filling pressure (which often decreases immediately after unclamping).

Ischaemic vasodilation and vasomotor paralysis in the lower extremities exacerbate the expected fall in systemic vascular resistance and create a reactive hyperaemia, thereby decreasing venous return and filling pressures. Any resulting fall in cardiac output added to the already decreased systemic vascular resistance causes pronounced arterial hypotension. This is largely preventable by appropriate volume loading, i.e. ventricular performance should be on the horizontal portion of the Frank–Starling curve.

Pulmonary artery occlusion pressure should be increased to 3–6 mmHg above preoperative level before the cross-clamp is released. Additional management includes discontinuation of vasodilators if these have been used during cross-clamping, decreasing anaesthetic depth and, occasionally, administration of a vasopressor. The surgeon can also assist by gradual release of the aortic cross-clamp.

Emergency abdominal aortic surgery

Patients present either with an expanding, tender, contained rupture and a stable haemodynamic profile, or with a ruptured aneurysm and unstable haemodynamics requiring immediate resuscitation.

Haemodynamically stable patients have the same anaesthetic considerations as already described. Anaesthesia is induced following preoxygenation and using cricoid pressure. Titration of hypnotic agents, opioids and muscle relaxant aims to avoid hypertension. Adjuvants used include esmolol, nitroglycerin and nitroprusside.

Haemodynamically unstable patients require ongoing resuscitative measures. Mortality is approximately 40% due to the high incidence of myocardial infarction, respiratory failure and coagulopathy.

Patients are best resuscitated in the operating theatre while preparations are made for laparotomy. The twin priorities of correction of hypovolaemia and surgical control of the proximal aorta are equally urgent. Restoration of intravascular volume and rapid surgical control are associated with a reduction in mortality[7].

Anaesthetic management

Preparation

- At least one, and ideally several, large-gauge peripheral i.v. catheters are placed.
- Blood is immediately sent for cross-matching (10–12 units), O-negative blood may be used if type-specific blood is unavailable.
- Autotransfusion equipment should be available.
- Crystalloid is infused until a systolic pressure of 80–100 mmHg is achieved.
- Monitoring is placed (ECG, non-invasive blood pressure measurement, praecordial stethescope); however, placement of arterial and pulmonary artery catheters can await intravascular volume resuscitation.
- The abdomen is prepared and draped before induction of anaesthesia, as this results in loss of abdominal tone and may cause free haemorrhage by releasing the retroperitoneal tamponade.

Induction

Following preoxygenation, induction proceeds with the surgeon standing by. An opioid-based technique can provide satisfactory cardiovascular haemodynamics, taking care to avoid truncal rigidity and decreased pulmonary compliance by appropriate administration of muscle relaxant (see Chapter 2 for regimens)[23]. However, any one of a number of induction techniques may be chosen with due regard to the priorities of minimizing cardiovascular instability while seeking to avoid hypertension, tachycardia and myocardial ischaemia.

Anaesthesia

Further intravenous access should be established. Central venous cannulation using the internal jugular or subclavian vein may be necessary, as hypovolaemia makes peripheral venous cannulation difficult. A pulmonary artery catheter introducer sheath is often valuable in this situation for rapid administration of fluid and blood. Subsequently, an arterial catheter should be placed. A bladder catheter and nasogastric tube can then be inserted.

The surgical priority is to control bleeding by cross-clamping the aorta. If rapid control of haemorrhage and stable haemodynamics can be quickly achieved (while monitoring devices are secured), the surgery proceeds as for elective aortic operations. Pulmonary artery catheterization can then be undertaken. However, if haemorrhage is not controlled and haemodynamic stability persists, attention should continue to be directed at volume replacement.

Postoperative care

The aims of the immediate postoperative period include:

- stabilization and optimization of haemodynamic, respiratory and renal functions
- normothermia
- normal oxygen carrying capacity
- correction of any coagulation defects
- control of blood glucose
- efficient analgesia
- recognition and treatment of new disturbances, e.g. bleeding, myocardial ischaemia, hypoxaemia and neurological deficits
- early detection of graft dysfunction by observation of the peripheral circulation.

Cardiovascular complications are the most frequent adverse events following aortic surgery. These include myocardial ischaemia and infarction, left ventricular failure, arrhythmias and pulmonary embolism. Less frequent complications include respiratory dysfunction, renal failure, paraplegia and intestinal dysfunction.

Recovery

Emergence from anaesthesia should follow similar principles to those applied at induction, i.e. minimal disturbance to haemodynamics and myocardial oxygenation. Postoperative analgesia is therefore of paramount importance. Epidural analgesia, if employed, should be established before emergence. This may entail administration of opioids well in advance of the anticipated end of surgery.

Extubation is not always desirable immediately after aortic surgery (Table 6.6). Elective ventilation for some hours is often undertaken until residual anaesthesia has worn off, haemodynamic stability is assured, a normal temperature has been achieved, adequate haemoglobin levels and urine output have been confirmed and adequate spontaneous ventilation is established.

Table 6.6 Indications for postoperative ventilation

Unstable cardiac or pulmonary function
Inadequate haemostasis/ongoing bleeding
Hypothermia ($<33°C$)
Inadequate analgesia/large opioid requirements

Transport to the intensive care unit

During transport to the intensive care unit, patients require close monitoring of ECG, arterial blood pressure, pulmonary artery pressure and oxygenation. Fluid administration and maintenance of oxygenation and normothermia continue. Drugs needed to manage haemodynamic problems and airway management equipment should accompany the patient.

Hypertension

Postoperative hypertension is one of the early problems, and is due to emergence from anaesthesia, hypoxaemia, noxious stimuli such as pain, bladder distension and the endotracheal tube, overhydration or excessive blood transfusion, postoperative hypothermia with vasoconstriction, rebound following vasodilator therapy and preoperative hypertension, and vascular reactivity.

The consequences of untreated postoperative hypertension in the aortic surgery patient include myocardial ischaemia, left ventricular failure and pulmonary oedema and vascular anastomotic leak.

Treatment should be directed at the underlying problem, and intravenous agents may also be indicated. Hydrallazine and sodium nitroprusside effectively lower arterial pressure but may precipitate tachycardia and myocardial ischaemia, and therefore nitroglycerin ($1-2\,\mu g/kg$ per min) may be a safer agent as it is a potent coronary vasodilator. Excess catecholamine release, tachycardia and increased cardiac output (causing a postoperative hyperdynamic state) and hypertension can effectively be treated with a beta-adrenergic blocking agent such as labetalol or esmolol if left ventricular function is adequate.

Postoperative analgesia

The preferred postoperative analgesia technique following aortic surgery is epidural analgesia, although analgesia can adequately be provided by several other means. In addition to those previously described[99], the benefits associated with epidural analgesia in the postoperative period include:

- early tracheal extubation
- better tolerance of physiotherapy
- improved lung volumes and oxygenation
- early ambulation.

References

1. Ross R. The pathogenesis of atherosclerosis–an update. *N Engl J Med* 1986; **314**: 488–500.
2. Guidelines for preoperative cardiovascular evaluation for non-cardiac surgery. Report of the American College of Cardiology/American Heart Association Task Force on Practice Guide. *Circulation* 1996; **93**: 1278–317.
3. Darling RC, Brewster DC. Elective treatment of abdominal aortic aneurysms. *World J Surg* 1980; **4**: 661.
4. Bernstein EF, Dalley RB, Goldberger LE *et al*. Growth rates of small abdominal aortic aneurysms. *Surgery* 1976; **80**: 765.
5. Sabawla PB, Strong MJ, Keats AS. Surgery of the aorta and its branches. *Anesthesiol* 1970; **33**: 229.
6. Darling RC. Ruptured arteriosclerotic abdominal aortic aneurysm. *Am J Surg* 1970; **119**: 397.
7. Wakefield TW, Whitehouse WM, Wu SC *et al*. Abdominal aortic aneurysm rupture: statistical analysis of factors affecting outcome of surgical treatment. *Surgery* 1982; **91**: 586–96.
8. Fielding JWL, Black J, Ashton F *et al*. Ruptured aortic aneurysms: postoperative complications and their aetiology. *Br J Surg* 1984; **71**: 487–91.
9. Szilaggi DE. Clinical diagnosis of intact and ruptured abdominal aortic aneurysms. In: Bergan JJ, Yao JST eds. *Aneurysms–Diagnosis and Treatment*. Grune and Stratton, 1982: 205–15.
10. Hollier LH, Plate G, O'Brien PC *et al*. Late survival after abdominal aortic aneurysm repair: influence of coronary artery disease. *J Vasc Surg* 1984; **1**: 290–9.
11. Soreide O, Leffestol J, Christensen O *et al*. Abdominal aortic aneurysms: survival analysis of four hundred and thirty-four patients. *Surgery* 1982; **91**: 188–93.
12. Gayliss H, Kessler E. Ruptured aortic aneurysms. *Surgery* 1980; **87**: 300–4.
13. Lawrie GM, Crawford ES, Morris GC *et al*. Progress in the treatment of ruptured abdominal aortic aneurysm. *World J Surg* 1980; **4**: 653–60.
14. Johansen K, Koepsell T. Familial tendency for abdominal aortic aneurysms. *JAMA* 1986; **256**: 1934–6.
15. Sicard GA, Freeman MB, Vander Woude JC *et al*. Comparison between the transabdominal and retroperitoneal approach for reconstruction of the infrarenal abdominal aorta. *J Vasc Surg* 1987; **5**: 19.
16. Crawford ES, Bomberger RA, Glaser DH *et al*. Aorto-iliac occlusive disease: factors influencing survival and function following reconstructive operation over a twenty five year period. *Surgery* 1981; **90**: 1055–67.

17. Hertzer NR. Fatal myocardial infarction following lower extremity revascularization: two hundred and seventy three patients followed six to eleven postoperative years. *Ann Surg* 1981; **193**: 492–8.

18. Downs A. Aortofemoral bypass. In: Rutherford RB ed. *Vascular Surgery*. WB Saunders, 1984: 566–72.

19. Vancanti CJ, Van Houten RJ, Hill RC. A statistical analysis of the relationship of physical status to postoperative mortality in 68 338 cases. *Anesth Analg* 1970; **49**: 564.

20. Harrison GC. Anaesthetic contributory death–its incidence and causes. *S Afr J Med* 1968; **192**: 514.

21. Brown OW, Hollier LH, Pairolero PC *et al.* Abdominal aortic aneurysm and coronary artery disease. A reassessment. *Arch Surg* 1981; **116**: 1484–7.

22. O Donnell TF, Darling RC, Linton RR. Is 80 years too old for aneurysmectomy? *Arch Surg* 1976; **111**: 1250–7.

23. Clark NJ, Stanley JH. Anesthesia for vascular surgery. In: Miller RD ed. *Anesthesia*. Churchill Livingstone, 1994: 1851–95.

24. Young AE, Sandburg GW, Couch NP. The reduction of mortality of abdominal aortic aneurysm resection. *Am J Surg* 1977; **134**: 585–91.

25. Diehl JT, Cali RF, Hertzer NR *et al.* Complications of abdominal aortic reconstruction. Analysis of perioperative risk factors in 557 patients. *Ann Surg* 1983; **197**: 49–56.

26. Cooperman M, Pflug B, Martin EW *et al.* Cardiovascular risk factors in patients with peripheral vascular disease. *Surg* 1978; **84**: 5–8.

27. De Bakey ME, Lawrie GM. Combined coronary artery and peripheral vascular disease: recognition and treatment. *J Vasc Surg* 1984; **1**: 605–7.

28. Ruby ST, Whitemore AD, Couch NP *et al.* Coronary artery disease in patients requiring abdominal aortic aneurysm repair. Selective use of a combined operation. *Ann Surg* 1985; **201**: 758–62.

29. Yeager RA, Weigel RM, Murphy ES *et al.* Application of clinically valid cardiac risk factors to aortic aneurysm surgery. *Arch Surg* 1986; **121**: 278.

30. Eagle KA, Coley CM, Newell JB *et al.* Combining clinical and thallium data optimizes preoperative assessment of cardiac risk before major vascular surgery. *Ann Int Med* 1989; **110**: 859.

31. Goldman L. Cardiac risks and complications of non-cardiac surgery. *Ann Int Med* 1983; **287**: 845–50.

32. Goldman L, Caldera DL, Nussbaum SR *et al.* Multifactorial index of cardiac risk in non-cardiac surgery procedures. *N Engl J Med* 1977; **297**: 845–50.

33. Goldman L. Multifactorial index of cardiac risk in non cardiac surgery – a 10 year status report. *J Cardiothoracic Anaesth* 1987; **1**: 237–44.

34. Jeffrey CC, Kunsman J, Cullen DJ *et al.* A prospective evaluation of cardiac risk index. *Anesthesiol* 1983; **58**: 464–4.

35. Domaingue CM, Davies MJ, Cronin KD. Cardiovascular risk factors in patients for vascular surgery. *Anaesth Int Care* 1982; **10**: 324–7.

36. Goldmann L. Cardiac risk in non-cardiac surgery: an update. *Anesth Analg* 1995; **80**; 810–20.

37. Slogoff S, Keats AS. Does perioperative myocardial ischaemia lead to postoperative myocardial infarction? *Anesthesiol* 1989; **70**: 19.

38. Cunningham AJ. Anaesthesia for abdominal aortic surgery–a review. Part I. *Can J Anaes* 1989; **36**: 426–44.

39. Cunningham AJ. Anaesthesia for abdominal aortic surgery–a review. Part II. *Can J Anaes* 1989; **36**: 568–77.

40. Meloche R, Pottecher J, Audet J *et al.* Haemodynamic changes due to clamping of the abdominal aorta. *Can Anaes Soc J* 1977; **24**: 20–34.

41. Silverstein PR, Caldera DL, Cullen DJ *et al.* Avoiding the hemodynamic consequences of aortic cross-clamping and unclamping. *Anesthesiol* 1979; **50**: 462–6.

42. Reiz S, Peter T, Rais O. Hemodynamic and cardiometabolic effects of infrarenal aortic and common iliac artery declamping in man–an approach to optimal volume loading.

Acta Anaesth Scand 1979; **23**: 579–86.

43. Gelman S. The pathophysiology of aortic cross–clamping and unclamping. *Anesthesiol* 1995; **82**: 1026–60.

44. Attia RR, Murphy JD, Snider M *et al.* Myocardial ischemia due to infrarenal aortic cross-clamping during aortic surgery in patients with severe coronary artery disease. *Circ* 1976; **53**: 961–4.

45. Dauchot PJ, De Palma R, Grum D *et al.* Detection and prevention of cardiac dysfunction during aortic surgery. *J Surg Res* 1979; **26**: 574–80.

46. Gooding JM, Archie JP, Mc Dowell H. Hemodynamic response to infrarenal aortic cross-clamping in patients with and without coronary artery disease. *Crit Care Med* 1980; **8**: 382–5.

47. Carroll RM, Laravuso RB, Schauble JF. Left ventricular function during aortic surgery. *Arch Surg* 1976; **111**: 740–3.

48. Kalman PG, Wellwood MR, Weisel RD *et al.* Cardiac dysfunction during abdominal aortic operation: the limitation of pulmonary wedge pressures. *J Vasc Surg* 1986; **3**: 773–9.

49. Gelman S, Mc Dowell H, Proctor J. Does cardiac index really decrease during infrarenal aortic cross-clamping? *Anesthesiol* 1986; **65**: A41.

50. Roizen MF, Beaupre PN, Albert RA *et al.* Monitoring with two-dimensional trans-esophageal echocardiography. *J Vasc Surg* 1984; **1**: 300–5.

51. O'Toole DP, Broe P, Bouchier-Hayes D *et al.* Perioperative haemodynamic changes during aortic vascular surgery: comparison between occlusive and aneurysmal disease states. *Br J Anaesth* 1988; **60**: 322.

52. Johnston WE, Balestrieri FJ, Plonk G *et al.* The influence of periaortic collateral vessels on the intraoperative hemodynamic effects of acute aortic occlusion in patients with aorto-occlusive disease or abdominal aortic aneurysms. *Anesthesiol* 1987; **66**: 386–9.

53. Franf RS, Moursi MM, Podrazik RM *et al.* Renal vasoconstriction and transient declamp hypotension after infrarenal aortic occlusion: role of purine degradation products. *Surg* 1988; **7**: 515–23.

54. Rittenhouse EA, Maixner BA, Knott HW. The role of prostaglandin E in hemodynamic response of aortic clamping and unclamping. *Surg* 1976; **80**: 137–42.

55. Utsunomiya T, Krausz M, Dunham B *et al.* Maintenance of cardiodynamics with aspirin during abdominal aortic aneurysmectomy. *Ann Surg* 1981; **91**: 322–8.

56. Krausz MM, Utsonomiya T, Dunham B *et al.* Modulation of cardiovascular function and platelet survival by endogenous prostacyclin release during surgery. *Surg* 1983; **93**: 554–9.

57. Utsunomiya T, Krausz MM, Dunham B *et al.* Depression of myocardial ATPase activity by plasma obtained during positive end expiratory pressure. *Surg* 1982; **91**: 322–8.

58. Damask MC, Weismann C, Rodriguez K *et al.* Abdominal aortic cross-clamping. Metabolic and hemodynamic consequences. *Arch Surg* 1984; **119**: 1332–7.

59. Kasiske BL, Kjellstrand CM. Perioperative management of patients with chronic renal failure and postoperative acute renal failure. *Urol Clin N Amer* 1983; **10**: 35–50.

60. Kwaan JHM, Connolly JE. Renal failure complicating aortoiliofemoral reconstructive procedures. *Am J Surg* 1980; **46**: 295–7.

61. Bush HL. Renal failure following abdominal aortic reconstruction. *Surgery* 1983; **93**: 107–9.

62. Port FK, Wagoner RD, Fulton RE. Acute renal failure after angiography. *Am J Roentgenol* 1974; **121**: 544–9.

63. Golden MA, Donaldson MC, Whittemore AD *et al.* Evolving experience with thoracoabdominal aortic aneurysm repair at a single institution. *J Vasc Surg* 1991; **13**: 792–7.

64. Nanson EM, Noble JG. The effect on the kidneys of cross-clamping of the abdominal aorta distal to the renal arteries. *Surgery* 1959; **46**: 288–92.

65. Abbott WM. Cooper JD, Qusten WG. The effect of aortic clamping and declamping on renal blood flow distribution. *J Surg Res* 1973; **14**: 385–92.

66. Gamulin Z, Forster A, Morel D *et al*. Effect of infrarenal cross clamping on renal hemodynamics in humans. *Anesthesiol* 1984; **61**: 394–9.
67. Gamulin Z, Forster A, Simonet F *et al*. Effects of renal sympathetic blockade on renal hemodynamics in patients undergoing major aortic abdominal surgery. *Anesthesiol* 1986; **65**: 688–92.
68. Cronenwett JL, Lindenaauer SM. Distribution of intrarenal blood flow following aortic clamping and declamping. *J Surg Res* 1977; **22**: 469–82.
69. Szilagyi DE, Hageman JH, Smith RF *et al*. Spinal cord damage in surgery of the abdominal aorta. *Surgery* 1978; **83**: 38–56.
70. Blaisdell FW, Cooley DA. The mechanism of paraplegia after temporary thoracic aortic occlusion and its relationship to spinal fluid pressure. *Surgery* 1962; **51**: 351–5.
71. Cunningham JN, Laschinger JC, Markin HA *et al*. Measurement of spinal cord ischemia during operations upon the thoracic aorta: initial clinical experience. *Ann Surg* 1982; **196**: 285–96.
72. Wadouh F, Lindeman EM, Arndt CF *et al*. The arteria radicularis magna anterior as a decisive factor influencing spinal cord damage during aortic occlusion. *J Thorac Cardiovasc Surg* 1984; **88**: 1–10.
73. Cormier JM. Colonic ischemia after aorto-iliac surgery. *Ann Gastroenterol Hepatol* 1986; **22**: 321–5.
74. Gelman S, Patel K, Bishop SP *et al*. Renal and splanchnic circulation during infrarenal aortic cross-clamping. *Arch Surg* 1984; **119**: 1394–9.
75. Fry RE, Huber PJ, Ramsey KL *et al*. Infrarenal aortic occlusion, colonic blood flow and the effect of nitroglycerin afterload reduction. *Surg* 1984; **95**: 479–86.
76. Svensson LG, Hess KR, Coselli JS *et al*. A prospective study of respiratory failure after high-risk surgery of the thoracoabdominal aorta. *J Vasc Surg* 1991; **14**: 271–82.
77. Tuman KJ, Roizen MF. Outcome assessment and pulmonary artery catheterization: why does the debate continue? *Anesth Analg* 1997; **84**: 1–4.
78. Mangano DT. Monitoring pulmonary artery pressure in coronary artery disease. *Anesthesiol* 1980; **53**: 364–70.
79. Rice CL, Hobelman CF, John DA *et al*. Central venous pressure or pulmonary capillary wedge pressure as the determinant of fluid replacement in aortic surgery. *Surgery* 1978; **84**: 437–40.
80. Kaplan JA, Wells PH. Early diagnosis of myocardial ischemia using the pulmonary artery catheter. *Anesth Analg* 1981; **60**: 789–93.
81. Divertie MB, Mc Michan JC. Continuous monitoring of mixed venous oxygen saturation. *Chest* 1984; **85**: 3423–8.
82. Freund PR. Transesophageal Doppler scanning versus thermodilution during general anesthesia. An initial comparison of cardiac output techniques. *Am J Surg* 1987; **154**: 490–4.
83. Jorgensen BC, Hoilund-Carlsen PF, Marving J *et al*. Left ventricular performance monitored by radionuclide cardiography during induction of anesthesia. *Anesthesiol* 1985; **62**: 278–86.
84. Waters DD, Da Luz P, Wyatt HL *et al*. Early changes in regional and global left ventricular function induced by graded reductions in regional coronary perfusion. *Am J Surg* 1977; **39**: 537–43.
85. Coles JG, Wilson GJ, Sima AF *et al*. Intraoperative detection of spinal cord ischemia using somatosensory cortical evoked potentials during thoracic aortic occlusion. *Ann Thorac Surg* 1982; **34**: 299–306.
86. Grundy BL. Intraoperative monitoring of sensory evoked potentials. *Anesthesiol* 1983; **58**: 72–87.
87. Levy WJ. Spinal evoked potentials from the motor tracts. *J Neurosurg* 1983; **58**: 38–44.
88. Levy WJ, York DH, McCaffrey M *et al*. Motor evoked potentials from transcranial stimulation of the motor cortex in humans. *Neurosurg* 1984; **15**: 287–302.
89. Cheng MK, Robertson C, Grossman RG *et al*. Neurological outcome correlated with

spinal evoked potentials in a spinal cord ischemia model. *J Neurosurg* 1984; **60**: 786–95.

90. Benefiel DJ, Roizen JL, Levine A *et al.* Morbidity after aortic surgery with sufentanil versus isoflurane anesthesia. *Anesthesiol* 1986; **66**: 259–61.

91. Friesen RM, Thompson IR, Hudson RJ *et al.* Fentanyl oxygen anaesthesia for abdominal aortic surgery. *Can Anaes Soc J* 1986; **33**: 719–22.

92. Hudson RJ, Thomson IR, Cannon JE *et al.* Pharmacokinetics of fentanyl in patients undergoing abdominal surgery. *Anesthesiol* 1986; **64**: 334–6.

93. Hudson RJ, Bergstrom RG, Thomson IR *et al.* Pharmacokinetics of sufentanil in patients undergoing abdominal aortic surgery. *Anesthesiol* 1989; **70**: 426–8.

94. Crosby ET, Miller DR, Hamilton PP *et al.* A randomized double-blind comparison of fentanyl and sufentanil–oxygen anesthesia for abdominal aortic surgery. *J Cardiothorac Anesth* 1990; **168**: 4–6.

95. Moffitt EA, Sethna DH. The coronary circulation and myocardial oxygenation in coronary artery disease. Effects of anesthesia. *Anesth Analg* 1986; **65**: 395–410.

96. Cousins MJ, Wright CJ. Graft, muscle and skin blood flow after epidural block in vascular surgical procedures. *Surg Gynecol Obstet* 1971; **133**: 59–65.

97. Rosseel P, Marichal P, Lauwers LF *et al.* A hemodynamic study of epidural versus intravenous anesthesia for aortofemoral bypass surgery. *Acta Anaesthesiol Belg* 1985; **36**: 345–7.

98. Lunn JK, Dannemiller FJ, Stanley TH. Cardiovascular responses to clamping of the aorta during epidural and general anesthesia. *Anesth Analg* 1979; **58**: 372–6.

99. Yeager MP, Glass DD, Neff RK *et al.* Epidural anesthesia and analgesia in high-risk surgical patients. *Anesthesiol* 1987; **66**: 641–4.

100. Her C, Kizelshteyn G, Walker V *et al.* Combined epidural and general anesthesia for abdominal aortic surgery. *J Cardiothorac Anesth* 1990; **552**: 4–7.

101. Tuman KJ, McCarthy RJ, Marcj RJ *et al.* Effects of epidural anesthesia and analgesia on coagulation and outcome after major vascular surgery. *Anesth Analg* 1991; **73**: 696–8.

102. Baron JF, Bertrand M, Barre E *et al.* Combined epidural and general anesthesia versus general anaesthesia for abdominal aortic surgery. *Anesthesiol* 1991; **75**: 611–14.

103. Bovill JG. Opioid analgesics in anesthesia, with special reference to their use in cardiovascular anesthesia. *Anesthesiol* 1984; **61**: 731–55.

104. Reier EC, George JM, Kilman JW. Cortisol and growth hormone response to surgical stress during morphine anesthesia. *Anesth Analg* 1973; **52**: 1003–9.

105. Thomson IR, Putnins CI, Friesen RM. Hyperdynamic cardiovascular responses to anesthetic induction with high-dose fentanyl. *Anesth Analg* 1986; **65**: 91–5.

106. Moffitt EA, Sethna DH, Gray RJ *et al.* Nitrous oxide added to halothane reduces coronary flow and myocardial oxygen consumption in patients with coronary disease. *Can Anaesth Soc J* 1983; **30**: 5–9.

107. Moffitt EA, Scovil JE, Barker RA *et al.* The effects of nitrous oxide on myocardial metabolism and hemodynamics during fentanyl or enflurane anesthesia in patients with coronary disease. *Anesth Analg* 1984; **63**: 1071–5.

108. Moffitt EA, Mc Intyre AJ, Glenn JJ *et al.* Myocardial metabolism and haemodynamic responses with fentanyl–halothane anaesthesia for coronary patients. *Can Anaesth Soc J* 1985; **32**: S86.

109. Moffitt EA, Mc Intyre AJ, Barker RA *et al.* Myocardial metabolism and hemodynamic responses with fentanyl–enflurane anesthesia for coronary artery surgery. *Anesth Analg* 1986; **65**: 46–52.

110. Merin RG. Is isoflurane dangerous for the patient with coronary artery disease? Another view. *Anesthesiol* 1987; **67**: 284–5.

111. Reiz S, Balfors E, Sorensen MB *et al.* Isoflurane–a powerful coronary vasodilator in patients with coronary artery disease. *Anesthesiol* 1983; **59**: 91–7.

112. Wade JG, Stevens WC. Isoflurane: anesthetic for the eighties. *Anesth Analg* 1981; **60**: 666–82.

113. Gelman S, Fowler KC, Smith LR. Regional blood flow during isoflurane and halothane

anesthesia. *Anesth Analg* 1984; **63**: 557–65.

114. Tarnov J, Markschies-Hornung A, Schulte-Sasse W. Isoflurane improves the tolerance to pacing-induced myocardial ischemia. *Anesthesiol* 1986; **64**: 147–56.

115. Eger EI. New inhaled anesthetics. *Anesthesiol* 1994; **80**: 906–22.

116. Klassen GA, Bramwell RS, Bromage PR *et al*. Effect of acute sympathectomy by epidural anesthesia on the canine coronary circulation. *Anesthesiol* 1980; **52**: 8–15.

117. Bunt TJ, Manczuk M, Varley K. Continuous epidural anesthesia for aortic surgery: thoughts on peer review and safety. *Surgery* 1987; **101**: 706–14.

118. Rao TKL, El-Etr AA. Anticoagulation following placement of epidural and subarachnoid catheters: an evaluation of neurologic sequelae. *Anesthesiol* 1981; **55**: 618–20.

119. McPeek B. Inference, generalizability and a major change in anesthetic practice. *Anesthesiol* 1987; **66**: 723–4.

120. Mangano DT, Browner WS, Hollenberg M *et al*. Association of perioperative myocardial ischemia with cardiac morbidity and mortality in men undergoing non-cardiac surgery. *J Gen Int Med* 1990; **323**: 211–19.

121. Mangano DT. Perioperative cardiac morbidity. *Anesthesiol* 1990; **72**: 153–84.

122. Bush HL, Lynn JH, Fischer E *et al*. Hypothermia during elective abdominal aortic aneurysm repair: the high price of avoidable morbidity. *J Vasc Surg* 1995; **21**: 392–402.

123. Boutros AR, Ruess R, Olson L *et al*. Comparison of hemodynamic, pulmonary and renal effects of use of three types of fluid after major surgical procedures on the abdominal aorta. *Crit Care Med* 1979; **7**: 9–13.

124. Toy PT, Strauss RG, Stehling LC *et al*. Predeposited autologous blood for elective surgery. A national multicentre study. *N Engl J Med* 1987; **316**: 517–20.

125. Stehling LC, Zaudeer HL. Acute normovolaemic hemodilution. *Transfusion* 1991; **31**: 857–68.

126. Willamson KR, Taswell HF. Intraoperative blood salvage: a review. *Transfusion* 1991; **31**: 663–75.

127. Simpson P. Perioperative blood loss and its reduction: the role of the anaesthetist. *Br J Anaesth* 1992; **69**: 498–507.

128. Hallett JW, Popovsky M, Ilstrup D. Minimizing blood transfusion during abdominal aortic surgery: recent advances in autotransfusion. *J Vasc Surg* 1987; **5**: 601–6.

129. Gelman S, Mc Dowell H, Varner PD *et al*. The reason for cardiac output reduction after aortic cross-clamping. *Am J Surg* 1988; **155**: 578–86.

130. Zaidan JR, Guffin AV, Perdue G *et al*. Hemodynamics of intravenous nitroglycerin during aortic cross-clamping. *Arch Surg* 1982; **117**: 1285–8.

131. Utsunomiya T, Kravsz MM, Shepro D *et al*. Induction of myocardial damage with nitroprusside. *J Surg Res* 1981; **31**: 195–200.

132. Fremes SE, Weisel RD, Baird RJ *et al*. The effects of postoperative hypertension and its treatment. *J Thorac Cardiovasc Surg* 1983; **86**: 47–52.

133. Sethna DH, Gray RJ, Moffitt EA *et al*. Dobutamine and cardiac oxygen balance in patients following myocardial revascularization. *Anesth Analg* 1982; **61**: 917–20.

134. Abbott WM, Austen WG. The reversal of renal cortical ischemia during aortic occlusion by mannitol. *J Surg Res* 1974; **16**: 482–9.

135. Flores J, Dibona DR, Beck CH *et al*. The role of cell swelling in ischemic renal damage and the protective effect of hypertonic solute. *J Clin Invest* 1972; **51**: 118–23.

136. Walsh JJ, Venuto RC. Acute oliguric renal failure induced by indomethacin: possible mechanism. *Ann Int Med* 1979; **91**: 47–9.

137. Colson P, Ribstein J, Seguin JR *et al*. Mechanisms of renal hemodynamic impairment during infrarenal aortic cross-clamping. *Anesth Analg* 1992; **75**: 18–23.

138. Paul MD, Mazer CD, Byrick RJ *et al*. Influence of mannitol and dopamine on renal function during elective infrarenal aortic clamping in man. *Am J Nephrol* 1986; **6**: 427–34.

139. Kouchoukos NT, Dougenis MD. Surgery of the thoracic aorta. *New Engl J Med* 1997; **336**: 1876–1888.

140. Hollier LH, Money SR, Naslund TC *et al*. Risk of spinal cord dysfunction in patients undergoing thoracoabdominal aortic replacement. *Am J Surg* 1992; **164**: 210–213.
141. Cambria RP, Davison JK, Zannetti S *et al*. Clinical experience with epidural cooling for spinal cord protection during thoracic and thoracoabdominal aneurysm repair. *J Vasc Surg* 1997; **25**: 234–43.
142. Crowson M, Fielding JWL, Black J *et al*. Acute gastrointestinal complications of infrarenal aortic aneurysm repair. *Br J Surg* 1984; **71**: 225–8.

7

Lower limb revascularization

Surgical considerations

Lower limb atherosclerotic disease is common in elderly patients, particularly those with a long history of smoking, but is asymptomatic in most. Of those who develop symptoms, intermittent claudication (IC–i.e. calf or leg pain on walking which resolves within minutes of rest) is the most frequent complaint, but other presentations include leg ulcers, gangrene, critical ischaemia or acute total ischaemia (white leg). The prevalence of IC in the population is very age-dependent, being unusual in patients under 60 years old, occurring in approximately 2% between 60–70 years old, and 2.7% when over 70[1].

Critical ischaemia of a leg refers to the situation when *resting* blood flow is insufficient to allow basic oxygenation of the limb, and usually presents as rest pain. There is normally disease or occlusion of the superficial femoral artery. Without surgical intervention, amputation is almost inevitable.

Peripheral vascular disease itself is rarely a cause of mortality, but its presence does indicate a severe degree of generalized atherosclerosis and patients with IC have a two- to four-fold increase in mortality when compared with matched patients without IC. The 10-year mortality rate for patients with IC is 45%, and most of these excess deaths result from coronary artery and cerebrovascular disease[1].

Types of operation

There is a multitude of different techniques used to bypass arterial stenoses in the lower limb. If required, blood flow to the femoral artery must first be established, and then bypass of the arterial stenosis in the leg performed.

Improvement of flow into the femoral artery. Occlusion or stenosis of the abdominal aorta, common iliac or external iliac arteries reduces blood flow to one or both common femoral arteries. Depending on the site and rate of progression of the occlusion, the thigh often remains reasonably well-perfused by collateral circulation via the obturator arteries from the ipsi- or contralateral internal iliac artery, with symptoms arising mainly in the calf. The iliac arteries are reasonably amenable to radiological procedures such as angioplasty or stent insertion, provided the radiologist can pass a wire across the obstruction from a femoral or brachial arterial puncture. These are normally performed with local anaesthesia. However, surgery is frequently necessary and may involve:

- aorto-bifemoral graft–this is described in Chapter 6
- ilio-femoral graft, normally via an extraperitoneal approach to the common iliac artery
- femoro-femoral crossover graft
- axillo-femoral or axillo-bifemoral graft.

These bypass procedures require large diameter grafts and are therefore normally performed with synthetic material, sometimes with vein 'cuffs' at the distal end (see below). The size and synthetic nature of the graft is such that early graft failure is unusual, and the influence of the anaesthetic technique on surgical outcome is less than that for more distal procedures.

Improvement of flow to the lower leg is achieved with either a femoro-popliteal graft or a femoro-distal graft to one of the three branches of the popliteal artery below the knee. These bypass grafts often require a long length of graft material of small calibre feeding into distal vessels (the 'run-off'), which are themselves diseased and therefore of high resistance. Types of graft used, some of which are shown in Figure 7.1, include the following.

- Synthetic grafts usually made from PTFE or woven dacron. They are of uniform size (making distal anastomosis to small vessels difficult), relatively thrombogenic compared with vein graft, and associated with a higher failure rate than equivalent grafts using vein.
- Synthetic grafts with a distal vein cuff such as a Miller cuff (Figure 7.1). Vein cuffs of various types are described which reduce the incidence of neo-intimal hyperplasia (and therefore stenosis) at the distal anastomosis.
- Reverse vein graft, in which the patient's own vein is harvested (usually from the leg, but arm veins may be used), turned around to remove the effect of the valves, and resited as an arterial conduit. Reversing the vein introduces a discrepancy in size at both ends, with the larger end of vein being anastomosed to the smaller artery and vice versa.
- *In situ* vein graft, when a portion of the long saphenous vein is identified near the arterial sites for bypass and anastomosed to the artery in its natural position. There is less size discrepancy, but valves must be rendered incompetent with a valve cutter and significant venous side branches identified and tied off to minimize arteriovenous fistulae.
- Arteriovenous fistulae may be created deliberately at the end of grafts onto distal tibial arteries, for example near the ankle, to substantially increase flow through the graft and thereby maintain patency, even though a proportion of the blood does not perfuse distal tissues.

Intraoperative measurement of graft flow may be performed using a Doppler-based flowmeter placed around the graft at the completion of surgery. Using the mean systemic arterial pressure (measured elsewhere), this allows the resistance distal to the graft to be calculated; a low resistance is

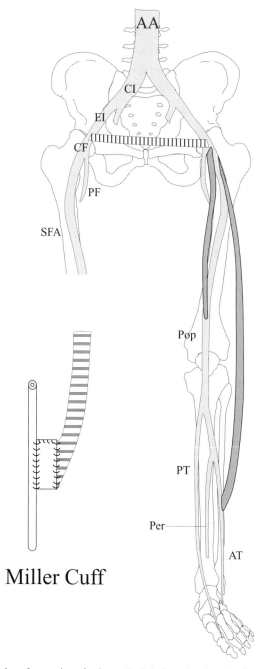

Miller Cuff

Figure 7.1 Examples of operations for lower limb ischaemia, showing femoro-femoral crossover graft with synthetic material, *in situ* femoro-popliteal graft and femoro-distal (anterior tibial) reverse vein graft, demonstrating the discrepancy in size between artery and vein at each end of the graft. Arteries shown are: AA, abdominal aorta; CI, common iliac; EI, external iliac; CF, common femoral; PF, profunda femoris; SFA, superficial femoral; Pop, popliteal; AT, anterior tibial; Per, peroneal; PT, posterior tibial.

known to be a good predictor of early graft success[2]. Flow and resistance measurement in this way allows identification and rectification of technical problems with the graft before completion of surgery.

Outcome with or without surgery

Utilization of lower limb revascularization for critical ischaemia is increasing. This increase is justified by studies showing that, compared with non-operative interventions, patients who undergo surgery are less likely to die in hospital, have a shorter hospital stay, survive longer, and consume less financial resources[3,4]. However, for the individual patient this overall advantage requires running significant risks as follows.

Mortality and morbidity of lower limb revascularization

In hospital mortality associated with femoro-popliteal or distal bypass grafts is around 3%[5,6], and increases with increasing age. Death results, in approximately equal proportions, from cardiac complications, stroke and multisystem failure[6]. Morbidity is much higher and includes many serious complications (incidence in parentheses)[6–8]:

- myocardial infarction (2–4.5%)
- clinical evidence of angina (1–8%)
- ECG evidence of ischaemia on continuous Holter monitoring (57%)
- heart failure (10–13%)
- respiratory complications (10%)
- renal impairment (increase of 150 µmol/l in postoperative creatinine) (6%).

Outcome without surgery[1]

The natural progression of patients presenting with intermittent claudication is that a substantial proportion will die of other cardiovascular diseases (5% per year or 45% at 10 years). Of the survivors, approximately one-fifth will develop gangrene or ischaemic pain at rest within 2–6 years and require surgical intervention. Diabetes, hypertension, increasing age and smoking all increase this deterioration in vascular disease, and with continued smoking the requirement for surgery increases to 80% within 6 years. Non-surgical treatment involves:

- stopping smoking
- exercise programmes–these double the walking distance before onset of IC, but the benefit only continues as long as the exercise continues, which becomes more difficult with increasing age
- adequate treatment of hypertension, hyperlipidaemia and diabetes mellitus
- aspirin, which reduces the rate of progression of peripheral atherosclerosis.

Non-surgical treatment of *critical* ischaemia is usually only instituted to allow time to investigate the patient's suitability for revascularization surgery, and to optimize their general condition prior to it. Close attention is paid to hydration, analgesia and cardiac status, whilst anticoagulants and peripheral vasodilators are administered intravenously.

Outcome following amputation

Amputation may become necessary, either following failed attempts at revascularization or as a primary procedure for pain or gangrene with arterial disease not suitable for bypass surgery. Following amputation mortality rates are extremely high, with a median survival of 2 years following one leg below knee amputation (BKA) and worsening to only 6 months following bilateral above knee amputations (AKA). This high mortality relates mainly to the association between peripheral arterial disease and other causes of cardiovascular death; a patient with disease severe enough to warrant two AKAs has a limited life expectancy generally. Nevertheless, the immobility associated with amputation may be quickly fatal in some cases. In addition, amputation is associated with a massive deterioration in quality of life, and a huge financial burden on healthcare budgets to facilitate long-term rehabilitation of amputees. The anaesthetic management of amputation is described on p. 237.

Failure of lower limb revascularization

Early graft failure is frequently caused by technical problems with the graft, such as kinks, valves, intimal flaps and external compression. Longer-term survival of the technically acceptable graft depends on the blood flow through the graft, blood coagulability and the propensity of the patient to develop atherosclerosis in the graft. Flow rate through the graft itself is dependent on Poiseuille's formula:

$$\text{Flow rate } = \frac{\text{Pressure gradient} \times \pi \times (\text{radius})^4}{8 \times \text{length} \times \text{viscosity}}$$

such that increasing length, and particularly decreasing diameter, have a large effect. There is little the anaesthetist can do to influence graft length and diameter, but some degree of manipulation is possible for other factors affecting graft flow:

- viscosity is directly related to haematocrit, so some degree of haemodilution may be helpful, and a haemoglobin concentration of 10–12 g/dl is probably optimal in that it reduces viscosity without significantly affecting oxygen delivery or cardiac output
- blood pressure should not be allowed to fall significantly (> 30%) below preoperative values
- vasodilatation of distal tissues will improve 'run-off' and lower the blood pressure distal to the graft, so improving flow
- some degree of anticoagulation is desirable immediately following the bypass graft, and is usually provided by not reversing the heparin used during arterial clamping

● platelet aggregation should be inhibited either before or shortly after surgery.

Practical methods of achieving these aims are described below.

Graft failure rates are very variable, depending on the extent of arterial disease, operation performed, medical condition of the patient, indication for surgery and perioperative management. Success of surgery is usually measured simply by amputation rate, although some vascular surgeons will undertake complex procedures to minimize the extent of amputation required, for example converting the need for a BKA to losing only a few toes, which represents a huge long-term benefit to the patient. Early amputation following either femoro-popliteal or femoro-distal bypass surgery occurs in less than 10% of patients, whilst in the long term (2 years) this figure is 10% or 20% respectively.

Early graft failure requires urgent investigation and surgical intervention. Late graft failure may be anticipated by non-invasive screening of graft blood flow, and appropriate intervention with either balloon angioplasty or further bypass surgery. However, redoing lower limb revascularization is much more complex than primary surgery and carries a substantially higher mortality and amputation rate.

Choice of anaesthetic technique

Many health care personnel underestimate the gravity of lower limb revascularization surgery, and it is therefore unsurprising that most patients are also unaware of the risks. Preoperative discussions with the patient concerning the risks and benefits of surgery are normally carried out by surgical staff, but it is important that vascular anaesthetists are involved. The anaesthetist is often better equipped to assess the implications of the patient's other medical problems on the perioperative course for that patient, and should contribute to ensuring that the patient is fully informed before consenting to surgery. In view of the outcomes described above with or without surgery, in a large majority of cases the patients have little choice but to 'risk' having surgery rather than contemplate amputation or further debilitating pain.

Is regional anaesthesia better than general anaesthesia?

This question has been debated extensively in the anaesthetic and surgical literature over the last few years, and the intensity of the debate indicates that there are no clear answers[9-13]. Before considering the evidence for or against a particular technique, it is necessary to consider the possible advantages and disadvantages of each[14]. These are presented in Table 7.1 and are theoretical only; that is, the advantages and disadvantages stated may not be proven in suitable clinical trials.

There are three physiological changes resulting from regional anaesthesia (RA) that may influence patient outcome:

Table 7.1 Theoretical advantages and disadvantages of regional and general anaesthesia for lower limb revascularization procedures[14]

Anaesthetic	Advantages	Disadvantages
Regional	<ul><li>self monitoring of angina, orthopnoea</li><li>better graft blood flow</li><li>vasodilatation so good tissue perfusion</li><li>stress response to surgery reduced</li><li>better respiratory function postoperatively</li><li>good analgesia postoperatively</li><li>possibly less DVTs</li></ul>	<ul><li>uncomfortable to perform</li><li>may be impossible or unsuccessful, particularly in patients with obesity, previous back surgery, kyphosis etc.</li><li>time-consuming to initiate</li><li>vasodilatation requires careful fluid management</li><li>hypotension common</li><li>respiratory problems with high blocks</li><li>patient discomfort with long procedures</li><li>risk of headaches</li><li>rare neurological complications; may be increased by use of anticoagulants</li></ul>
General	<ul><li>100% reliable</li><li>comfortable for patient during surgery</li><li>cardiovascular control relatively easy during surgery</li></ul>	<ul><li>inadequate analgesia and postoperative cardiovascular instability more common</li><li>nausea and vomiting</li><li>sedation and respiratory complications</li><li>hypercoagulable post-operatively</li></ul>

- sympathetic block results in vasodilatation of peripheral vessels, which necessitates increased fluid infusion to create a 'low pressure, high flow' circulation in the lower body
- conduction block leads to complete analgesia in most cases
- endocrine stress-response to surgery is attenuated, probably as a result of the conduction blockade[15].

Whether or not these changes do in practice influence outcome beneficially is only partially clear.

Mortality

Table 7.2 presents a summary of studies that have directly compared general anaesthesia (GA) with regional anaesthesia (RA). Comparison of studies in this way is fraught with difficulties, not least of which are differences in the patients studied and the actual techniques used, which are indicated in the final column of the table. Earlier studies, particularly that of Yaeger *et al.*[17], indicated a large benefit in RA techniques, but this study included all patients

Table 7.2 Summary of studies comparing outcome following general anaesthesia (GA) or regional anaesthesia (RA) for lower limb vascular reconstruction

Study	Numbers		Perioperative mortality (%)		Cardiovascular complications (%)		Respiratory complications (%)		Notes
	GA	RA	GA	RA	GA	RA	GA	RA	
Cook et al. 1986[16]	51	50	5.9	2.0	7.8	4.0	33	16	RA = Spinal
Yaeger et al. 1987[17]	25	28	16	0	52	14	32	3.4	Includes all forms of major surgery
Tuman et al. 1991[18]	40	40	0	0	27	10	12	2.5	RA = Epidural and general. All types of vascular surgery (45 lower limb surgery)
Christopherson et al. 1993[7]	51	49	3.9	4.1	7.8	8.2	27	12	RA = Epidural and sedation
Bode et al. 1996[6]	138	285	2.9	3.1	19	23	–	–	RA = 149-epidural, 136-spinal

Cardiovascular complications include myocardial infarction or significant worsening or new occurrence of heart failure, and in some studies changes in ST segments.

having major surgery, including non-vascular abdominal and thoracic procedures, and so cannot really be extrapolated to lower limb revascularization. The three larger and more recent studies have each found no difference in mortality between RA and GA, irrespective of whether epidural or spinal is used, with or without general anaesthesia as well.

Morbidity

As described above, major complications are common following lower limb revascularization. Table 7.2 shows the relative occurrence of cardiovascular and respiratory complications with RA and GA techniques. It is fairly clear that respiratory problems occur less frequently following regional anaesthesia, an observation which is more difficult to explain for leg surgery than for surgery involving the abdomen or chest. However, this may result from better surgical outcomes (see below) and analgesia resulting in earlier mobility and return to normal activities.

Cardiovascular complications are difficult to define, varying from severe clinical heart failure to transient changes in ST segment on continuous ECG monitoring, which explains the wide variations in occurrence seen in Table 7.2. There are many possible explanations for an effect of RA, all of which probably arise from the attenuation of the stress hormones, catecholamines in particular:

- reduced myocardial work by reduction of afterload with sympathetic blockade
- improved global and regional left ventricular function as a direct effect of sympathetic block[9]
- less periods of hypertension during and after surgery[19]
- reduction in hypercoagulability normally seen following vascular surgery[18].

Though the general trend of figures shown in Table 7.2 is for higher complication rates in GA patients, the two most recent studies have shown little difference between RA and GA. This failure to find a difference in more recent studies almost certainly results from improved cardiovascular management of the patients in both groups when compared with earlier studies.

It therefore seems likely that the anaesthetic technique has little effect on cardiovascular outcome provided there is appropriate, usually invasive, management of the circulation throughout the perioperative period[10–12].

Graft patency

Regional analgesia continued into the postoperative period may reduce the incidence of early graft failure, as indicated by the requirement for thrombectomy, regrafting or amputation. Two studies showed a highly significant difference in graft failure rates between GA only groups (20%) and RA groups with or without GA (4%)[7,18]. Other studies have found no difference[16,20], so it is necessary to look at the mechanisms more closely. There are two ways in which RA may influence graft patency:

- improved graft flow due to reduction of vascular resistance distal to the graft by direct sympathetic nerve blockade[21] and improved analgesia reducing both sympathetic activity and circulating catecholamines
- reduced tendency to graft thrombosis.

The effects of epidural analgesia on coagulation have been studied mainly in non-vascular patients, and include inhibition of platelet aggregation[22], attenuation of the postoperative rises in serum fibrinogen, factor VIII and von Willebrand factor[23], and an increase in postoperative plasminogen activator, which will improve thrombolysis. Patients having vascular surgery are already hypercoagulable preoperatively with increased α angle and MA (p. 140) on thromboelastography, and epidural analgesia reduces these almost to normal[18].

With this clear scientific evidence of improved graft blood flow and reduced coagulability with RA, why are the outcome studies unclear? The answer once again probably lies in methodological differences between studies in terms of the indications for surgery, type of grafts used, distal vessel disease, etc. Thus for patients having lower limb revascularization the difference in surgical outcome between RA and GA is small, and the use of epidural analgesia is most likely to be of benefit in those with the highest risk of early graft failure. In our unit, use of an epidural (either as the sole anaesthetic or as an adjunct to GA) is therefore regarded as specifically indicated in patients having femoro-distal grafts or in patients having repeat revascularization procedures, and is regarded as more optional in other patients. For the former group, patients are specifically told that the epidural is to improve graft blood flow postoperatively and that the analgesic effects are secondary. Once the decision to use an epidural to improve graft blood flow is taken, it is important to maximize the vasodilation effects by using some form of dilute local anaesthetic solution (e.g. bupivacaine 0.1%) and to continue the technique for as long as possible into the postoperative period, usually until the patient is ready to mobilize 24–48 hours postoperatively.

Surgical factors affecting the choice of anaesthetic technique

Duration of surgery plays an important role in this decision. Increasing complexity of lower limb revascularization procedures has inevitably led to an increase in the duration of operations, the *average* duration for femorodistal bypass being 5 hours in one recent study[6]. Long operations do not prevent the use of RA, as continuous epidural infusions, spinal catheters or long-acting local anaesthetic solutions are available. However, patients may have difficulty keeping still throughout the operation and usually require continuous sedation and possibly conversion to general anaesthesia if required. Confusion or agitation in the patient during surgery may well result from simple intolerance of the surroundings, but before further sedation or GA is given the anaesthetist should consider whether or not confusion is a sign of developing complications such as hypothermia, hypoxia, acidosis or other medical problems. Indeed, one of the main advantages of RA is the use of the patients as their own monitors, reporting chest pain or shortness of breath often before problems are detected by monitoring.

Surgical requirements. Technically difficult operations of predictably long duration, such as repeat lower limb revascularization, may be best performed with GA and RA combined. In addition, the use of arm veins for vascular reconstruction renders RA alone impossible and communication between surgeon and anaesthetist prior to surgery is therefore vital. Indications that arm veins may be required can be identified by the anaesthetist during the preoperative assessment by a history of coronary artery bypass grafting, previous vein graft in the leg or varicose vein surgery, which usually involve stripping the veins used for revascularization.

Patient factors affecting the choice of anaesthetic technique

Contraindications to either RA or GA in a patient will assist the decision on the preferable anaesthetic technique. There are many contraindications to RA, which are discussed in detail below, whilst a patient who cannot have a carefully performed GA is extremely rare.

Choice is important for patients in the modern healthcare system. Some degree of personal choice can be offered, particularly in the absence of any significant evidence of benefit with one technique or another.

Medical problems can have a large influence on whether to use GA, RA or both. Patients with severe respiratory disease will benefit from RA, but may find it difficult to tolerate prolonged surgery awake. Lying flat may be difficult, and although femoral artery access is possible with a small degree of upper body elevation, this may make a regional anaesthetic alone impossible. In addition, patients with respiratory disease often have a permanent cough, which makes delicate surgery simply impossible. Similarly, patients with cardiovascular disease (particularly those with cardiac failure and orthopnoea) will be difficult to manage awake. However, in patients with uncomplicated angina which is carefully controlled, RA is perfectly acceptable.

Preoperative assessment for lower limb revascularization

Thorough preoperative assessment (as described in Chapter 3) is essential in all vascular patients. Medical problems should be optimally treated prior to surgery in all but the most urgent of cases, preferably by the involvement of other specialists in the management of cardiac disease, diabetes mellitus and renal disease. In patients for lower limb arterial surgery, cardiovascular disease is so frequent and often so severe that it is sometimes impossible fully to 'treat' their heart failure or angina. Therapy must be optimal before surgery, but this often still means undertaking surgery in patients with significant symptoms.

During preoperative assessment, it is important to be wary of patients who seem to have minimal cardiovascular disease. The advent of angioplasty means that nowadays surgery for lower limb ischaemia is limited to those with severe arterial disease and symptoms, so patients presenting for operation can rarely walk more than a few yards. Some will continue to report shortness of breath or angina with this small amount of exercise, and some will report symptoms at rest or with emotional upset, but many will deny symptoms of heart disease. Other forms of exercise to induce angina have been investigated for patients unable to walk (such as the arm ergometer, a large handle offering variable resistance which patients must turn at an increasing rate), but there has been little success in attaining the work rate needed to achieve a significant cardiovascular challenge. Pharmacological methods are available, such as stress echocardiography in which dobutamine and/or atropine are administered to 'stress' the heart whilst observing for symptoms or echocardiographic signs of wall motion abnormalities (p. 99), but this technique is invasive and expensive.

The anaesthetist should provide the patient with a detailed explanation of perioperative events before surgery. This should include discussion about the types of anaesthesia proposed and the relative merits and drawbacks of each. When this is agreed upon, in-depth explanations are given for all proposed procedures, including the siting of epidural, venous, arterial, central venous and urinary catheters as appropriate and the implications of these for patient comfort and activity in the postoperative period. Once a decision has been taken about the environment for postoperative care (e.g. recovery, intensive care, high dependency, ward), the patient should be informed of what to expect in each area. Most patients benefit greatly from being told what to expect following the surgery with respect to pain, immobility and limitation of oral intake and the duration of these disturbances. It remains a common finding on postoperative rounds that patients' expectations of their recovery are very unrealistic, and are usually equally divided between those who feel better than they expected and vice versa.

All decisions about perioperative management are best taken a few days before surgery. Provision of a vascular pre-assessment clinic facilitates this, as well as allowing a more relaxed environment in which to undertake the discussions described previously.

Prior to surgery, it is important to note baseline recordings of blood pressure and heart rate, preferably when the patient is relaxed and settled into the new environment in hospital. The patient should be asked about angina whilst in hospital, and if this has occurred, investigate the blood pressure and pulse rate at the time. It is traditional to use the minimum (resting) blood pressure reading from the preoperative chart as a target figure during anaesthesia, but observation of charts on any vascular ward will reveal massive variations in blood pressure, particularly systolic values. This approach probably remains correct, as recent work has failed to find an association between a high blood pressure reading on admission to hospital ('white coat hypertension') and cardiovascular death, whilst a past history of hypertension remains an important risk factor for cardiovascular complications and death[24].

Premedication for lower limb revascularization surgery is a matter of personal choice for the anaesthetist concerned, but is normally unnecessary if adequate time has been spent allaying the patients fears about the surgery and anaesthesia. On the rare occasions when anxiety remains to such an extent that there is a possibility of cardiovascular disturbances such as hypertension or angina, then an oral benzodiazepine is often used, for example temazepam.

Preoperative optimization of the cardiovascular system is advocated by some centres. In a relatively small study of 89 patients, half received aggressive cardiovascular monitoring (including Swan–Ganz catheterization) to guide fluid, inotrope and vasodilator therapy over the 12 hours preoperatively. All patients received standard GA, and the mortality rate was considerably lower in the preoperatively optimized group (1.55 versus 9.5%)[25]. This form of therapy is expensive and not without its own risks, and cannot be advocated as routine practice on the basis of this one small study, but may be worth considering in high-risk patients.

Conduct of general anaesthesia

Monitoring. On arrival in the anaesthetic room or operating theatre, basic monitoring of ECG, pulse oximetry and non-invasive blood pressure should be instituted, although interpretation of the blood pressure value obtained at this time requires caution. If required, cannulae for invasive monitoring can be inserted either using local anaesthesia prior to induction or after the patient is asleep. The major argument in favour of siting lines prior to induction is the improved monitoring obtained during the significant cardiovascular stress of induction and tracheal intubation, whilst against this is the cardiovascular stress involved in having the cannulae inserted when awake. The latter problem is minimized with a good rapport between the anaesthetist and patient, established prior to arrival in theatre, and attention to detail when providing local anaesthesia for cannulae insertion. When to institute invasive monitoring is therefore a matter for the anaesthetist to decide in each case, but the threshold for commencing monitoring whilst awake will be reduced in patients with greater cardiovascular risk. Insertion of an arterial line is relatively easy with local anaesthesia and allows close monitoring of blood pressure during induction, following which the more uncomfortable central lines may be inserted; this technique provides a compromise between full or minimal monitoring during induction.

Vascular surgical units now commonly use invasive cardiovascular monitoring[14] via a radial artery cannula and central venous pressure (CVP) monitoring with an internal jugular or subclavian vein multilumen catheter. Invasive monitoring is advisable in all patients having distal limb revascularization surgery, and in any patient for lower limb revascularization who has significant myocardial ischaemia, heart failure or renal impairment, which in practice means the majority of patients. Invasive cardiovascular monitoring is helpful during prolonged surgery with insidious blood loss, arterial clamping and reperfusion of ischaemic limbs, but is also particularly beneficial in the postoperative period.

More detailed assessment of left ventricular function is required in a patient with poorly controlled heart failure, previous episodes of pulmonary oedema, or poor left ventricular function on preoperative echocardiography. In this situation, either a Swan–Ganz catheter or oesophageal Doppler is suitable, depending on the anaesthetist's preference (Chapter 4).

Induction of anaesthesia with intravenous agents requires care. Although etomidate in theory causes the least cardiovascular instability, postoperative nausea and vomiting limits its use to all but the sickest of patients. Propofol or thiopentone are acceptable alternatives, provided the patient's age and medical condition is taken into account when deciding on the dose required and speed of injection. Use of an opioid will further reduce the requirement for, and therefore cardiovascular depression with, the induction agent. There are many intravenous opioids now available, all with little direct effect on cardiovascular function (p. 71), and the choice depends mainly on the likely duration of surgery and the analgesia method chosen. Fentanyl (1–3 µg/kg) or alfentanil (30–50 µg/kg) are suitable for use during induction, but will not have sufficient duration of action for maintenance analgesia following a single dose.

The duration of lower limb revascularization operations normally requires the trachea to be intubated and the lungs ventilated by intermittent positive pressure ventilation (IPPV). Prolonged spontaneous ventilation during general anaesthesia in elderly patients, particularly in the presence of significant doses of opioids, will lead to the development of atelectasis and increasing oxygen requirements throughout surgery and into the postoperative period. If intraoperative analgesia is provided by a regional block, then opioid requirement will be minimal and spontaneous respiration is more feasible, but even then it offers little benefit over IPPV.

Maintenance. Anaesthesia is easily maintained with either inhalational agents or intravenous infusions, depending on personal preference, supplemented if required by intravenous opioids. Once again, the advanced age and poor cardiac state of many vascular patients requires careful titration of anaesthetic dose to prevent undue depression of cardiac output and blood pressure. The dose requirement for volatile anaesthetic agents, or minimal alveolar concentration (MAC), declines logarithmically with age (Figure 7.2) such that at 80 years old required doses are consistently 77% of those at age 40 years[26].

Most operations for lower limb revascularization can be performed without muscle relaxation, except for procedures requiring access to the aorta or iliac arteries. However, muscle relaxants are often needed to facilitate prolonged IPPV with 'light' general anaesthesia.

Analgesia is often achieved using a regional anaesthetic in addition to the GA, and the techniques are described below. In cases where RA is not possible or in operations that require the harvesting of arm veins, long-acting opioid analgesics are required (for example morphine), which will continue to be effective into the postoperative period. Perioperative use of non-steroidal anti-inflammatory agents for analgesia is best avoided because of their propensity to cause renal impairment. This is most likely to occur in older patients, following hypovolaemia, and in those with pre-existing renal impairment (for example secondary to renal vascular disease or hypertension)[27], and so places patients having lower limb vascular surgery at risk.

Patient temperature falls progressively during surgery, with many detrimental effects (p. 136), particularly on the cardiovascular system. Maintenance of a near normal body temperature will avoid unstable blood pressure and pulse rate as well as preventing postoperative confusion or respiratory depression, and can be achieved by using:

- maintenance of appropriate operating theatre temperature
- warmed humidified gas for ventilation
- a warming mattress under the patient

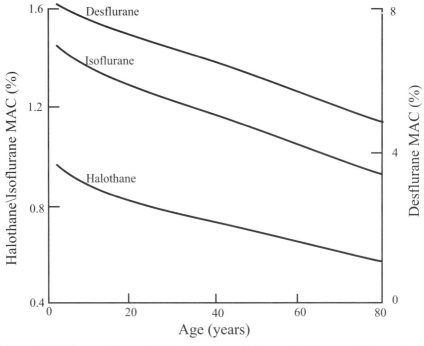

Figure 7.2 Influence of age on MAC of common volatile anaesthetic agents. Redrawn from data in Mapleson 1996[26].

- a forced-air warming blanket (e.g. Bair Hugger) over any part of the patient not being operated upon
- a fluid warming system.

Use of forced-air warming systems has greatly improved the ability of anaesthetists to maintain patient temperature during prolonged surgery, with few complications[28]. Although there are no published cases of complications, manufacturers of forced-air warming systems advise against their use on ischaemic tissues during surgery, for example on the legs during aortic, iliac or femoral artery clamping. Air temperature with active warming systems is as high as 43°C and may theoretically cause skin burns or accelerate anaerobic metabolism in the ischaemic tissue and thereby intensify metabolic disturbances on reperfusion.

Emergence and recovery for lower limb revascularization surgery does not differ greatly from other forms of surgery. Muscle relaxants should be reversed if necessary, normally by using a combination of neostigmine and glycopyrollate to minimize the resulting tachycardia. Reversal can often be avoided by the use of medium-duration non-depolarizing relaxants such as atracurium and vecuronium, along with continuous infusion administration and suitable monitoring.

Fluid management

Administration of intravenous fluids for patients having lower limb revascularization presents the usual challenges associated with any group of high-risk patients. Normal or even supranormal circulating volume is beneficial in minimizing cardiovascular and renal disturbances, both of which are common and serious complications of vascular surgery, but many patients also have impaired left ventricular function and are at increased risk of developing pulmonary oedema. Maintaining a patient in this sometimes narrow window between opposing complications requires close attention to fluid management, aided by suitable monitoring, normally including arterial and central venous pressure along with urinary output.

There are three sources of fluid loss to be considered:

1 *Maintenance fluid* must be replaced throughout surgery at approximately 70–100 ml/hour, normally with a crystalloid. In addition, patients need to receive maintenance fluid for the period of 'nil-by-mouth' prior to surgery, which may be several hours if there have been delays with previous operations. The volume of fluid required may again be calculated as approximately 70 ml/hour, and therefore often represents a greater than 1 l deficit. As this represents a deficit on arrival in theatre it may be given rapidly either prior to, during or shortly after induction, though it is normally necessary to correct this deficit before establishing RA block if catastrophic reductions in blood pressure are to be avoided (see below). Patients with actual or potential renal impairment, including those who have recently received radiological contrast, should be given intravenous maintenance fluid as soon as the preoperative fast begins to prevent the development of oliguria before surgery even starts.

2 *Third space* fluid loss is a term used to describe fluid requirements as a result of intraoperative losses from:

- ventilation–minimized by adequate humidification of inspired gases
- the gastrointestinal system–particularly if paralytic ileus develops
- evaporation from the wound
- 'stress response' fluid shifts from the circulation into the extracellular and intracellular spaces.

Lower limb revascularization represents a moderate degree of third space loss in that it may require multiple or large wounds, but does not involve opening a major body cavity (pleura, peritoneum or pericardium). Quantifying third space loss is clearly difficult, once again signalling the need for invasive monitoring, but approximately 5 ml/kg per hour of crystalloid during surgery is an acceptable starting point.

3 *Blood replacement* with colloid is also required. Blood loss during lower limb revascularization is insidious, and can amount to significant losses over a few hours. Replacement with synthetic colloid solutions should be instituted early, and blood replacement commenced when estimated blood loss exceeds the reserve available based on preoperative haemoglobin (approximately 400 ml blood loss per gram of Hb above the desired postoperative Hb).

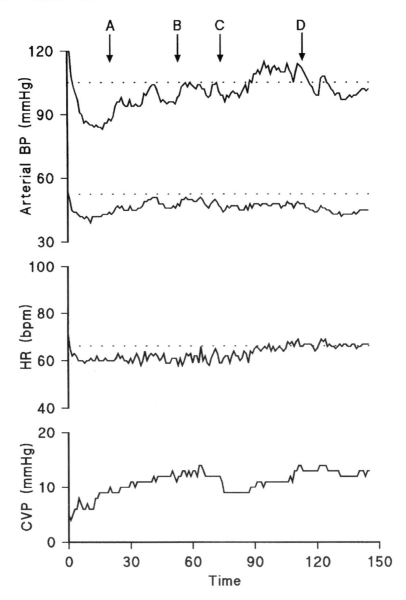

Figure 7.3 Cardiovascular monitoring data from a patient undergoing an femoro-popliteal *in situ* vein graft under general anaesthesia. The patient's normal resting blood pressure (systolic and diastolic) and heart rate (HR) are marked on the *y*-axes with dotted lines. The patient initially has a low central venous pressure (CVP) from preoperative fasting, so the pressor response to intubation quickly declines, but the small degree of hypotension is corrected when surgery starts (A). The infusion of 1.5 l of saline in the first 60 min establishes a high–normal CVP by the time the femoral artery is clamped (B). During valvulotomy, blood loss of approximately 500 ml occurs (C) which requires 1 l colloid to maintain the CVP at over 12 mmHg. Reperfusion of the leg (D) is then associated with only a minimal change in blood pressure. In spite of changes in CVP, note how the normal signs of hypovolaemia (hypotension and tachycardia) were absent as a result of preoperative beta blockers and calcium antagonist therapy for angina.

Based on the equation on page 202, a reduction in blood viscosity will increase blood flow through the bypass graft. The main determinant of blood viscosity is Hb concentration, so some degree of anaemia may be beneficial for high-risk grafts although this will reduce oxygen delivery to all tissues including those supplied by the graft. A compromise Hb of 10 g/dl is therefore regarded as optimal, but in vascular surgery patients' care must be taken not to undershoot this target as myocardial ischaemia may be exacerbated.

An example of the cardiovascular management of a femoro-popliteal graft is shown in Figure 7.3 for a patient receiving GA alone, as RA was contraindicated by infected bed sores in the lumbar region.

Conduct of regional anaesthesia

Before deciding to proceed with any form of regional anaesthetic the contraindications must be considered. Fortunately most of these are only relative contraindications, and the risks of proceeding with RA are balanced carefully against the benefits (see above).

Contraindications to RA are numerous, but only the first four are absolute:

● lack of consent
● local infection or sepsis, for example from infected bed sores
● raised intracranial pressure
● lack of a suitably experienced anaesthetist
● lack of patient co-operation, which prevents the patient keeping still in a suitable position–e.g. a patient with dementia or acute confusion. This does not preclude use of RA in conjunction with a GA provided that consent to surgery, however given, includes consent to the RA
● severe cardiovascular disease, which prevents an increase in cardiac output in response to the reduction in vascular resistance (e.g. aortic stenosis)
● hypovolaemia, along with time considerations, prevents the use of RA with arterial disruption such as leaking anastomoses postoperatively
● neurological disease (e.g. multiple sclerosis) is a contraindication more for legal than medical reasons, in case of deterioration in neurological function for which the RA may be blamed
● technical problems such as previous back surgery, scoliosis etc. RA is often possible in these circumstances, but is still avoided by many anaesthetists for the same reasons as for neurological disease
● coagulopathy is discussed separately below.

Anticoagulants and use of regional anaesthesia

A patient with impaired haemostasis having either a spinal or epidural injection is theoretically at risk of developing a haematoma in the spinal canal, leading to spinal cord compression and potential permanent and disastrous neurological sequelae. This is estimated to occur at a rate of 0.6 per 100 000 spinal or epidural injections, with slightly greater risk following epidural injection[29]. These risks may be considerably increased when haemostasis is impaired, and this can occur in four situations in patients for vascular surgery.

1 *Aspirin* is commonly administered preoperatively in patients presenting for vascular surgery, as prophylaxis against the progression of coronary, cerebral or peripheral arterial disease. Though low doses are used, platelet aggregation is disturbed for several days, as evidenced by the efficacy of aspirin in preventing many arterial diseases.
2 *Intravenous heparin* may be administered preoperatively for the treatment of acute arterial thrombosis or embolism, normally in high doses to fully anticoagulate the blood.
3 *Preoperative deep vein thrombosis prophylaxis* with heparin or low molecular-weight heparin (LMWH) is now routine practice for almost all patients undergoing major surgery, including arterial surgery.
4 *Heparin* may be administered during surgery to prevent thrombosis during arterial clamping.

Any of these situations should cause the anaesthetist to question the relative risks and advantages of RA, but this requires information on the actual, rather than the theoretical, risk to the patient from a haematoma. A majority of reported haematomata following diagnostic lumbar puncture[30] or spinal/epidural injection[31,32] occur in patients who have significant impairment of haemostasis. RA should therefore be avoided in these patients, including those receiving continuous heparin infusions preoperatively unless this can be stopped in advance and return of coagulation to normal values confirmed prior to surgery. In the case of LMWH for thromboembolism prophylaxis, spinal haematoma has been reported when an epidural was performed shortly after its administration[32]. Therefore current advice, based on the pharmacokinetics of LMWH, is that spinal/epidural injection is safe when performed more than 12 hours after the last dose of LMWH[29].

Administration of intravenous heparin after insertion of spinal or epidural catheters has been reported as safe. A study of 4000 patients having RA as part of the anaesthetic for lower limb revascularization reported no spinal haematomas[33], but strict precautions were observed:

- patients with pre-existing coagulopathies were not included in the study
- heparin was not given until at least 60 minutes after the RA catheter was inserted
- the operation was postponed for 24 hours if frank blood was seen in the needle or catheter at insertion
- anticoagulation was closely monitored
- catheters were removed only when heparin activity was low.

This study was also undertaken some years before the widespread use of aspirin for vascular disease.

In practice patients commonly have more than one defect of haemostasis, for example LMWH and aspirin preoperatively, and an increased risk of epidural haematoma is therefore likely and must be accepted as a risk of the technique. This risk must be offset against the potential benefits of RA use in each patient as described above. In the absence of pathological haemostatic defects, we will use RA techniques for lower limb revascularization cases receiving aspirin and/or LMWH provided that:

- intravenous heparin can be stopped early enough to allow spontaneous correction of coagulation
- LMWH is administered the night before surgery
- heparin is not given until 60 minutes after the epidural is sited
- ACT can be monitored and maintained at $< 2 \times$ baseline
- the patient can be observed closely postoperatively for neurological signs of epidural haematoma, such as unexpected weakness, numbness or bowel/bladder dysfunction.

Perioperative thrombolysis, normally using tissue plasminogen activator (TPA), may be performed before or during surgery for acute arterial thrombosis or embolism. Its use is theoretically hazardous even when RA was performed some hours earlier, as clots formed at the time may be lysed. Unexpected use of TPA during surgery when RA is already established cannot be avoided, and in spite of the theoretical risks we know of no reported cases of subsequent problems.

Epidural analgesia

Siting of the epidural catheter is performed once venous access and appropriate monitoring have been established. When combined with a general anaesthetic there is debate about whether the epidural should be sited before or after induction of anaesthesia. Advantages of siting the catheter prior to induction include the ability to have the patient sitting up, feedback on needle position based on nervous sensation, better information following a test dose (see below), and being able to establish and confirm success of the RA before proceeding with GA and surgery. Disadvantages include discomfort or pain for the patient with resulting cardiovascular instability immediately prior to surgery. If the anaesthetist wishes to minimize the likelihood of spinal haematoma with intraoperative heparin administration by abandoning surgery following a 'bloody tap', then the epidural must be sited first to avoid an unnecessary GA. Advantages of siting the epidural after induction include a still patient, maximal spinal flexion in the lateral position and no requirement for patient co-operation and therefore less likelihood of sudden movement during needle insertion and consequent trauma. Once again, the choice is a personal one for the anaesthetist. If the RA is the primary anaesthetic technique being used then we advocate the establishment of an adequate block before giving sedation or a light GA, but if the RA is secondary to a GA, for example simply to improve limb blood flow following distal revascularization, then the epidural may be inserted when the patient is asleep.

Epidural injection by any technique is more challenging in vascular patients than in the obstetric patients that most trainee anaesthetists have become used to before joining the vascular team. In the elderly patient back flexion is reduced, intervertebral spaces are narrowed and ligaments calcified, making identification of the epidural space difficult. Experience is the only answer to this, although it is helpful to be proficient in both midline and paramedian (lateral) approaches[34].

For lower limb revascularization insertion of the catheter in the mid-lumbar region (L2–3 or L3–4) is acceptable, although high lumbar or low thoracic (L1–2 to T11–12) may be required for access to the iliac vessels through an extraperitoneal lower abdomen incision.

Test doses are used to detect inadvertent intravascular or subarachnoid placement of the epidural catheter, which occurs in approximately 2% and 0.5% respectively of epidural insertions[35]. The drug and dose requirements for a test dose are complex[35], but it usually involves giving a local anaesthetic (LA) in sufficient quantity to allow detection of neural block with subarachnoid but not epidural placement, and a beta-adrenergic receptor stimulant (such as adrenalin or isoprenaline) to produce tachycardia with intravenous injection. A suitable test dose is 3 ml of 1.5% or 2% lignocaine with 1:200 000 adrenalin (15 µg)–an intravenous injection produces an increase of 20 bpm in the heart rate lasting approximately 60 seconds, whilst intrathecal injection will produce significant sensory blockade, normally in the sacral region, within 2 minutes. In patients taking beta blockers the adrenalin test will be unreliable. Similarly, general anaesthesia attenuates the tachycardic response such that an increase in heart rate of only 8 bpm signifies intravascular placement[35]. Detection of intrathecal placement during GA is even more difficult as sensory signs cannot be elicited, but intrathecal injection of lignocaine is very likely to cause significant hypotension during GA, which should be actively sought during an otherwise stable period of the operation.

If there is any doubt about the validity of a test dose, it is prudent to establish the epidural block using incremental doses of 3–5 ml of LA until a satisfactory block is obtained. Though time-consuming, particularly with a long-acting (slow onset) drug such as bupivacaine, this remains the safest technique.

Local anaesthetics are normally used for intraoperative epidural nerve block. Use of progressively increasing doses causes conduction block in autonomic nerves, sensory nerves and finally motor nerves, so choice of suitable concentration and volume of LA solution allows control over the resulting neural block. Larger doses of LA are required initially to establish the block, which can then be maintained with smaller doses by infusion for longer periods. Its long duration of action in the epidural space has resulted in almost universal popularity for bupivacaine, and suitable dose regimes for lumbar epidurals are suggested below. As with all anaesthetic agents, it is vital to tailor the dose to the individual patient needs based on size, age and medical conditions, but the following regimes are a suitable starting point for a typical patient for lower limb vascular surgery.

- Surgery with RA only (± sedation). Establish block with 10–15 ml 0.5% bupivacaine, followed by 5–10 ml per hour of 0.25% bupivacaine. This will result in total sensory and motor block, the latter being very helpful when RA is used as the sole anaesthetic technique.
- RA for analgesia only, supplemented with GA. Establish block with 10–15 ml 0.25% bupivacaine, followed by 5–10 ml per hour of 0.167%

bupivacaine. Motor block is unlikely to be total and in this case is unnecessary.

- RA only, to improve graft blood flow. Establish block with 5–10 ml 0.25% bupivacaine, followed by 5–10 ml per hour of 0.1% bupivacaine. This will result in autonomic block of the lower thoracic region and produce a variable amount of analgesia, requiring careful titration of analgesic dose as part of the GA to avoid excessive narcosis postoperatively.

Opiates are used increasingly in the epidural space, where they have analgesic effects and so reduce the stress response to surgery without having the same motor and autonomic nerve effects as LAs. In practice, this results in a synergism between epidural opiates and LA, allowing a reduction in the required dose of both. However, when using RA for lower limb revascularization motor block and autonomic block may both be regarded as desirable during surgery, and epidural opiates are used more widely in the postoperative period (Chapter 9) and for aortic aneurysm surgery (Chapter 6).

Spinal (subarachnoid) anaesthesia

The principles of spinal anaesthesia are similar to those for epidural block. Duration of action for spinal anaesthetics has become a limiting factor in lower limb vascular surgery as operations have become more complex and, consequently, of longer and more unpredictable duration. Some answers to this problem have become available, but spinal anaesthesia is less popular than epidural for this type of surgery. Technical difficulty in identification of the subarachnoid space is less common than with epidurals due to the smaller and sharper needle. Relatively large rigid spinal needles can be used (24 or 22 G) compared to obstetric practice, as headaches following spinal injection are uncommon in vascular patients because of their age and fairly slow postoperative mobilization.

Single shot techniques with bupivacaine 0.5% 2–3 ml will produce good operating conditions for up to 2 hours. Use of hyperbaric bupivacaine and suitable positioning of the patient allows specific blocks to be established, of which a unilateral block is the most useful as this limits the effects on blood pressure mediated by autonomic disturbance (see below). This technique is therefore very suitable for short arterial procedures such as localized repairs of the femoral artery or embolectomy, although it is important to establish anaesthesia of the whole leg if arterial clamping is proposed, or ischaemic pain during surgery will be intense.

Spinal anaesthesia in the USA is enhanced by the availability of tetracaine, which has much longer duration of action than bupivacaine. A dose of 1.5–2.0 ml of 1% tetracaine combined with 3–5 mg of phenylephrine injected in the lumbar region produces adequate anaesthesia for surgery, lasting up to 5 hours[6].

Spinal catheters allow continuous infusion of LA to facilitate prolonged anaesthesia. Although an attractive idea, technical problems with the catheters have reduced their acceptance by anaesthetists. There is a design conflict between size and function–catheters must be very small to allow insertion through a suitable size needle, yet remain strong enough to prevent breakage, kinking or compression during a prolonged stay in the ligaments of the spine, where huge forces may be applied to the catheter. These problems are slowly being surmounted, but at present spinal catheters are not widely used in vascular surgery.

Combined epidural and spinal techniques utilize a spinal injection to establish a reliable and rapid onset of sensory blockade and then an epidural catheter to continue the block, should the surgery outlast the spinal or block be required into the postoperative period. Combination RA has gained popularity in obstetric practice (where in some situations the rapid establishment of RA for caesarian section is beneficial), but the technique has little to offer for vascular surgery where a gradual onset of RA is better for the unfit patient.

Cardiovascular changes with RA

There are two mechanisms by which RA affects the cardiovascular system:

- reduction of surgical stimulus by effective sensory blockade
- sympathetic nerve block (Figure 1.10), including both vasomotor nerves (T1–12) and cardioaccelerator nerves (T1–4).

Lack of surgical stimulus causes reductions in both nervous activity in the sympathetic system and circulating catecholamines, both of which lead to a reduction in heart rate, cardiac output and blood pressure. With combined RA and GA, it is useful to think of the RA 'unmasking' the deleterious effects of general anaesthesia on the cardiovascular system, effects that are normally counteracted by pain. Sympathetic blockade reduces blood pressure by effects on both arterial and venous systems, with the latter predominating. Arteriolar vasodilation reduces vascular resistance, whilst venodilation reduces venous return and hence cardiac output. Small unmyelinated sympathetic nerve fibres are blocked by LA at low concentrations, so sympathetic blockade usually extends two to six segments higher than the sensory block, particularly with spinal anaesthesia. Lumbar epidurals with the block centred around T12/L1 are therefore unlikely to result in blockade of cardioaccelerator nerves or total sympathetic block, and usually only cause sympathetic block in the pelvis, legs and lower abdomen. This situation is ideal for lower limb revascularization, as it maximizes blood flow to the legs without causing severe cardiovascular disturbance.

Acceptable limits for intraoperative blood pressure and pulse rate are controversial[19], but pulse rates of between 40–100 bpm and blood pressures ranging between ±20% of preoperative resting values are unlikely to be associated with excess perioperative morbidity. In patients undergoing arterial surgery, achieving these targets requires an aggressive approach.

Management of the reduction in blood pressure and heart rate with RA requires:

- appropriate 'depth' of GA for a pain-free patient
- gradual onset of RA, if possible

- optimal fluid therapy, as described for GA. Hypovolaemia from preoperative fasting is the usual cause of dangerous reduction of blood pressure with RA and should be aggressively treated. Invasive monitoring will facilitate pre-emptive or rapid fluid therapy
- vasopressors.

Vasopressor agents such as ephedrine and phenylephrine should only be administered when optimal fluid therapy is either well underway or complete. Ephedrine is a combined adrenergic agonist, with both direct and indirect effects on sympathetic nerves and their receptors. Thus its action in RA-induced hypotension includes vasoconstrictor effects via alpha receptors, beta$_2$-mediated vasodilatation in some tissues, and both inotropic and chronotropic effects on the heart mediated by all adrenoreceptors. Effects on the heart are a significant part of the increase in blood pressure seen with ephedrine, and this aspect of the response will be poor in patients with hypovolaemia or poor left ventricular function. Conversely, the chronotropic effects of ephedrine are useful in patients with pre-existing bradycardias, such as those taking beta blockers or calcium antagonists. Phenylephrine is a direct alpha agonist, so has effects predominantly on the vasculature, and is a more appropriate drug in situations where cardiac activity is believed to be already adequate.

Intraoperative events

Vein harvesting normally involves identifying and removing the long saphenous vein from the same leg that requires arterial reconstruction. If this vein has been removed because of varicosities or already used as an arterial conduit in the heart or legs, then the short saphenous veins or contralateral long saphenous vein may be used. Finally, when all these possibilities are exhausted, arm veins may be required from one or both arms. In this situation, venous access for both intraoperative and postoperative periods should be assured using a CVP line, and lower limb regional analgesia supplemented with systemic analgesics.

Anticoagulation is normally required before arterial clamping, but a few minutes after any synthetic or venous conduit has been tunnelled by blunt dissection to minimize haemorrhage along the tunnel. Heparin is administered intravenously, normally in a dose of 3000–5000 units for adults. Monitoring of coagulation, for example with ACT (p. 139) is helpful, and if possible a baseline measurement should be performed before heparin is given. During arterial clamping, an ACT of 1.5–2 × baseline, or 200 seconds, is required, and additional heparin doses should be given as necessary. It is worth remembering that the half-life of heparin varies between patients and with the dose given, so monitoring is advisable, particularly when regional anaesthesia is used. Reversal of heparin with protamine is not normally performed, as a small degree of anticoagulation into the postoperative period is believed to be beneficial for graft survival. If required because of persistent bleeding, protamine should be administered slowly (over at least 2 minutes) and in small doses (5–20 mg), preferably with measurement of ACT to monitor its effect.

Arterial clamping for lower limb revascularization rarely presents problems with vascular resistance. Most operations are performed for severe occlusive disease, and the arterial clamps make little difference. Should changes occur on clamping they should be managed in the same way as for aortic clamping (p. 186).

Cardiovascular and respiratory changes on reperfusion are less dramatic than those seen with aortic unclamping because of the smaller amount of ischaemic tissue involved. However, cardiovascular changes are still seen relatively commonly, and the magnitude of these depends on:

● extent and metabolism of unperfused tissue
● duration of ischaemia–this is often greater in lower limb revascularization than for aortic surgery because of the small vessels and complexity of bypass grafts
● amount of collateral circulation present, which relates mainly to the duration of the arterial disease
● degree of preoperative ischaemia, particularly in the case of acute occlusion of leg arteries when each additional hour of waiting for surgery will worsen the responses to reperfusion.

The mechanisms of reperfusion injury are identical to those described following aortic surgery (p. 176). Management is also similar, and relies in particular on achieving an ideal (slightly supranormal) circulating volume before releasing the clamps (Figure 7.3), avoiding sudden reperfusion by spacing the release of each major arterial branch (e.g. profunda femoris and superficial femoral arteries), and administering inotropes such as ephedrine or calcium only if these manoeuvres fail. Use of RA seems to reduce the severity of cardiovascular instability with unclamping, possibly because RA produces maximal dilatation of the lower limb vessels long before unclamping, and thereby forces the anaesthetist to increase the circulating volume.

Observation of legs 24 hours after successful revascularization frequently reveals a very warm hyperaemic distal limb, particularly when there was prolonged preoperative ischaemia. It is easy to see how this can result in a systemic inflammatory response syndrome, resulting in renal, pulmonary or even multisystem failure in the first few days following surgery, a situation which is associated with significant mortality even with intensive care.

References

1. McDermott MM, McCarthy W. Intermittent claudication–the natural history. *Surg Clin North Am* 1995; **75(4)**: 581–91.
2. Davies AH, Magee TR, Baird RN *et al.* Intraoperative measurement of vascular graft resistance as a predictor of early outcome. *Br J Surg* 1993; **80**: 854–7.
3. Cheshire NJ, Wolfe JHN, Noone MA *et al.* The economics of femorocrural reconstruction for critical leg ischaemia with and without autologous vein. *J Vasc Surg* 1992; **15**: 167–75.
4. Harris PL, Da Silva AF, Holdsworth J. Criticial limb ischaemia: management and outcome. Report of a national survey. *Eur J Vasc Endovasc Surg* 1995; **10**: 108–13.

5. Manolio TA, Beattie C, Christopherson R *et al*. Regional versus general anesthesia in high-risk surgical patients: the need for a clinical trial. *J Clin Anesth* 1989; **1**: 414–21.
6. Bode RH, Lewis KP, Zarich SW *et al*. Cardiac outcome after peripheral vascular surgery. Comparison of general and regional anaesthesia. *Anesthesiology* 1996; **84**: 3–13.
7. Christopherson R, Beattie C, Frank SM *et al*. Perioperative morbidity in patients randomized to epidural or general anesthesia for lower extremity vascular surgery. *Anesthesiology* 1996; **79**: 422–34.
8. Krupski WC, Layung EL, Reilly LM *et al*. Comparison of cardiac morbidity between aortic and infra-inguinal operations. *J Vasc Surg* 1992; **15**: 354–65.
9. Tuman KJ, Ivankovich AD. Pro: Regional anesthesia is better than general anesthesia for lower extremity revascularization. *J Cardiothorac Vasc Anesth* 1994; **8**: 114–7.
10. Kahn RA, Hollier L. The epidural space: is it the place to be during vascular surgery? *J Cardiothorac Vasc Anesth* 1997; **11**: 127–8.
11. Gelman S. General versus regional anesthesia for peripheral vascular surgery–is the problem solved? *Anesthesiology* 1993; **79**: 415–8.
12. Go AS, Browner WS. Cardiac outcomes after regional or general anesthesia–do we have the answer? *Anesthesiology* 1996; **84**: 1–2.
13. Bode RH, Lewis KP. Con: Regional anesthesia is not better than general anesthesia for lower extremity revascularization. *J Cardiothorac Vasc Anesth* 1994; **8**: 118–21.
14. Ellis JE, Klock A, Klafta JM *et al*. Choice of anesthesia and intraoperative monitoring for lower extremity revascularization. *Surg Clin North Am* 1995; **75(4)**: 665–78.
15. Breslow MJ, Parker SD, Frank SM *et al*. Determinants of catecholamine and cortisol responses to lower extremity revascularization. The PIRAT study group. *Anesthesiology* 1993; **79**: 1202–9.
16. Cook PT, Davies MJ, Cronin KD *et al*. A prospective randomized trial comparing spinal anaesthesia using hyperbaric cinchocaine with general anaesthesia for lower limb vascular surgery. *Anaesth Intensive Care* 1986; **14**: 373–80.
17. Yaeger M, Glass DD, Neff RK *et al*. Epidural anesthesia and analgesia in high-risk surgical patients. *Anesthesiology* 1987; **66**: 729–36.
18. Tuman KJ, McCarthy RJ, March RJ *et al*. Effects of epidural anesthesia and analgesia on coagulation and outcome after major vascular surgery. *Anesth Analg* 1991; **73**: 696–704.
19. Christopherson R, Glavan NJ, Norris EJ *et al*. Control of blood pressure and heart rate in patients randomized to epidural or general anesthesia for lower extremity vascular surgery. *J Clin Anesth* 1996; **8**: 578–84.
20. Pierce ET, Pomposelli FB, Stanley GD *et al*. Anesthesia type does not influence early graft patency or limb salvage rates of lower extremity arterial bypass. *J Vasc Surg* 1997; **25**: 226–33.
21. Hickey NC, Wilkes MP, Howes D *et al*. The effect of epidural anaesthesia on peripheral resistance and graft flow following femoro-distal reconstruction. *Eur J Endovasc Surg* 1995; **9**: 93–6.
22. Henny CP, Odoom JA, Cate HT *et al*. Effects of extradural bupivacaine on the haemostatic system. *Br J Anaesth* 1986; **58**: 301–5.
23. Steele SM, Slaughter TF, Greenberg CS *et al*. Epidural anesthesia and analgesia: implications for perioperative coagulability. *Anesth Analg* 1991; **73**: 683–5.
24. Howell SJ, Sear YM, Yeates D *et al*. Hypertension, admission blood pressure and perioperative cardiovascular risk. *Anaesthesia* 1996; **51**: 1000–4.
25. Berlauk JF, Abrams JH, Gilmour IJ *et al*. Preoperative optimization of cardiovascular hemodynamics improves outcome in peripheral vascular surgery. *Ann Surg* 1991; **214**: 289–97.
26. Mapleson WW. Effect of age on MAC: a meta-analysis. *Br J Anaesth* 1996; **76**: 179–85.
27. O'Callaghan CA, Andrews PA, Ogg CS. NSAIDs in the postoperative period–many factors threaten renal function. *BMJ* 1993; **307**: 257.
28. Bennet J, Ramachandra V, Webster J *et al*. Prevention of hypothermia during hip surgery: effect of passive compared with active skin surface warming. *Br J Anaesth* 1994; **73**:

180–3.

29. Horlocker TT, Heit JA. Low molecular-weight heparin: biochemistry, pharmacology, perioperative prophylaxis regimens and guidelines for regional anaesthetic management. *Anesth Analg* 1997; **85**: 874–85.

30. Owens EL, Kaston GW, Hessel EA. Spinal subarachnoid haematoma after lumbar puncture and heparinization: a case report, review of the literature, and a discussion of anaesthetic implications. *Anesth Analg* 1986; **65**: 1201–7.

31. Vandermeulen EP, Van Aken H, Vermylen J. Anticoagulants and spinal-epidural anesthesia. *Anesth Analg* 1994; **79**: 1165–77.

32. Dahlgren N, Tornebrandt K. Neurological complications after anaesthesia: a follow up of 18 000 spinal and epidural anaesthetics performed over 3 years. *Acta Anaesthesiol Scand* 1995; **39**: 872–80.

33. Rao TL, El-Etr AA. Anticoagulation following placement of epidural and subarachnoid catheters; an evaluation of neurologic sequelae. *Anesthesiology* 1981; **55**: 618–20.

34. Wildsmith JAW, Armitage EN. *Principles and Practice of Regional Anaesthesia.* Churchill Livingstone, 1987.

35. Mulroy MF, Norris MC, Liu SS. Safety steps for epidural injection of local anesthetics: review of the literature and recommendations. *Anesth Analg* 1997; **85**: 1346–56.

8

Miscellaneous vascular operations

Endovascular aortic aneurysm surgery

A less invasive method of treating abdominal aortic aneurysm (AAA) than traditional surgery has been sought for a long time, and has become a reality in the last 4 years[1]. There are many techniques now being developed by several different manufacturers, most of which require a combined approach by both a vascular surgeon and a radiologist. An example is shown in Figure 8.1, based on the Vanguard™ device manufactured by Maedox® (Boston Scientific Corporation).

An open arteriotomy of one femoral artery (in this case the right) is performed and a guide wire passed through the aneurysm, over which a stent device is threaded into the suprarenal aorta (Figure 8.1a). The stent device has three components:

- an outer sheath, containing
- a Y-graft made of polyester fabric strengthened with wire mesh, inside which there is
- a catheter with a smooth-ended obturator to allow insertion of the device with an aortic angioplasty balloon proximal to this.

Once the device is positioned immediately below the renal arteries, the outer sheath is withdrawn and the wire mesh expands by a technique of 'thermal memory' (the polymer automatically takes on a predesigned shape on being warmed to blood temperature) (Figure 8.1b). Small hooks on the proximal stent attach the top of the graft to the aortic wall, and the remainder of the outer sheath is withdrawn whilst the graft continues to expand to its preformed shape. The inner catheter is then slowly removed and the angioplasty balloon inflated to fully expand the graft (Figure 8.1c) and seal it with the distal implantation stent within the right common iliac artery (Figure 8.1d), leaving a 'stump' of graft orientated towards the left common iliac artery. A percutaneous puncture of the left femoral artery then allows a wire to be threaded through the stump of the graft into the aorta (Figure 8.1d). A smaller tube graft is then inserted in exactly the same way to connect the aortic graft stump to the left common iliac artery (Figure 8.1e), expanding the aortic end into the conical-shaped graft stump to ensure a tight connection. Finally, the distal end of the graft limb is sealed in the left common iliac

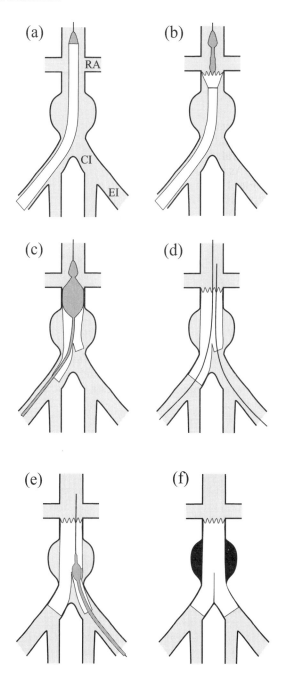

Figure 8.1 Schematic diagram showing the technique for an endovascular repair of an abdominal aortic aneurysm. The technique shown is based on the *Maedox® Vanguard*™ bifurcated graft, and is described in detail in the text. RA, renal artery; CI, common iliac artery; EI, external iliac artery.

artery, thus excluding the aneurysm sac from the circulation (Figure 8.1f). The inferior mesenteric artery, if patent, may need to be radiologically embolized prior to endovascular stenting, to prevent this maintaining contact between the aneurysm and the circulation.

Following endovascular exclusion of the aneurysm most patients experience a post-implantation syndrome, involving fever, malaise and back pain for a few days postoperatively with raised levels of inflammatory cytokines[2]. The aetiology is uncertain, but probably follows manipulation of the device within the aneurysm and resorption of the blood within the aneurysm, which is excluded by the graft.

Only 25% of AAAs are suitable for endovascular treatment, which requires a non-tortuous aorta, 15 mm of normal aorta between the aneurysm neck and renal arteries, and a similar distance of normal vessel below (either aorta or common iliac). Data on the success and risks of endovascular AAA repair are difficult to interpret because most units are still low down on the learning curve for a very new procedure, using a multitude of different techniques and equipment. Early reports indicate that the procedure is successful in excluding the aorta in 80% of cases[3], and that mortality rates initially are between 6 and 10%[4]. The need to convert to an open operation may occur in up to 35% of cases[5], and in this situation the mortality is high.

In these early stages of the technique it is not certain whether endovascular repair should be used mainly in high- or low-risk patients requiring AAA repair. Use in low-risk patients will undoubtedly give better results for endovascular repair, but will also expose patients to unquantified risks unnecessarily when an open repair would be relatively simple. Conversely, high-risk patients have the most to gain from avoiding a laparotomy, but are also more likely to succumb to the complications of endovascular repair when they occur. These factors make assessment of the place of endovascular repair difficult, and render large randomized clinical trials vital to the future of the technique. In the meantime, the attractions of a less invasive technique for patients at high risk from open repair are already becoming overwhelming.

Questions remain about the long-term performance of endovascular grafts. Late graft failures (either from leakage of blood into the aneurysm sac or displacement of the graft) are already described, but the frequency with which these occur using different manufacturers' systems is unknown. The necessity for open surgery at a later date in only a small proportion of cases may substantially affect the risk–benefit analysis for endovascular repair.

Anaesthetic considerations[3]

Site for procedure. Throughout the procedure repeated angiograms are performed to check positioning of the device, and suitable quality angiograms may only be obtainable in the X-ray department. It is therefore necessary to establish a suitable environment for anaesthesia for major surgery within this normally remote site, with all the equipment, drugs and personnel which would be used in the theatre suite, including those necessary to deal with major complications such as aortic rupture, femoral artery repair and embolectomy.

Duration of the procedure may be long, particularly during the early stages of the 'learning curve' for radiologists or surgeons. For this reason, it is advisable to use a general anaesthetic until the team is suitably experienced. A general anaesthetic should include full provision for maintaining normal body temperature (p. 211) in a room that may be maintained at a cool temperature for technical reasons relating to the radiographic equipment.

Angiography is frequently performed, and requires apnoea to obtain suitable quality pictures. The anaesthetist should also closely monitor urine output and preferably maintain a high flow of dilute urine to minimize the renal effects of intravenous contrast in these patients, who normally have pre-existing renal impairment.

Arrhythmias may occur during the procedure, particularly ventricular tachycardia as a result of the very long guide wire slowly being introduced further into the patient until it eventually crosses the aortic valve and enters the left ventricle. Withdrawal of the wire should resolve the arrhythmia, and periodic checking of the wire tip radiologically is easily performed.

Anticoagulation with intravenous heparin is used prior to clamping the femoral artery for the arteriotomy to insert the device. The same dose and monitoring requirements are used as for other types of arterial surgery involving the femoral artery (p. 221).

Femoral occlusion begins on one side as soon as the arteriotomy is performed to insert the stent, and continues until the wire is removed on completion of the graft insertion and the arteriotomy is closed. This may amount to prolonged ischaemia if graft deployment is in any way complicated, and the resulting reperfusion response should be treated in the usual way (p. 222). The other leg should be exposed only to minimal ischaemia as perfusion can continue through the graft (Figure 8.1d) and during percutaneous puncture, with short ischaemic episodes during balloon dilation of the left leg limb of the graft (Figure 8.1e).

Aortic occlusion occurs only intermittently with inflation of the angioplasty balloon for periods of approximately 30 seconds, which are associated with transient changes in blood pressure.

Bleeding is insidious, but may amount to a substantial volume over time. Insertion and manipulation of the device through an arteriotomy results in a continual and sometimes brisk loss of blood from the insertion site.

Anaesthetic technique. If endovascular repair is successful, then regional analgesia is unnecessary postoperatively; pain from the femoral arteriotomy can then easily be treated with oral analgesics and the patient quickly mobilized. In addition, the unpredictable duration of the procedure and potential risks of regional anaesthesia (p. 204) have led some workers to recommend general anaesthesia[3]. The usual monitoring is instituted, and a routine general anaesthetic administered including tracheal intubation and IPPV. It is advisable to use the same invasive monitoring for endovascular aortic repair as for open surgery, including measurement of direct arterial pressure, CVP, temperature, urine output, and pulmonary arterial catheterization if required.

When successful, endovascular repair of AAA really does appear to be 'minimally invasive', with patients returning to normal activity soon afterwards with a significantly smaller degree of stress response to the surgery compared with open repair[2]. However, the technique is in its infancy, with an as yet ill-defined place in the management of AAA and uncertainty about the incidence and outcome of complications and the long-term reliability of currently available devices.

Arterial embolectomy

Acute arterial embolism occurs most commonly in the leg, but is occasionally seen in the arms, and is strongly associated with atrial fibrillation. It is an acute surgical emergency, requiring intervention within a few hours if permanent limb damage or amputation are to be avoided. The advent of intra-arterial thrombolysis has significantly reduced the proportion of cases requiring surgery, but the result of this is that those patients presenting for surgery have more complex arterial problems and have waited longer before surgery, so have a more severe ischaemic insult and reperfusion injury. The in-hospital mortality following embolectomy has been reported to be almost 50%, with immediate heparinization, early intervention and an absence of previously documented peripheral vascular disease all being associated with improved limb salvage rates[6].

Local anaesthesia. Immediate preoperative treatment consists of intra-venous fluids and heparin. Local anaesthesia may be used for open femoral arteriotomy and embolectomy. Local infiltration by the surgeon is a suitable technique in a co-operative patient with a clear history of embolism and a short ischaemic time. Even in these circumstances full anaesthetic involvement is mandatory, to monitor the patient throughout, deal with problems which may arise during surgery (such as blood pressure instability, arrhythmias, angina, hypoxia etc.) and, finally, to be available if embolectomy is unsuccessful and further, more extensive reconstructive surgery becomes necessary.

General anaesthesia. If there is any doubt about the feasibility of a procedure under local anaesthesia, then it should not be attempted. General anaesthesia for an embolectomy or for revascularization will almost always require invasive cardiovascular monitoring, and is described in detail in Chapter 7. However, unlike for elective surgery, preoperative preparation of the patient may be poor with dehydration, limited cardiovascular investigations and suboptimal treatment of cardiovascular disease, all of which will therefore require careful management during surgery. Finally, cardiovascular instability following reperfusion may be severe following acute embolism, as collateral circulation will be minimal compared with chronic limb ischaemia.

Intra-arterial thrombolysis is used to treat acute ischaemia caused by arterial thrombosis, and is normally performed in the X-ray department. Using local anaesthesia, a percutaneous arterial puncture allows arteriography to define the position and extent of the thrombus, following which an arterial catheter is placed immediately proximal to the thrombus through which either streptokinase or tissue plasminogen activator (TPA) can be infused. Clinical assessment of the limb and repeat angiography will then allow a decision about the necessity for reconstructive surgery and the operation required. In spite of the short half-life of TPA, regional anaesthesia by spinal or epidural block should not be used (see p. 215) in the event of surgery being required.

Visceral revascularization

'Intestinal angina' refers to a rare condition characterized by postprandial abdominal pain, fear of eating and weight loss. The arterial supply to the large and small bowel is via a combination of the coeliac axis and the superior mesenteric and inferior mesenteric arteries, which may develop atherosclerotic stenosis in the same way as any other medium-sized artery. Symptoms are uncommon until at least two of the three vessels are affected. As with the legs and heart, resting blood flow is normally adequate, but the massive increase in mesenteric blood flow which normally follows eating cannot be accommodated and bowel ischaemia develops.

Revascularization may involve reimplantation of visceral arteries (which is uncommon as aortic disease is almost inevitable) or bypass grafting of the artery, and carries a significant mortality rate of up to 25% in some series[7]. The surgical technique will therefore vary from clamping only the visceral artery concerned, through side-clamping the aorta, to fully clamping the aorta above the coeliac axis. Anaesthetic considerations are mostly considered in Chapter 6, and include:

- cardiovascular management with supracoeliac aortic clamping
- spinal cord preservation techniques
- renal protection
- reperfusion injury following bowel and liver ischaemia
- possibility of sepsis secondary to bacterial translocation across ischaemic bowel mucosa.

Thoracoscopic cervical sympathectomy

Thoracoscopic cervical sympathectomy has now almost completely replaced the more major operation of open surgical cervical sympathectomy, and is performed for palmar hyperhidrosis (a rare condition resulting in profuse sweating, usually from both hands). Medical treatment of palmar hyperhidrosis has only moderate success rates, so surgical intervention is now the treatment of choice in severe cases. Patients requesting surgery are normally fit, healthy young adults in whom an imminent life event such as school examinations, marriage or a new job renders dripping wet hands no longer tolerable.

Surgery involves collapse of the lung with CO_2 insufflation into the pleural space, and insertion of two or three trocars through which diathermy is used to divide the sympathetic chain between T2 and T5, depending on the clinical presentation. In the largest study to date of thoracoscopic sympathectomy, involving 602 patients[8], treatment was successful in 99% of cases with symptoms recurring later in less than 1%. Complications of surgery are rare but include:

- pneumothorax
- haemothorax
- damage to other chest structures, most commonly intercostal arteries
- prolonged postoperative pain, often reported as 'back pain'

- Horner's syndrome
- compensatory hyperhidrosis elsewhere on the body, which may be gustatory (related to eating).

Anaesthesia[9,10]

Palmar hyperhidrosis is a socially and psychologically debilitating condition, but can in no way be described as life- or limb-threatening. Therefore, during preoperative assessment, the anaesthetist needs to be certain that the patient understands and accepts the risks of surgery. These patients normally require none of the usual preoperative investigations required for other types of vascular surgery, but a baseline chest X-ray is advisable to allow comparison in the event of postoperative chest complications.

General anaesthesia is required, and should include muscle relaxants to facilitate control of the airway and ventilation as described below.

Airway maintenance can be satisfactorily achieved using either a tracheal[11] or endobronchial tube. Tracheal intubation is inexpensive, simple, and less likely to cause hypoxia than one lung ventilation (OLV), but gives less clear surgical access and may be associated with a greater incidence of pulmonary trauma[11]. A well positioned endobronchial tube will allow complete deflation of the lung with less likelihood of lung trauma and good surgical access, but is more expensive and time-consuming, may require fibreoptic confirmation of positioning and can lead to hypoxia during OLV. The type and side of tube used is a matter of personal preference; right-sided tubes are easy to position but may occlude the right upper lobe bronchus producing hypoxia during OLV, whilst left-sided tubes are harder to position but avoid occlusion of the segmental bronchi. The author's preference is to use a left-sided endobronchial tube to maximize surgical effectiveness and safety, whilst overcoming any hypoxia by simple techniques used in any patient undergoing OLV (see below).

Carbon dioxide insufflation requires co-operation between surgeon and anaesthetist. Whichever type of airway maintenance is used, the lungs must be deflated fully when the surgeon inserts the insufflation needle into the chest cavity. With endobronchial intubation the correct lung should be disconnected from the ventilator and the bronchial tube opened to the atmosphere, whilst with a tracheal tube the patient should be allowed a full expiration with breathing system expiratory valves fully open to prevent the formation of any positive pressure in the lung. The visceral and parietal pleura will not separate until gas is introduced into the pleural space, but these respiratory manoeuvres will allow the visceral pleura to fall away from the chest wall as soon as some CO_2 is introduced, so minimizing the chance of pulmonary trauma.

With tracheal intubation the capnogram may be used to confirm correct needle placement when CO_2 is first injected into the pleural space[11], and this is illustrated in Figure 8.2. During the prolonged expiration allowed for needle insertion, the normal trace (Figure 8.2a) should change to a slow upsloping CO_2 concentration with a plateau no higher than end-tidal CO_2 (Figure 8.2b) as the lung on the operative side is deflated. With needle placement outside the pleural cavity or pleural adhesions preventing lung collapse this will not occur (Figure 8.2c), and if the needle is within the

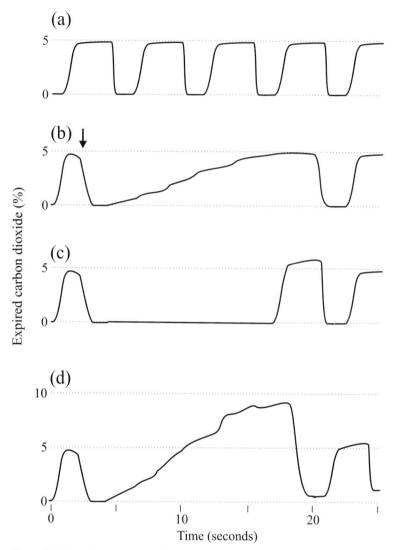

Figure 8.2 Use of capnogram to detect incorrect needle placement during insufflation of CO_2 for thoracoscopic cervical sympathectomy using tracheal intubation. Arrow indicates the point at which respiration is suspended in expiration during needle insertion. (a) Normal trace; (b) correct needle placement; (c) needle not within pleural cavity or adhesions preventing lung deflation; (d) intrapulmonary injection of CO_2. See text for details. Reproduced from Olsfanger et al. 1995[11] with permission of the authors and the publishers of British Journal of Anaesthesia.

lung a high concentration of CO_2 will develop in the expired gas (Figure 8.2d).

Initially, 0.5 to 1.0 l of CO_2 is insufflated into the pleural cavity, following which the thoracoscope camera is inserted to check that the lung is deflated. More gas may then be used, but it is important to use a pressure-limited CO_2

insufflator set to 5 mmHg, and if surgical access is inadequate at this pressure efforts must be made to collapse the lung more completely rather than simply increasing the intrathoracic pressure. The recommended maximum permissible volume of gas to be insufflated is variable, estimates ranging between 1–2 l[12], but in practice this is difficult to assess as there will inevitably be loss of gas from leaks around the trocar and from the trocar seals when instruments are inserted and removed.

Deliberate or accidental increases in intrathoracic pressure cause physiological changes consistent with a tension pneumothorax. These changes include severe hypotension, bradycardia and hypoxia as a result of reduced venous return, cardiac filling, coronary perfusion and compression or kinking of bronchi. This complication occurred in 2 of 58 cases in one study, and was immediately reversed by removal of gas from the chest cavity[10].

Cardiac complications during surgery are rare, and are usually related to intrathoracic pressure changes as previously described. However, denervation of T2–T4 sympathetic ganglia will result in partial denervation of the sympathetic supply to the heart and possibly an increased risk of arrhythmia. Reversible depression of ST segments has been described[12], as have two cases of successfully treated cardiac arrest[13], so careful monitoring of the ECG during surgery is mandatory.

Intraoperative hypoxia occurs mainly as a result of OLV. A detailed discussion of the physiology of OLV is beyond the scope of this book, but the main cause of hypoxia is pulmonary shunting as a result of blood flow through pulmonary tissue that is not ventilated. When the non-ventilated lung collapses, pulmonary capillaries are compressed and less shunting occurs; thus the worst situation is seen when a non-ventilated lung remains fully inflated. Attempts should therefore be made to minimize this time by insufflating CO_2 as rapidly as possible whilst paying close attention to intrathoracic pressure and cardiovascular disturbances, and by ensuring the non-ventilated lung is open to atmospheric pressure with no obstruction to air outflow. Once the lung has collapsed, hypoxia may still occur. In theory, hypoxic pulmonary vasoconstriction (HPV) should further reduce blood flow through pulmonary vessels in the non-ventilated lung, but there is conflicting evidence about the effectiveness of HPV during anaesthesia. If unacceptable hypoxia persists when the lung is maximally collapsed, further measures are required, one or more of which is usually successful:

- Increase the inspired O_2 concentration. This has no effect on the shunt fraction but may improve oxygenation from the ventilated lung and has the advantage of causing little harm over a short period of time.
- Apnoeic oxygenation of the non-ventilated lung involves placing a small catheter down the endobronchial tube with a continuous flow of 1–3 l/min of O_2. The catheter must not occlude free flow of gas from the lung, as this will result in lung inflation during the procedure.
- Intermittent small inflations of the non-ventilated lung will often correct hypoxia for several minutes, and can be performed at appropriate stages of the procedure.

If serious and persistent hypoxia occurs at any stage the surgery must be halted and the lung reinflated before further attempts may be made, possibly using a tracheal intubation technique as an alternative to OLV.

Temperature monitoring during surgery is a useful guide to successful nerve division. A peripheral temperature probe is sited on each hand before surgery commences, and sympathectomy should give rise to an immediate increase in temperature.

Residual pneumothorax (technically a capnothorax) can be avoided by reinflating the lung under direct vision with the thoracoscope, which is not removed until the lung can be seen against the chest wall. Full reinflation of pulmonary atelectasis requires prolonged positive pressure breaths, for example using inflation pressures of $30 \, cmH_2O$ sustained for 10 seconds three times, with normal breathing between. This manoeuvre should only be performed once the chest is fully closed, to prevent herniation of lung into the trocar sites. Chest drains are not normally used postoperatively, in order to reduce analgesic requirement.

All patients have a small ($< 5 \, mm$) apical pneumothorax and approximately 10% have a more significant volume of pleural gas, with little difference seen between anaesthetic techniques[9]. Only 1 in 10 of these will require a chest drain, normally for expanding pneumothorax following unrecognized pulmonary injury, which must always be considered. Otherwise, the decision whether or not to insert a drain depends on the clinical circumstances for each patient, but one is definitely required if the pneumothorax is associated with dyspnoea, hypoxia or significant pulmonary collapse on X-ray.

Postoperative pain may be severe in the first few hours, and is normally perceived in the back of the chest or lower neck rather than from the surgical incisions. The pain therefore probably arises from the cut sympathetic nerves, or from residual CO_2 in the pleura. Three analgesic methods are available:

- opiates used during surgery and continued postoperatively
- non-steroidal anti-inflammatory agents (NSAIs) may be particularly effective for treating pain of pleuritic origin
- intrapleural local anaesthetic has been used with some success, but may be associated with bilateral phrenic nerve block.

Surgery for thoracic outlet syndrome

Thoracic outlet syndrome (TOS) results from compression of the subclavian artery or vein as they pass over the first rib between the anterior and middle scalene muscles. Symptoms relate either to nerve compression (parasthesia, pain and, rarely, muscle wasting and weakness) or vascular damage (poststenotic dilatation, arterial emboli or subclavian vein thrombosis). The C8/T1 nerve root is most commonly affected. Many patients develop a neurogenic component to their symptoms, commonly following shoulder trauma (for example after road traffic accidents), and this is believed by some groups to be widely under-diagnosed[14]. Surgical treatment is reserved for severe cases for whom more conservative measures have failed, and is required in less than 1 in 20 cases.

Operations performed for TOS are variable, but are all aimed at increasing the space available between the clavicle and the first rib:

- removal of a cervical rib if present via a supraclavicular route
- transaxillary first rib resection, usually involving removal of most of the first rib from directly underneath the subclavian artery
- supraclavicular first rib resection to remove an anterior portion of first rib
- scalenectomy to remove part of the tendinous insertion of the anterior and/or middle scalene muscles
- supraclavicular approach to repair subclavian aneurysm.

Surgery is reported to be very successful, with good results in 80% of patients irrespective of the operation used[15].

Anaesthetic considerations

These must be tailored to the proposed surgery, which can vary from a short procedure through a small incision to remove a cervical rib to a large procedure involving resection of the clavicle and arterial reconstruction.

Intravenous access and monitoring. The subclavian artery and vein are almost as large as the femoral vessels but are considerably more difficult to access, particularly via the transaxillary route. Even if it is proposed only to operate on structures around the artery (e.g. in a first rib resection), wide-bore intravenous cannullae and immediate availability of blood are required in case of arterial damage which may be difficult to control. If arterial reconstruction is proposed then an arterial line is advisable. All vascular access should be sited in the non-operative arm, as both subclavian artery and vein may be occluded intermittently during surgery.

Analgesic requirements. Patients with long standing TOS often suffer from chronic pain for which they may already be receiving substantial quantities of one or more analgesic drugs, and this must be fully evaluated preoperatively. First rib resection is often a painful procedure and will commonly require the use of opiates postoperatively, including the use of patient-controlled analgesia systems.

Venous surgery

Surgery for varicose veins remains a common procedure for vascular surgery units. In young patients, surgery is usually performed for symptoms such as pain, swelling, itching and eczema, or for cosmetic reasons. In the elderly, varicose veins may require surgery to attempt to heal chronic leg ulcers. Widespread use of preoperative Doppler-based scans now allows the underlying cause of varicose veins to be easily elucidated, and surgery is targeted at correcting incompetent communications between the deep and superficial venous systems as well as removing the varicosities. This approach is associated with a greatly reduced recurrence rate[16], but often makes surgery more prolonged and complex. Corrective procedures performed include:

- saphenofemoral junction ligation and stripping of the long saphenous vein, performed through a small groin incision in the supine position

- saphenopopliteal junction ligation, requiring the patient to be in the lateral or prone position to gain access to the popliteal fossa
- thigh or calf perforator ligation, which may require the patient to be prone depending on where the perforator is located, identified by preoperative scanning. In some centres, subfascial endoscopic procedures are now being performed to ligate all venous perforators. These procedures may initially require prolonged anaesthesia until the surgeon becomes more familiar with the technique.

The possibility of trauma to major veins, particularly the femoral and popliteal veins, should not be forgotten and, though rare, may be associated with significant blood loss.

Anaesthesia

Most patients requiring varicose vein surgery are fit and well, so the choice of anaesthetic technique is an individual one made between the anaesthetist and patient. Elderly patients need more assessment, and a regional or local anaesthetic technique may be more appropriate.

General anaesthesia is uncomplicated and requires only moderate amounts of analgesia with, for example, short-acting opiates, local anaesthetic infiltration of incisions and oral analgesics shortly after waking. Stripping of the long saphenous vein is the most painful component of the surgery. Surgeons prefer the patient to be 'head down' during surgery to reduce venous pressure in the legs and so minimize blood loss. Intermittent positive pressure ventilation (IPPV) may theoretically increase venous pressure but will also control arterial CO_2 better, so preventing venodilation from this cause. In a head-down patient the choice of ventilatory mode probably has little effect on blood loss, and is therefore at the discretion of the anaesthetist. For patients requiring surgery only in the supine position, we use a technique of spontaneous respiration via a laryngeal mask airway. In obese patients or those requiring a prone position for part of the surgery, we use muscle relaxants, intubation and IPPV.

Regional or local anaesthesia is an attractive technique for venous surgery, as it may reduce hospital stay to just a few hours. Local infiltration is suitable for saphenofemoral or perforator ligation, but is not feasible for vein stripping or large numbers of phlebectomies. Spinal anaesthesia by any standard technique is excellent for varicose vein surgery, but may be associated with an unacceptable incidence of complications for outpatient surgery[17]. Femoral and genitofemoral nerve block produces anaesthesia of the groin and anteromedial aspects of the thigh and lower leg and so is ideal for long saphenous vein stripping[17], but will not provide anaesthesia for other procedures, which would require a more difficult sciatic nerve block. Choice of spinal anaesthesia, nerve block or local infiltration is therefore mainly determined by the proposed surgery.

Prevention of thromboembolism[18]

Whether or not varicose vein surgery constitutes a high-risk procedure for the development of postoperative deep vein thrombosis (DVT) is controversial[18,19]. Intuitively it may be expected that these patients would have disturbed venous flow and therefore possibly be more at risk of DVT, but varicose vein surgery involves only minimal trauma and patients mobilize quickly. Patients with varicose veins who undergo abdominal or pelvic surgery have an increased risk of developing postoperative deep vein thrombosis, but this finding cannot be extrapolated to varicose vein surgery itself. The incidence of pulmonary embolism in over 1063 varicose vein operations has been quoted as 0.56%[19], which is similar to that following laparotomy. This controversy is reflected in a recent survey of vascular surgeons in the UK, which found wide variations in the provision of DVT prophylaxis[20]. Preoperative heparin (usually low molecular-weight heparin), infusion of dextran solutions and antiembolism stockings may all be used for prevention. Some of these methods were used for all patients for varicose vein surgery in only 12% of units, whilst almost three-quarters of units used DVT prophylaxis in selected patients, including those for recurrent varicose vein surgery, the obese and the patient with a history of previous DVT.[20]

Agreement needs to be reached between surgeons and anaesthetists in each unit about appropriate prophylactic measures. Where heparin is used, the anaesthetist should consider the potentially increased risk of complications with spinal anaesthesia (p. 215) in an otherwise healthy patient undergoing what is generally a non-essential operation.

Amputation

Amputation is an inevitable part of surgery for peripheral vascular disease and, although performed less frequently than in the past, it remains a common operation in vascular units. In some patients amputation may be the primary surgical treatment as overwhelming gangrene and infection and severely diseased distal arteries leave no other option, but in many cases attempts will have been made to revascularize the leg.

Leg amputation normally leads to poor quality of life, particularly in the early stages, and in many cases is associated with a shorter life expectancy (p. 202). From the patient's point of view, amputation may be seen as desirable to bring to an end a prolonged period of unremitting severe ischaemic pain. For the majority pain relief is rapid and permanent, but for some the pain continues in spite of the loss of a limb.

Phantom pain

Following amputation, 'phantom limb' refers to any sensations perceived to be from the absent limb, whilst 'phantom pain' is any form of pain from the absent limb. Phantom limb is common immediately after surgery, and over a few months the perceived limb reduces in size and withdraws toward the stump. Sensations of phantom limb could in theory arise anywhere in the neural pathway between the cut nerves in the stump and the sensory cortex. Psychological and emotional aspects of a phantom limb have led Professor Melzack, one of the leading workers in this field, to conclude that the phantom limb has its origins in the higher centres of the brain rather than the spinal cord or periphery[21].

In the first few weeks following amputation phantom pain occurs in over 75% of patients[22,23], and by 2 years later it is still present in 60%[22]. Phantom pain is more common in patients either with long-standing pre-amputation pain (greater than 1 month), or in those with severe pain immediately prior to amputation[22]. As with phantom limb, the phantom pain is initially very similar to the pre-amputation pain, but the character and perceived site change with time. There are purported to be over 50 types of treatment described for phantom pain[24]; this in itself indicates the general lack of success of any of them, and treatment of phantom pain remains a major challenge to pain specialists. As a form of analgesia for ischaemic leg pain amputation can therefore occasionally be strikingly unsuccessful, and for this reason it is important to consider any possible therapeutic avenues to prevent the development of phantom pain[24].

Anaesthetic technique and phantom pain. A possible link between anaesthetic technique and the incidence of phantom pain was first described in 1988[25] and involved a study of only 25 patients, all of whom had preoperative limb pain. Eleven patients received an epidural infusion of bupivacaine and morphine for 3 days prior to surgery with epidural anaesthesia, whilst the remainder received standard analgesia preoperatively and epidural or spinal anaesthesia for surgery. A similar study was reported more recently[23], this time with 24 patients, 11 of whom received general anaesthesia and 13 epidural anaesthesia with bupivacaine, diamorphine and clonidine for 24 hours preoperatively. The results of both studies are shown in full in Table 8.1.

It is clear that from these studies that establishing an epidural infusion preoperatively can reduce the long-term incidence of phantom limb pain, but the findings of these studies are not universally accepted because:

- a very small number of patients were involved, and in one study were unrandomized[23]
- many patients were excluded from the studies, including those with a contraindication to epidural anaesthesia and those in whom epidural anaesthesia became ineffective at any stage

Table 8.1 Results of studies into the prevention of phantom limb pain by preoperative epidural analgesia

Study	1 week		6 months		1 year	
	Epidural	Control	Epidural	Control	Epidural	Control
Bach *et al.*, 1988[25]	3/11	9/14	0/10	5/13	0/8	3/11
Jahangiri *et al.*, 1994[23]	3/13	9/11	1/11	8/11	1/11	8/11
Combined	6/24	18/25	1/21	13/24	1/19	11/22
Percentage with phantom pain	25	72	5	54	5	50

All figures refer to prevalence of phantom pain at specified times following amputation. Epidural refers to preoperative epidural analgesia with different regimes for each study; control refers to groups given standard analgesic treatment. Numbers in each group decline with time due to deaths from unrelated causes.

- all patients included had severe preoperative pain
- neurological origins of phantom limb may be above spinal cord level[21], so it is difficult to explain how epidural analgesia can modulate a phantom limb sensation
- complete analgesia must be established at least 24 hours preoperatively, and was continued for 3 days post-surgery in one study[23]. This is sometimes impractical in sick patients.

Although there is currently no evidence from large, randomized, controlled trials that phantom pain can be prevented, these studies do indicate that some patients may benefit from preoperative epidural analgesia, and if this can be provided safely for at least 24 hours before surgery it should be considered[24]. It is likely to be of most benefit for those patients with significant preoperative pain.

Anaesthetic technique

Preoperative assessment should address some specific problems.

Pain control must be optimal before surgery, unless there are over-whelming reasons for immediate amputation. A lumbar epidural should be sited at least 24 hours preoperatively, and a block established with a combination of local anaesthetic and opiates. A suitable regime involves establishing the block with 10–15 ml of 0.25% bupivacaine and 2–3 mg diamorphine with the patient sitting at about 45°, and then an infusion of 5–10 ml/hour of 0.167% bupivacaine with 10 mg diamorphine in 250 ml. For surgery, the epidural should be topped up with 0.5% bupivacaine and the same infusion regime continued for 1 or 2 days postoperatively. Throughout this period the patient should be in a high dependency unit (HDU), to allow rapid recognition and treatment of the side-effects of epidural infusions (p. 247).

If epidural anaesthesia is contraindicated (p. 215), then analgesia should be optimized using other methods, normally involving opiate administration. Peripheral nerve blocks such as femoral or sciatic blocks may be useful, but there is no evidence that they have the same efficacy as central neural blockade in reducing subsequent phantom pain.

Systemic toxicity as a result of extensive gangrene or infection may lead to potentially serious organ failure prior to amputation. Patients may develop sepsis syndrome with one or more organ failures, and become dehydrated, oliguric, cardiovascularly unstable and confused. Rehydration, antibiotics and cardiovascular control must be achieved before surgery, if necessary in the HDU. Complete resolution of metabolic complications is unlikely to be achieved until the leg is amputated, so the timing of surgery is often a compromise that must be agreed upon between anaesthetist and surgeon. Diabetes is very common in this group of patients and almost always requires frequent blood sugar monitoring, with a sliding scale intravenous infusion of insulin for adequate control.

Regional anaesthesia is an excellent technique for lower limb amputation. A preoperative epidural for use during surgery has already been described. Spinal anaesthesia may be achieved using any standard technique. Traditional techniques involve the use of local anaesthetic alone to allow early establishment of a suitable postoperative analgesic regime, but the use of spinal opiates is becoming more widespread and provides more prolonged analgesia. It is normally possible to position the patient on the side with the operative leg down to allow injection of hyperbaric bupivacaine 0.5% (2–2.5 ml), following which the patient remains on that side for 15 minutes until the block is almost fully established. This normally results in a mostly unilateral block, which has little effect on the cardiovascular system. Provided the patient begins the operation adequately hydrated, this technique requires the infusion of minimal amounts of intraoperative fluid, and the patient can return to oral fluid intake soon afterwards.

If using regional anaesthesia, the patient should be sedated or receive a supplemental general anaesthetic to reduce any perception and memory of the noises associated with the surgery of amputation. Small doses of intravenous midazolam (1 mg increments) or nitrous oxide/oxygen by facemask are suitable techniques to provide short-acting sedation for this group of patients.

General anaesthesia is the default technique if regional methods are impossible. The technique of choice is essentially a personal one for the anaesthetist, but muscle relaxants are not required for surgery. Postoperative pain may require the use of on-demand opiates. If a preoperative epidural has not been used, there is no evidence that the type of anaesthesia (regional versus general) affects the incidence of phantom limb pain.

Intraneural block[26,27] is effected with a small (18–20 G) catheter inserted within the neural sheath of major leg nerves at the time of surgery. The catheter is inserted several centimetres along either the sciatic (above knee amputation) or anterior tibial (below knee) nerves. Local anaesthetic solutions such as bupivacaine 0.25% 10 ml/hour or bupivacaine 0.5% 2–6 ml/hour are infused for up to 3 days, and complications are rare. Analgesia is unlikely to be complete with this technique, mainly due to involvement of areas of leg supplied by the femoral nerve and its branches, but opiate requirement is usually significantly reduced. There is some evidence that this technique may also reduce the incidence of phantom pain, so it should be considered for use in all patients not receiving epidural analgesia[26,27].

Regional anaesthesia in amputees

There have been many reports of the development of phantom limb pain in otherwise pain-free amputees during spinal or epidural anaesthesia performed for operations unrelated to their previous amputation[28]. This observation has supported the concept of phantom pain originating in the brain and being 'switched off' by spinal cord sensory input, which is abolished by a regional block. Irrespective of the mechanism, the acute onset of perioperative phantom pain may be very distressing. Many successful forms of treatment are described, including intravenous benzodiazepines or opiates and intrathecal opiates, but these are not effective in all cases and general anaesthesia may be required[29]. The frequency with which this type of phantom pain occurs in amputees is not known—a handful of case reports over several years indicates a probably small incidence, but the anaesthetist should be aware of the possibility when deciding on a regional technique for any patient with a previous amputation.

References

1. Collin J. Transluminal aortic aneurysm replacement. *Lancet* 1995; **346**: 457–8.
2. Norgren L, Swartbol P. Biological responses to endovascular treatment of abdominal aortic aneurysms. *J Endovasc Surg* 1997; **4**: 169–73.
3. Grieff JMC, Thompson MM, Langham BT. Anaesthetic implications of aortic stent surgery. *Br J Anaesth* 1995; **75**: 779–81.
4. May J, White G, Yu W *et al*. Endoluminal grafting of aortic aneurysms: causes of failure and their prevention. *J Endovasc Surg* 1994; **1**: 44–52.
5. Baranowski AP, Adiseshiah M. Aortic stent surgery. *Br J Anaesth* 1996; **76**: 882–3.
6. Burgess NA, Scriven MW, Lewis MH. An 11-year experience of arterial embolectomy in a district general hospital. *J R Coll Surg Edinb* 1994; **39**: 93–6.
7. Stanton PE Jr, Hollier PA, Seidel TW *et al*. Chronic intestinal ischaemia: diagnosis and therapy. *J Vasc Surg* 1986; **4**: 338–44.
8. Gothberg G, Drott C, Claes G. Thoracoscopic sympathectomy for hyperhidrosis–surgical technique, complications and side-effects (602 patients). *Eur J Surg Suppl* 1994; **572**: 51–3.
9. Fredman B, Olsfanger D, Jedeikin R. Thoracoscopic sympathectomy in the treatment of palmar hyperhidrosis: anaesthetic implications. *Br J Anaesth* 1997; **79**: 113–19.
10. Jedeikin R, Olsfanger D, Schachor D *et al*. Anaesthesia for transthoracic endoscopic sympathectomy in the treatment of upper limb hyperhidrosis. *Br J Anaesth* 1992; **69**: 349–51.
11. Olsfanger D, Jedeikin R, Fredman B *et al*. Tracheal anaesthesia for transthoracic endoscopic sympathectomy: an alternative to endobronchial anaesthesia. *Br J Anaesth* 1995; **74**: 141–4.
12. Parry-Jones AJD. Thoracoscopic sympathectomy. *Br J Anaesth* 1997; **79**: 688–92.
13. Lin CC, Mo RL, Hwang MH. Intraoperative cardiac arrest: a rare complication of T2, 3 sympathectomy for the treatment of hyperhidrosis palmaris. *Eur J Surg Suppl* 1994; **572**: 43–5.
14. Turgut M, Ayberk G, Ozcan OE *et al*. Thoracic outlet compression syndrome: clinical evaluation and surgical results of 94 cases. *Acta Chir Belg* 1996; **96**: 211–16.
15. Sanders RJ. Results of the surgical treatment for thoracic outlet syndrome. *Semin Thorac Cardiovasc Surg* 1996; **8**: 221–8.
16. Neglen P, Einarsson E, Eklof B. The functional long-term value of different types of treatment for saphenous vein incompetence. *J Cardiovasc Surg* 1993; **34**: 295–301.
17. Vloka JD, Hadzic A, Mulcare R *et al*. Femoral and genitofemoral nerve blocks versus spinal anesthesia for outpatients undergoing long saphenous vein stripping surgery. *Anesth Analg* 1997; **84**: 749–52.
18. Campbell B. Thrombosis, phlebitis, and varicose veins. *BMJ* 1996; **312**: 198.
19. Bounameaux H, Huber O. Postoperative deep vein thrombosis and surgery for varicose veins. *BMJ* 1996; **312**: 1158.
20. Campbell WB, Ridler BM. Varicose vein surgery and deep vein thrombosis. *Br J Surg* 1995; **82**: 1494–7.
21. Melzack R. Phantom limbs. *Scientific American* April 1992, pp. 120–6.
22. Jensen TS, Krebs B, Nielsen J *et al*. Immediate and long-term phantom pain in amputees: incidence, clinical characteristics and relationships to pre-amputation pain. *Pain* 1985; **21**: 267–78.

23. Jahangiri M, Bradley JWP, Jayatunga AP *et al*. Prevention of phantom pain after major lower limb amputation by epidural infusion of diamorphiine, clonidine and bupivacaine. *Ann R Coll Surg Engl* 1994; **76**: 324–6.
24. Thompson HM. Pain after amputation: is prevention better than cure? *Br J Anaesth* 1998; **80**: 415–16.
25. Bach S, Noreng MF, Tjellden NU. Phantom limb pain in amputees during the first 12 months following limb amputation, after preoperative lumbar epidural blockade. *Pain* 1988; **33**: 279–301.
26. Elizaga AM, Smith DG, Sharar SR *et al*. Continuous regional analgesia by intraneural block: effect on postoperative opioid requirements and phantom limb pain following amputation. *J Rehabil Res Dev* 1994; **31**: 179–87.
27. Fisher A, Meller Y. Continuous postoperative regional analgesia by nerve sheath block for amputation surgery–a pilot study. *Anesth Analg* 1991; **72**: 300–3.
28. Uncles DR, Glynn CJ, Carrie LES. Regional anaesthesia for repeat Caesarean section in a patient with phantom limb pain. *Anaesthesia* 1996; **51**: 69–70.
29. Murphy JP, Anandaciva S. Phantom limb pain and spinal anaesthesia. *Anaesthesia* 1984; **39**: 188.

9

Postoperative care

The principles of postoperative care of the vascular patient are the same as those of any patient. This chapter is an attempt to highlight specific problems in the postoperative period of special relevance to vascular surgical patients, and is not intended as a complete outline of postoperative surgical care. The specific points in the postoperative management of vascular patients for various operations are mainly covered in the relevant chapters.

Vascular patients have an increased likelihood of serious cardiovascular disease and may have undergone prolonged operations, with the possibility of large blood loss. This potentially large insult on top of a poor preoperative condition can make the postoperative management of these patients particularly difficult. One study of 1361 mixed surgical patients found a 69% complication rate in the vascular patients postoperatively[1]. Complications of all grades of severity led to an increase in the duration of hospital stay. Another study of 8702 patients undergoing vascular surgery showed that patients developing complications were at an increased risk of dying and had a significantly increased length of hospital stay[2]. These figures highlight the potential benefits to the patient and savings to the hospital that would be achieved if the complication rate could be reduced. The provision of high quality postoperative care is one factor that can hopefully help to reduce the relatively high complication rate following vascular surgery.

Immediate postoperative care

The initial management of the patient in the post-anaesthetic care unit (PACU) is the same for all patients.

Airway must be kept clear and maintained until the patient is awake enough to protect and maintain it alone.

Breathing must be adequate to ensure oxygenation of the blood. In the presence of added oxygen, the minute volume needed to maintain high arterial saturation may in fact be quite low. If there is any doubt about the adequacy of ventilation, blood gases should be taken and the $Paco_2$ checked.

Circulation may be inadequate due to poor cardiac function or bleeding and hypovolaemia.

Neurological status should be assessed, and may be obtunded due to hypothermia, opiates, or neurological damage following a carotid endarterectomy. It is particularly important that neurological status be regularly assessed after a carotid endarterectomy as any sudden deterioration may indicate thrombosis of the internal carotid artery, necessitating immediate re-exploration.

Fluid status should be checked, and the peroperative intravenous fluids checked against the estimated blood loss and preoperative haemoglobin. A urinary catheter, if present, should be draining an appropriate amount of urine. A full blood count and urea and electrolytes can easily be sent at this stage to provide a baseline result for planning a postoperative fluid regimen. Measurements of central venous pressure, if a central line is *in situ*, can give a guide to fluid status.

Analgesia is important, and the postoperative analgesic regimen should be checked to see that it is correct and working (epidural or patient-controlled analgesia). The patient should be assessed before discharge to the ward to ensure that analgesia is adequate.

Monitoring in the PACU should include electrocardiograph (ECG), pulse oximetry and blood pressure, invasive or non-invasive as appropriate. Respiratory rate, urine output, pain scores and temperature should also be charted. If necessary central venous pressure may also be measured, and blood sugar checked if the patient is diabetic. Drains that have been inserted should be monitored for excessive blood loss, and the incision checked for abnormal amounts of oozing. A chest X-ray can be taken at this time to check the position of any central lines and ensure the absence of a pneumothorax.

Site of postoperative care of the vascular patient

Vascular patients can be looked after on the normal surgical wards, on a high dependency unit or on an intensive care unit.

High dependency unit

A high dependency unit (HDU) is defined as 'an area for patients who require more intensive observation, treatment and nursing care than can be provided on a general ward. It would not normally accept patients requiring mechanical ventilation, but could manage those receiving invasive monitoring'[3]. HDUs are usually used for the management of patients with single system failure (not respiratory failure), who may have been planned admissions after elective operations or who are deteriorating on the ward and needing a 'step up' in their level of care. They can also be used as a 'step down' unit from intensive care for those patients not requiring ventilation but still too ill for general ward care. It is intended that the surgical team that admitted the patient is responsible for that patient's care and management while on the HDU.

From the above definition it can be seen that many vascular postoperative patients will comfortably fit the entry criteria for HDU care, and many HDUs have a high proportion of vascular patients. One HDU reported that vascular surgical patients occupied 24% of their beds by 1994/5[4]. Many vascular patients have severe cardiac, respiratory or renal disease that may decompensate in the postoperative period, and need close monitoring of the vital signs to prevent deterioration and organ failure. Some patients would benefit from invasive arterial pressure monitoring for an extended period of time, such as carotid endarterectomy patients who are most unstable in the 12 hours postoperatively. Some HDUs do not accept arterial lines, but in theory arterial lines can be safely managed on an HDU provided the level of nursing cover is adequate (i.e. at least one nurse for every two patients) and nurses are fully trained in the management and potential complications of these lines. Patients with epidurals *in situ* need close monitoring to prevent potentially disastrous complications, and many hospitals will only allow epidural analgesia on an HDU or ICU. The higher levels of nursing care and monitoring also allow other analgesic techniques such as spinal catheters or spinal opioids, which would be unsafe on the general ward.

Provision of an HDU may have certain advantages over the alternative of having one or two 'HDU' beds on a general ward. It allows concentration of equipment and nursing expertise, avoiding unnecessary duplication of equipment and making nursing training easier. Protocols can be established, patient care can be optimized and research can be undertaken more easily.

The main problem is the lack of HDUs across the country. The Royal College of Anaesthetists recently reported a total of only 39 hospitals in the United Kingdom with designated HDUs[5]. Anaesthetists involved in the care of vascular surgical patients usually have to chose between the intensive unit or ward care for their patients postoperatively.

Intensive care units

Intensive care can be defined as 'a service for patients with potentially recoverable conditions who can benefit from more detailed observation and invasive treatment than can safely be provided on the general wards or high dependency areas'[6]. This includes patients requiring multiple organ support and mechanical ventilation. Unlike HDUs, intensive care units (ICUs) require 24-hour dedicated medical staffing and have allocated sessional consultant medical cover. All organ system failures can be supported, especially respiratory, circulatory and renal.

Many hospitals have a chronic shortage of intensive care beds, and the anaesthetist must decide preoperatively which patients can be anaesthetized without an intensive care bed being available postoperatively. This may lead to the cancellation of surgery in the high-risk patients if no intensive care bed is available. Hospitals vary in their policies; some will admit all patients to intensive care following aortic aneurysm surgery, while others will operate and send selected patients back to the ward.

Vascular patients likely to benefit from ICU care include the following:

- patients with unstable cardiac or pulmonary function postoperatively
- patients with inadequate haemostasis/ongoing bleeding
- patients with hypothermia ($< 33°C$)
- patients needing postoperative ventilation after aortic surgery

- patients with postoperative neurological complications following carotid endarterectomy
- patients with unanticipated surgical problems
- patients requiring specialized monitoring
- patients requiring significant vasoactive infusions
- patients in hospitals where HDU facilities do not exist and who need more intensive monitoring than can be provided on the ward.

Principles of postoperative care of vascular surgical patients

The mainstays of postoperative care of vascular patients include attention to oxygenation, fluid balance and analgesia.

Oxygenation

Adequate oxygenation of the blood is essential to maintain oxygen delivery to the tissues. Vascular patients often have pre-existing chest disease from cigarette smoking which is exacerbated by the drop in functional residual capacity on induction of anaesthesia. This leads to basal atelectasis with resulting V/Q abnormalities, which can persist into the postoperative period and lead to hypoxaemia. Retention of secretions (for example because of poor analgesia) can predispose to postoperative chest infections.

Hypoxaemia can be, but is not always, associated with myocardial ischaemia in the postoperative period. Although the exact relationship between the two is unknown it is important to ensure that hypoxaemia is avoided, and patients should receive oxygen, especially at night, for the first 5 days after the operation. It has been documented that hypoxaemia can occur up to at least 5 days postoperatively following abdominal vascular surgery[7]. Oxygen can be supplied via an MC mask or nasal cannula, depending on the patient's preference.

Aortic aneurysm surgery is especially likely to lead to postoperative respiratory complications. The incision is almost the full length of the abdomen up to the xiphisternum, and good postoperative analgesia is required to ensure that adequate tidal volumes are achieved. The abdomen may also be distended with an ileus, which will splint the diaphragm and further impair respiration. Approach to the aneurysm can be achieved by a transverse abdominal incision. This may have advantages in terms of postoperative respiratory function, and also makes it easier to block the afferent fibres with an epidural as far fewer dermatomes are involved.

Fluids

Provision of adequate and appropriate fluid replacement in the postoperative period is the most important factor for the maintenance of an effective cardiovascular system and functioning kidneys. This is one area where HDUs can improve patient management, with increased levels of monitoring and frequent updates of fluid delivery guided by measurement of the central venous pressure and hourly urine output. This level of care is just not possible with the levels of staffing on a general ward.

Postoperative patients can lose large volumes of fluid into the gut if an ileus is present, or from bleeding into drains or onto dressings. This relative hypovolaemia may manifest itself as a reduced urine output during the first postoperative night, and is more likely to be treated by frusemide than by extra intravenous fluid. It is not uncommon for elective aneurysm patients to be 3–4 litres in 'positive' fluid balance at the end of the first postoperative day. This is an indication of the fluid lost, and generous replacement is needed to maintain intravascular volume. Patients with poor cardiac function may have a 'rigid' cardiovascular system, and there may be only a narrow line between hypovolaemia and cardiac failure. In these patients, pulmonary artery catheters are often needed for optimal fluid replacement. Regular full blood counts and urea and electrolyte measurements can guide the details of the fluid regime for each patient, and the cardiovascular and renal function can be assessed by measuring blood pressure, heart rate and urine output. In the intensive care unit, measurement of cardiac output, pulmonary artery occlusion pressure and calculations of systemic vascular resistance can be used as a logical guide to the best fluid and/or inotropic therapy.

Analgesia

Good quality analgesia is not only humanitarian, but may benefit the patient in many other ways. A reduction in the tachycardia and hypertension associated with pain will reduce myocardial workload. Deeper breaths can be taken if not limited by pain on inspiration, and collapsed areas of lung can be re-expanded and secretions coughed up more easily. Blocking the 'stress response' to surgery with an effective epidural will reduce the surges in catecholamines and other hormones, and may reduce the cardiac workload, increased coagulability of the blood and hyperaggregability of platelets that is seen in the postoperative period when general anaesthesia is used alone[8–10]. There is some evidence of a reduced rate of re-operation for reduced tissue perfusion in patients having epidural anaesthesia for peripheral vascular surgery[11].

Epidurals are frequently employed for postoperative pain relief in the vascular patient, and the disadvantages and advantages are shown in Table 7.1. Strictly speaking, epidurals should ideally be managed on an ICU or HDU as there are potentially serious complications that can arise from their use. In practice facilities are limited, and many anaesthetists prefer to send a patient with an epidural *in situ* back to a ward where the staff have been adequately trained, rather than miss out on the advantages of epidural analgesia if no HDU/ICU bed is available. One study of epidural anaesthesia in 2000 patients on general surgical wards showed a low level of reversible complications in the postoperative patients studied. Pain relief in the vascular patients after lower limb surgery was especially good[12]. It is essential in these circumstances for the ward staff to have adequate training in the management and monitoring of epidural analgesia, and the anaesthetists must satisfy themselves of this before allowing patients to return to a ward with an epidural *in situ*. Either the anaesthetist who inserted the epidural or an anaesthetist on-call in the hospital must be available to help with advice or sorting out problems with the management of the epidural. The patient should be visited regularly and supervised by an anaesthetist until the epidural is removed.

For peripheral vascular surgery, epidural analgesia is usually continued for only 24–36 hours as these patients are rapidly mobilized. After aortic surgery, a working epidural is often advantageous for 3–5 days post-operatively. The epidural must be assessed regularly as infection at the site is possible, and an epidural abscess, although very rare, is a potentially disastrous complication which can lead to paralysis. Signs to watch for include increasing pain in the back, fever, and a reddened epidural skin site with exudation of pus from the catheter site. Magnetic resonance imaging followed by emergency decompression will be necessary if an epidural abscess occurs.

Various concentrations of local anaesthetics and mixtures of local anaesthetics with opioids are used for analgesia, and the choice is an individual one. Many hospitals will have a set regimen to make it easier for nursing, medical and pharmacy staff, and to avoid confusion. Combinations of a local anaesthetic given epidurally and an intravenous morphine patient-controlled analgesia (PCA) system can also be used.

Possible regimens include:

- epidural bupivacaine 0.1%, 6–10 ml/hr for peripheral surgery
- epidural bupivacaine 0.167%, with diamorphine 5–10 mg per 250 ml bag, 6–12 ml/hr for aortic surgery
- epidural bupivacaine 0.167%, 6–12 ml/hr, plus morphine PCA intra-venously, for aortic surgery.

Problems in the early postoperative period

Hypothermia

Anaesthetized patients at the normal theatre temperature of 20–24°C will lose heat from conduction, convection, radiation and evaporation, and as the basal metabolic rate is reduced and hypothalamic regulatory mechanisms are altered they will be at risk of cooling down peroperatively. As vascular operations can take a long time, hypothermia may result if steps are not taken to keep the patient warm. Temperatures below 35°C are significant, and can lead to problems in the postoperative period.

Problems related to hypothermia include:

- vasoconstriction and increased blood viscosity
- shivering, with resultant large increases (up to 500% rise) in oxygen consumption[13]
- association with postoperative myocardial ischaemia[14]
- impairment of coagulation and increased risk of bleeding
- decreased metabolism of drugs, causing prolonged action
- progressive depression of consciousness
- vasodilatation on rewarming, leading to hypotension if extra fluid is not given.

Steps that can be taken to avoid hypothermia include:

- warming all fluids peroperatively, especially blood
- warmed-air 'blankets' over exposed parts of the patient, e.g. 'Bair Hugger'
- use of heat and moisture exchangers in the breathing circuit
- heated mattresses to lie on during the operation
- keeping the operating theatre as warm as possible
- use of silver foil leggings and hats.

Postoperatively, a cold patient should be covered with a warmed-air blanket and given oxygen and warmed fluids. Warm-air blankets should not be used on ischaemic peripheries peroperatively, as hypothermia is protective to the ischaemic limbs. Core temperature should be measured orally, nasally, rectally or from the tympanic membrane using an infrared thermometer. Shivering can be treated with 10–20 mg of pethidine, with good results.

Bleeding

Arterial surgery is associated with an incidence of postoperative bleeding which can result in the patient returning to theatre for re-exploration. After an aortic aneurysm repair, bleeding may be suspected if:

- the abdomen is enlarging and becoming tense
- large amounts of fluid and blood are needed to maintain blood pressure
- there is a drop in haemoglobin concentration in the face of continuing transfusion
- there is excessive drainage of blood into drainage bottles.

Drains can become blocked, and no drainage does not mean that there is no bleeding. Bleeding and the consequences of bleeding following carotid endarterectomy are covered on p. 161. Most bleeding occurs in the immediate postoperative period. Bleeding occurring 7–14 days postoperatively, for example a graft that suddenly 'blows', is usually associated with infection at the site.

Ultimately, re-exploration for bleeding may be indicated. In one reported series of 654 aneurysm patients there was a 3% incidence of re-operation for bleeding, and generally re-operation rates should be less than 5–6%[15]. In this study it was more common in patients undergoing emergency repair of aortic aneurysm, operations requiring a larger blood transfusion first time around, and in patients who were hypothermic after their first operation. The vast majority of patients had a coagulopathy after the first operation and lower platelet counts than a matched case-control group. The operative findings were: multiple small bleeding points (11/17), one discrete bleeding point (4/17), and no active bleeding points (2/17). There was a significantly increased mortality rate associated with re-operation for bleeding. This emphasizes the importance of checking and normalizing the clotting status of the patient postoperatively.

Drops in platelet count are common in the postoperative period following aortic aneurysm surgery; this occurred in 91% of patients in one study[16]. The drop was found to be significantly related to the duration of the aortic cross-clamp. However, at 10 days postoperatively all patients developed thrombo-cytosis and 74% developed hyperfibrinogenaemia, both of which persisted for several weeks, and this may obviously predispose to thrombotic complications in the postoperative period.

Thrombosis

In the postoperative period there is an increase in the coagulability of the blood and in the adhesiveness and aggregability of the platelets. In vascular patients this occurs even in the face of a decrease in platelet count and with aspirin and heparin therapy[17]. Abdominal aortic surgical patients also have decreased levels of antithrombin III and protein C postoperatively, which can predispose to thrombosis[18]. Vascular surgical patients are often hyper-coagulable preoperatively as well. In a study looking at peripheral revascularization, 80 vascular surgical patients were hypercoagulable compared to 40 matched controls, using thromboelastography[10]. Another study has reported that 26% of 234 patients presenting for vascular surgery had antiphospholipid antibodies, a condition known to predispose to arterial and venous thromboses[19].

The reported incidence of postoperative deep vein thrombosis following aortic and lower limb surgery in patients given heparin prophylaxsis has been reported as 8% and 3.4% respectively, as measured by Doppler[20]. Another prospective study of 142 vascular surgical patients reported an incidence of deep venous thrombosis of 9.8%, with one patient developing a pulmonary embolism, despite heparin prophylaxsis of 5000 i.u. three times a day[21]. This is still a significant incidence in patients supposedly receiving adequate prophylaxsis.

Thrombotic thrombocytopenic purpura (TTP) is a rare condition charac-terized by encephalopathy, thrombocytopenia and haemolytic anaemia. It is probably due to platelet aggregation in the capillaries following endothelial damage and subsequent release of humoral factors. It can occur after vascular or cardiac surgery, and can be treated with exchange plasmaphoresis. If not spotted early, there is a high mortality[22].

Infection

Wound infection is a serious complication, and can lead to limb loss or death. There is an approximate incidence of 5%, and this is usually in the groin[23]. Factors associated with an increased incidence include:

- diabetes
- increasing age
- pre-existing rest pain with critically ischaemic limbs.

Frequently cultured organisms include *S. aureus* and *epidermidis*. Most units seem to use either a cepholosporin or penicillin on induction of anaesthesia as prophylaxis. Some units also include aerobic cover, and most continue the antibiotic for three doses postoperatively[24].

Other infections that can occur include respiratory tract infections, urinary tract infections, cholecystitis and intra-abdominal abscesses. Blood cultures should be taken frequently and if any organ dysfunction occurs, then sepsis should be suspected[25]. Infection in the arterial graft is a serious complication, and the incidence of this should run at less than 2%.

Myocardial infarction/ischaemia

Myocardial infarction and ischaemia are the largest causes of postoperative mortality and morbidity following vascular surgery, accounting for approximately two-thirds of all deaths. The factors involved and the characteristics of postoperative infarction and ischaemia are more fully discussed on p. 86, but in summary they are as follows.

Preoperative factors involved:

- Recent myocardial infarction
- Congestive cardiac failure
- Unstable angina
- Age
- Diabetes
- Preoperative 'silent' ischaemia
- Emergency surgery
- Aortic surgery, especially if the cross-clamp time > 70 minutes[26].

Features of perioperative myocardial infarction:

- Often painless
- Occurs on day 1–4 postoperatively
- Associated with a high mortality (50–70%).

Diagnosis of perioperative myocardial infarction may be difficult and depends on how hard it is looked for, using the following tests:

- ECG changes over consecutive days
- Raised CK–MB fraction
- A raised cardiac troponin 1 level is possibly more sensitive and specific than CK–MB[27].

Possible mechanisms postoperatively:

- Increased myocardial oxygen demand
- Decreased myocardial oxygen delivery
- Increased coagulability of the blood.

Postoperative adverse outcomes possible:

- Sudden cardiac death
- Myocardial infarction

- Serious arrhythmia
- Unstable angina
- Congestive cardiac failure.

Possible areas for improved treatment:

- ? Preoperative beta blockade
- ? Improved monitoring postoperatively with aggressive treatment of ischaemia
- ? Local anaesthesia to block the stress response to surgery.

Renal failure

Renal failure in the postoperative vascular patient is associated with a high morbidity and mortality. Following elective aortic surgery the incidence is about 1–6%, with a mortality of 40%. After emergency aortic surgery the incidence is about 10–40%, with 60–70% mortality. It can occur on its own but is also a feature of multi-organ failure, when the mortality then approaches 100%. Maintenance of an adequate intravascular volume and normal perfusion pressure of the kidneys is of utmost importance. Factors associated with an increased risk of postoperative renal failure include:

- elevated preoperative creatinine
- recent preoperative radiographic contrast media
- clamping of the aorta
- renal vein ligation during aortic surgery
- peroperative hypotension/hypovolaemia
- peroperative cardiac failure
- rhabdomyolysis.

Dopamine

The use of 'renal' dopamine (2–3 µg/kg per min) is widely used in order to support the kidneys peroperatively. This regime may slightly improve diuresis and natriuresis[28], but has not been shown to significantly alter the rate of renal failure postoperatively and is no substitute for a 'well-filled' cardiovascular system, good cardiac output and adequate blood pressure. Some studies have shown no clinical effect of low-dose dopamine after abdominal vascular surgery[29]. The inotropic and vasoconstrictor effects of dopamine can, however, help to maintain blood pressure when a thoracic epidural is in use and working. In these circumstances there is a tendency to low blood pressure with a reduced cardiac index, and the dopamine can be increased above 'renal' levels to counteract these drops in blood pressure.

Mannitol

Mannitol is often used in aortic surgery to induce a diuresis and for its role as a 'free radical scavenger', in the hope that it may reduce complications related to reperfusion injury. Once again evidence of a significant reduction in postoperative renal failure is lacking, but there is some evidence that it may reduce subclinical renal damage[30]. Mannitol does increase renal cortical blood flow.

Diuretics

Loop diuretics are sometimes given to maintain urine output peroperatively. This should only be contemplated after adequate fluid replacement has been achieved.

Atrial natriuretic peptide

Atrial natriuretic peptide is a naturally occurring peptide that is released in response to increased atrial filling pressures, resulting in vasodilatation and increased urine output. In a small study of seven patients undergoing abdominal aortic graft insertion, atrial natriuretic peptide (ANP) was found to increase urine output and sodium excretion[31]. This was in the face of reduced cardiac index and cardiac filling pressures. The clinical applications of this are not yet clear.

Renal artery occlusive disease

Atheromatous disease of the renal arteries is common in vascular patients, and is significantly associated with complications in the postoperative period[32]. One study reported a renal artery disease rate of 44.9%, with serious disease present in 15.7% of all vascular patients[33]. The presence of renal artery disease was significantly related to the severity of the peripheral vascular disease and to increased postoperative mortality. This study recommends performing renal artery angiography at the time of peripheral angiography to identify high-risk patients.

Respiratory failure

Respiratory failure after vascular surgery (especially abdominal vascular surgery) is relatively common, and leads to an increase in mortality and large increases in length of hospital stay. Mortality was 28.9% in one study of patients with cardiac and pulmonary complications, 11% if cardiac or pulmonary complications occurred alone, and 3.7% in those patients with no complications[2]. Respiratory complications caused a greater increase in length of hospital stay than cardiac complications, presumably related to a prolonged 'weaning' period on the intensive care unit. Factors associated with a period of postoperative ventilation include[34,35]:

- long history of cigarette smoking
- lower preoperative Pao$_2$
- large intraoperative blood loss
- congestive cardiac failure.

Not all studies have identified a low preoperative FEV$_1$ as a predictive factor for the development of postoperative respiratory failure[34] although others have found it to be so[36], especially if it drops below 2.0 litres.

Compartment syndrome

Ischaemia of the limbs can cause rhabdomyolysis, resulting in locally increased capillary permeability, fluid accumulation and swelling of the tissue. When blood supply is restored a reperfusion injury can occur due to complement activation and production of oxygen-derived free radicals, which increases the damage. In muscle compartments with stiff fascial boundaries, such as the leg, resulting oedema will increase the pressure in the compartment to levels that will occlude capillaries and arterioles and lead to widespread muscle death and release of cell contents. High plasma levels of creatine kinase will be present (more than five times the normal level) and myoglobinaemia can cause acute tubular necrosis and renal failure if the urine is acidic. Patients with long duration arterial occlusion of the limbs are especially likely to develop this complication. In an appropriate patient the diagnosis is based on finding high pressures in the various compartments of the leg, which can be measured with a needle attached to an invasive pressure monitoring line, and by finding urine positive for haeme but not red blood cells. The limb affected is classically very painful, especially to passive stretching, and the urine is often dark and of low volume. Peripheral pulses can still be present, as the pressure in the compartment may not exceed arterial pressure but can still occlude capillaries. Treatment is based on reducing pressure in the compartments by performing fasciotomies if appropriate, and avoiding renal failure due to the myoglobin. The standard method employed is to induce a diuresis (of 300 ml of urine per hour) with a urinary pH >6.5, because the myoglobin forms haematin when the pH is <5.6 and it is this that is nephrotoxic. This is achieved by infusing large volumes of crystalloid together with sodium bicarbonate to alkalinize the urine, and mannitol to induce a diuresis. Careful monitoring of central venous pressures or pulmonary artery pressures should be performed because of the risk of fluid overload and pulmonary oedema, and this treatment should be carried out on an intensive care unit[37].

Nutrition

Adequate nutrition is important in the postoperative period. Malnutrition is common in hospital patients, and supplementary nutrition has been found to improve wound healing in patients undergoing below-knee amputations[38]. In this study 90% of patients were classed as malnourished preoperatively, and supplementary nutrition given postoperatively improved healing (but not overall mortality).

Nutrition should be provided entrally at the earliest opportunity, and there is a move to early feeding (2–3 days) after aortic surgery. Entral feeding is associated with less serious complications than parentral feeds and increases gut blood flow. If not tolerating entral feeds, intravenous feeding should be considered after about 1 week.

Gastrointestinal complications

Gastrointestinal complications related to vascular surgery usually occur after abdominal aortic aneurysm surgery. They are relatively rare, but carry an overall mortality of 40–50%. This is greatly increased if the following complications occur after emergency aortic surgery[39]:

- wound dehiscence
- small bowel obstruction
- perforated duodenal ulcer/diverticulitis.

Ischaemic colitis[40] is most common after aortic surgery, and presents with left-sided abdominal pain and diarrhoea. Septic shock and a metabolic acidosis will result if this condition is not spotted and emergency laparotomy performed. It is associated with a high mortality, and occurs more commonly in patients with:

- preoperative shock
- large intraoperative blood loss.

It is diagnosed clinically, by colonoscopy or at laparotomy.

Neurological complications

Complications following carotid artery surgery are covered on pp. 159. Neurological complications following vascular surgery may be related to the effect of low blood pressure in a patient with critical carotid stenosis, and this can result in stroke, either in the immediate postoperative period or up to 72 hours later. The incidence is low, at less than 1%[35,41].

Spinal cord ischaemia is possible in operations involving cross-clamping of the aorta. The blood flow to the anterior spinal cord is precarious, depending to a large extent on the artery of Adamkiewicz, usually arising from the left intercostal artery at T9 (although it can arise from T8–L2). The incidence of spinal cord damage following elective abdominal aortic surgery is approximately 0.2%[42]. Death or severe disability is a likely outcome[43]. Neurological testing should be carried out in the early postoperative period following aortic cross-clamping to identify this complication.

Postoperative delirium is also common postoperatively, and in one study[44] was related to:

- age over 70 years
- alcohol abuse
- poor cognitive status
- markedly abnormal preoperative glucose, sodium or potassium
- aortic aneurysm surgery.

In this study, postoperative delirium led to longer hospital stays and a greater incidence of complications.

Aortic aneurysm surgery

Aortic aneurysm surgery, with the need for a large incision, aortic cross-clamping and the potential for large fluid shifts, imposes a larger physiological insult to the body than most types of surgery. As it is also usually performed in an elderly population, there is no surprise that there is a relatively large morbidity and mortality[45].

Elective

Elective aortic aneurysm surgery should be performed with an overall mortality of less than 5–7%[46]. The main cause of mortality is cardiac-related, but it also occurs from respiratory failure and renal failure, often occurring together as part of a multi-organ failure following sepsis. Renal failure is also more likely if the left renal vein needs to be tied off during aneurysm repair[47]. Other more rare complications include:

- ischaemic colitis
- acute graft occlusion
- peripheral embolism.

Emergency

Patients presenting for emergency aortic aneurysm repair have a much higher mortality than elective patients (45–60% in most series)[46]. This has seemingly changed little in the past 40 years[48]. The overall mortality for ruptured aortic aneurysm is > 70%, as many patients do not survive to reach hospital. Pre- and peroperatively, the following have all been linked to early mortality[49,50]:

- cardiac arrest
- acidosis
- loss of consciousnes
- age > 80 years
- transfusion > 15 units
- hypotension despite fluids
- admission haematocrit < 25
- female gender.

The postoperative complication profile is similar to that occurring after elective surgery, but all complications occur more commonly, and prolonged respiratory support is more likely. Cardiac, respiratory and renal failure remain the major causes of death, often occurring together as part of a multi-organ failure syndrome.

Varicose vein surgery

Serious complications following varicose vein surgery are rare. One of the most common is hypovolaemia, especially in a patient undergoing bilateral surgery, when the amount of blood lost can go unappreciated. If adequate fluid replacement has not been provided the patient may become hypotensive, and feel faint when trying to get up later.

Other complications include:

- cutaneous nerve lesions due to the multiple avulsions, especially of the lateral popliteal nerve as it winds around the neck of the fibula
- lesions of the saphenous nerve from below-knee stripping
- haematomas
- femoral vein lesions
- femoral artery lesions (very rare, but could lead to limb loss).

Endoluminal aortic stent grafts

In general, the results from aortic stent grafts compare well with results from 'open' operations. In one group of 100 patients, factors associated with increased mortality included multi-organ failure, renal failure, anaemia <8 g/dl and length of surgery >4 hours[51]. Another study of 30 patients reported a successful procedure in 93% of cases, and two deaths[52]. The long-term results of this therapy are still to be discovered.

Audit and quality of care

Most hospitals have their own databases of surgical practice and results, and hold regular audit and morbidity and mortality meetings. The overall goal of these systems is to identify problems that are occurring in the delivery of high quality surgical care. These areas can then be targeted for improvement and changes implemented, and hopefully this will lead to an improvement in outcome. Scoring systems can be used to provide data to enable the comparison of different units.

Possum

In 1991, the **P**hysiological and **O**perative **S**everity **S**core for the en**U**meration of **M**ortality and morbidity was described[53]. This was an attempt to provide a simple scoring system for surgical patients for use in audit. The system identifies 12 physiological variables that at the time of surgery have significant impact on the risk of morbidity and mortality for that patient (Tables 9.1 and 9.2). The surgical procedure being performed also has an impact on outcome, and so an operative severity score was produced. Each of these categories was assigned a score, increasing exponentially with the degree of abnormality. Morbidity and mortality can be predicted with a high degree of accuracy using logistic regression analysis and the physiological and operative severity scores. The advantage over the APACHE scoring system is that 24 hours of observation are not needed, and morbidity as well as mortality is predicted.

Since its introduction it has been shown to accurately reflect morbidity and mortality in vascular, general and colorectal surgery. There is, however, a

Table 9.1 Possum physiological score

Physiological variable	Score			
	1	*2*	*4*	*8*
Age (years)	<60	61–70	>70	
Cardiac signs	No failure	Diuretic, digoxin, antianginal or hypertensive therapy	Peripheral oedema, warfarin therapy	Raised jugular venous pressure
Chest X-ray			Borderline cardiomegaly	Cardiomegaly
Respiratory history	No dyspnoea	Dyspnoea on exertion	Limiting dyspnoea (one flight)	Dyspnoea at rest, rate > 30 per min
Chest X-ray		Mild COAD	Moderate COAD	Fibrosis or consolidation
Blood pressure systolic (mmHg)	110–130	131–170 100–109	>171 90–99	<89
Pulse (bpm)	50–80	81–100 40–49	101–120	>121 <39
Glasgow coma score	15	12–14	9–11	<8
Haemoglobin (g/100/ml)	13–16	11.5–12.9 16.1–17	10–11.4 17.1–18	<9.9 >18.1
White cell count ($\times 10^{12}$/l)	4–10	10.1–20 3.1–4	>20.1 <3	
Urea (mmol/l)	<7.5	7.6–10	10.1–15	>15.1
Sodium (mmol/l)	>136	131–135	126–130	<125
Potassium (mmol/l)	3.5–5	3.2–3.4 5.1–5.3	2.9–3.1 5.4–5.9	<2.8 >6
Electrocardiogram	Normal		Atrial fibrillation	Any other abnormal rhythm or >5 ectopics per min, Q waves or ST/T wave changes

Table 9.2 Operative severity score

	Score			
	1	2	4	8
Operative severity	Minor	Moderate	Major	Major +
Multiple procedures	1	2	More than 2	
Total blood loss (ml)	Less than 100 ml	101–500	501–999	>1000
Peritoneal soiling	None	Minor (serous fluid)	Local pus	Free bowel content, pus or blood
Presence of malignancy	None	Primary only	Nodal metastases	Distant metastases
Mode of surgery	Elective		Emergency resuscitation of more than 2 h possible Operation <24 h after admission	Emergency (immediate surgery needed)

tendency to overpredict morbidity and mortality in a fit patient undergoing minor surgery[54].

There is still a need to standardize reporting with specific reference to vascular surgery. In his presidential address to the International Society for Cardiovascular Surgery in 1996, Robert Rutherford outlined the problems and proposed some solutions[55]. He emphasized the need to report outcomes in a standard fashion, but also that reports must include all the relevant data that is known to affect the outcome. Overall this means that:

- all patient factors involved in the case mix must be collected
- a scoring classification for varying severity of vascular disease should be developed
- a procedural severity score that is operation specific is needed
- all complications should be classified
- outcome measures should be standardized.

This is no easy task, but if meaningful comparisons are to be made between different treatments and different institutions this problem has to be addressed. The cost of these treatments also has to be incorporated if cost-effective high-quality patient care is to be delivered.

Further reading

Hambly PR, Sainsbury MC. *Perioperative Management for House Surgeons*. Bios Scientific, 1996.

References

1. Ardvidsson S, Ouchterlony J, Nilsson S *et al*. The Gothenburg study of perioperative risk. 1. Preoperative findings, postoperative complications. *Acta Anaesthesiol Scand* 1994; **38**: 679–90.
2. Kazmers A, Jacobs L, Perkins A. The impact of complications after vascular surgery in Veterans Affairs Medical Centres. *J Surg Res* 1997; **67**: 62–6.
3. Association of Anaesthetists of Great Britain and Ireland. Post-anaesthetic recovery facilities. *Recommendations of a Working Party* (Chairman Marks RL). Association of Anaesthetists of Great Britain and Ireland, 1991.
4. Coggins R, de Cossart L. Improving postoperative care: the role of the surgeon in the high dependency unit. *Ann R Coll Surg Engl* 1996; **78**: 163–7.
5. The Royal College of Anaesthetists. *National ITU Audit*. London: Royal College of Anaesthetists, 1992/1993.
6. NHS Executive. *Report of the Working Group on Guidelines on Admission to and Discharge from Intensive Care and High Dependency Units*. Department of Health, 1996.
7. Reeder MK, Goldman MD, Loh L, Muir AD, Foex P, *et al*. Postoperative hypoxaemia after major abdominal vascular surgery. *Br J Anaesth* 1992; **68**: 23–6.
8. Naesh O, Haljamae H, Hindberg I *et al*. Epidural anaesthesia prolonged into the postoperative period prevents stress response and platelet hyperaggregability after peripheral vascular surgery. *Eur J Vasc Surg* 1994; **8**: 395–400.

9. Parker SD, Breslow MJ, Frank SM *et al.* Perioperative Ischemia Randomized Anesthesia Trial Study Group. Catecholamine and cortisol responses to lower extremity revascularization: correlation with outcome variables. *Crit Care Med* 1995; **23**: 1954–61.

10. Tuman KJ, McCarthy RJ, March RJ *et al.* Effects of epidural anaesthesia and analgesia on coagulation and outcome after major vascular surgery. *Anesth Analg* 1991; **73**: 696–704.

11. Christopherson R, Beattie C, Frank SM *et al.* Perioperative Ischemia Randomized Anesthesia Trial Study Group. Perioperative morbidity in patients randomized to epidural or general anaesthesia for lower extremity vascular surgery. *Anesthesiology* 1993; **79**: 422–34.

12. Rygnestad T, Borchgrevink PC, Eide E. Postoperative infusion of morphine and bupivacaine is safe on surgical wards. Organization of the treatment, effects and side effects in 2000 consecutive patients. *Acta Anaesthesiol Scand* 1997; **41**: 868–76.

13. Bay J, Nunn JF, Prys-Roberts C. Factors influencing arterial P_{O_2} during recovery from anaesthesia. *Br J Anaesth* 1968; **40**: 398–407.

14. Frank SM, Beattie C, Christopherson R *et al.* The Perioperative Ischemia Randomized Anesthesia Trial Study Group. Unintentional hypothermia is associated with postoperative myocardial ischemia. *Anesthesiology* 1993; **78**: 468–76.

15. Milne AA, Murphy WG, Bradbury AW *et al.* Postoperative haemorrhage following aortic aneurysm repair. *Eur J Vasc Surg* 1994; **8**: 622–6.

16. Bradbury A, Adam D, Garrioch M *et al.* Changes in platelet count, coagulation and fibrinogen associated with elective repair of asymptomatic abdominal aortic aneurysm and aortic reconstruction for occlusive disease. *Eur J Vasc Endovasc Surg* 1997; **13**: 375–80.

17. Reininger CB, Reininger AJ, Steckmeier B *et al.* Increased pre- and postoperative thrombocyte activity in vascular surgery patients (German). *Vasa* 1994; **23**: 217–27.

18. Gibbs NM, Crawford GP, Michalopoulos N. A comparison of postoperative thrombotic potential following abdominal aortic surgery, carotid endarterectomy, and femoropopliteal bypass. *Anaesth Intensive Care* 1996; **23**: 11–14.

19. Taylor LM Jr, Chitwood RW, Dalman RL *et al.* Antiphospholipid antibodies in vascular surgery patients. A cross-sectional study. *Ann Surg* 1994; **220**: 544–50.

20. Farkas JC, Chapuis C, Combe S *et al.* A randomized controlled trials of a low molecular-weight heparin (enoxaprin) to prevent deep vein thrombosis in patients undergoing vascular surgery. *Eur J Vasc Surg* 1993; **7**: 554–60.

21. Fletcher JP, Batiste P. Incidence of deep vein thrombosis following vascular surgery. *Int Angiol* 1997; **16**: 65–8.

22. Chang JC, Shipstone A, Llenado-Lee MA. Postoperative thrombotic thrombocytopenic purpura following cardiovascular surgeries. *Am J Hematol* 1996; **53**: 11–17.

23. van Himbeeck FJ, van Knippenberg LA, Niessen MC *et al.* Wound infection after arterial surgical procedures. *Eur J Vasc Surg* 1992; **6**: 494–8.

24. Winslet MC, Obeid ML. A national audit of antimicrobial prophylaxsis in vascular surgery. *Eur J Vasc Surg* 1993; **7**: 638–41.

25. Parsson H, Swartbol P, Andersson R *et al.* The role of septic complications in aortic aneurysm surgery. *Int Angiol* 1994; **13**: 129–32.

26. Johnston KW, Scobie TK. Multicenter prospective study of nonruptured abdominal aortic aneurysms. I. Population and operative management. *J Vasc Surg* 1988; **7**: 69–81.

27. Adams JE III, Sicard GA, Allen BT *et al.* Diagnosis of perioperative myocardial infarction with measurement of cardiac troponin 1. *New Engl J Med* 1994; **330**: 670–4.

28. de Lasson L, Hansen HE, Juhl B *et al.* A randomized clinical study of the effects of low-dose dopamine on central and renal haemodynamics in infrarenal aortic surgery. *Eur J Vasc Endovasc Surg* 1995; **10**: 82–90.

29. Baldwin L, Henderson A, Hickman P. Effect of postoperative low-dose dopamine on renal function after elective major vascular surgery. *Ann Intern Med* 1994; **120**: 744–7.

30. Nicholson ML, Baker DM, Hopkinson BR *et al.* Randomized controlled trial on the effect of mannitol on the reperfusion injury during aortic aneurysm surgery. *Br J Surg* 1996; **83**:

1230–3.
31. Bergman A, Odar-Cederlof I, Theodorsson E *et al*. Renal effects of atrial natriuretic peptide in patients after major vascular surgery. *Acta Anaesthesiol Scand* 1994; **38**: 667–71.
32. Martin LF, Atnip RG, Holmes PA *et al*. Prediction of postoperative complications after elective aortic surgery using stepwise logistic regression analysis. *Am Surg* 1994; **60**: 163–8.
33. Missouris CG, Buckenham T, Cappuccio FP *et al*. Renal artery stenosis: a common and important problem in patients with peripheral vascular disease. *Am J Med* 1994; **96**: 10–14.
34. Jayr C, Matthay MA, Goldstone J *et al*. Preoperative and intraoperative factors associated with prolonged mechanical ventilation. A study in patients following major abdominal vascular surgery. *Chest* 1993; **103**: 1231–6.
35. Johnston KW. Multicenter prospective study of nonruptured abdominal aortic aneurysm. Part II. Variables predicting morbidity and mortality. *J Vasc Surg* 1989; **9**: 437–47.
36. Kispert JF, Kazmers A, Roitman L. Preoperative spirometry predicts perioperative pulmonary complications after major vascular surgery. *Am Surg* 1992; **58**: 491–5.
37. Ferreira TA, Pensado A, Dominguez L *et al*. Compartment syndrome with severe rhabdomyolysis in the postoperative period following major vascular surgery. *Anaesthesia* 1996; **51**: 692–4.
38. Eneroth M, Apelqvist J, Larsson J *et al*. Improved wound healing in trans-tibial amputees receiving supplementary nutrition. *Int Orthop*1997; **21**: 108–4.
39. Franko E, Cohen JR. General surgical problems requiring operation in postoperative vascular patients. *Am J Surg* 1991; **162**: 247–50.
40. Piotrowski JJ, Ripepi AJ, Yuhas JP *et al*. Colonic ischemia: the Achilles heel of ruptured aortic aneurysm repair. *Am Surg* 1996; **62**: 557–60.
41. Harris EJ Jr, Moneta GL, Yeager RA *et al*. Neurologic deficits following noncarotid vascular surgery. *Am J Surg* 1992; **163**: 537–40.
42. Szilagyi DE, Hageman JH, Smith RF *et al*. Spinal cord damage in surgery of the abdominal aorta. *Surgery* 1978; **83**: 38–56.
43. Dimakakos P, Arapoglou B, Katsenis K *et al*. Ischemia of the spinal cord following elective operative procedures of the infrarenal abdominal aorta. *J Cardiovasc Surg* 1996; **37**: 243–247.
44. Marcantonio ER, Goldman L, Mangione CM *et al*. A clinical prediction rule for delirium after elective non-cardiac surgery. *JAMA* 1994; **271**: 134–9.
45. Sayers RD, Thompson MM, Nasim A *et al*. Surgical management of 671 abdominal aortic aneurysms: a 13 year review from a single centre. *Eur J Vasc Endovasc Surg* 1997; **13**: 322–7.
46. Kazmers A, Jacobs L, Perkins A *et al*. Abdominal aortic aneurysm repair in Veteran Affairs medical centers. *J Vasc Surg* 1996; **23**: 191–200.
47. AbuRahma AF, Robinson PA, Boland JP *et al*. Elective resection of 332 abdominal aortic aneurysms in a southern West Virginia community during a recent five-year period. *Surgery* 1991; **109**: 244–51.
48. Chen JC, Hilderbrand HD, Salvian AJ *et al*. Progress in abdominal aortic aneurysm surgery: four decades of experience at a teaching centre. *Cardiovasc Surg* 1997; **5**: 150–6.
49. Harris LM, Faggioli GL, Fiedler R *et al*. Ruptured abdominal aortic aneurysms: factors affecting mortality rate. *J Vasc Surg* 1991; **14**: 812–8.
50. Johansen K, Kohler TR, Nicholls SC *et al*. Ruptured abdominal aortic aneurysm: the Harborview experience. *J Vasc Surg* 1991; **13**: 240–5.
51. Baker AB, Lloyd G, Fraser TA *et al*. Retrospective review of 100 cases of endoluminal aortic stent-graft surgery from an anaesthetic perspective. *Anaesth Intensive Care* 1997; **25**: 378–84.
52. Kretschmer G, Holzenbein T, Lammer J *et al*. The first 15 months of transluminal abdominal aortic aneurysm management: a single centre experience. *Eur J Vasc Endovasc Surg* 1997; **14**: 24–32.

53. Copeland GP, Jones D, Walters M. POSSUM: a scoring system for surgical audit. *Br J Surg* 1991; **78**: 356–60.
54. Wijesinghe LD, Mahmood T, Scott DJA *et al*. Comparison of POSSUM and the Portsmouth predictor equation for predicting death following vascular surgery. *Br J Surg* 1998; **85**: 209–12.
55. Rutherford RB. Presidential address: Vascular surgery–Comparing outcomes. *J Vasc Surg* 1996; **23**: 5–17.

Index

Essentials of Cardiac and Thoracic Anaesthesia

John W. W. Gothard FRCA
Consultant Cardiothoracic Anaesthetist, Royal Brompton National Heart and Lung Hospital, London UK

Andrea Kelleher FRCA
Consultant Anaesthetist, Royal Brompton National Heart and Lung Hospital, London, UK.

* A succinct, practical guide incorporating both cardiac and thoracic anaesthesia in one book
* A guide for the trainee with little previous experience of cardio-thoracic anaesthesia
* Written in a didactic style with all the essential information clearly presented
* Covers pre-operative assessment, intra-operative care and post-operative management and special procedures

CONTENTS:
Pre-operative assessment: cardiac surgery; Anaesthesia: cardiac surgery; Anaesthesia for specific cardiac and allied operations; Cardiopulmonary bypass; The early postoperative management of patients undergoing cardiac surgery; Pre-operative assessment of the thoracic surgical patient; Anaesthesia: thoracic surgery; Intra-operative management of specific thoracic procedures; Post-operative management - thoracic surgery.

1998   224pp   22 line illustrations   234 x 156 mm
Paperback   0 7506 2033 1   £22.50

Anaesthesia A-Z
An Encyclopaedia of Principles and Practice

S. Yentis BSc MB BS MD FRCA
Consultant Anaesthetist, Chelsea and Westminster Hospital, London, UK

G. Smith BM FRCA
Consultant Anaesthetist and Director of Intensive Care Services, Portsmouth Hospital, Portsmouth, UK

N.P. Hirsch MB BS FRCA
Consultant Anaesthetist and Honorary Senior Lecturer, The National Hospital for Neurology and Neurosurgery, Queen Square, London, UK

Now available in revised paperback format, this is an encyclopaedic source of information on all aspects of anaesthesia and pain control in a concise, alphabetical format. It has over 1800 entries and over 500 x-references. It is aimed primarily at anaesthetic trainees and their lecturers as a reliable, up-to-date source of information.

Reviews:
'..a huge amount of easily accessible and readable factual information on all aspects of anaesthesia in a single volume.' *Anaesthesia*

'The information presented is up-to-date, practical and clinically relevant... anaesthetists in general and examination candidates in particular may find [it] valuable as a spot check for current knowledge'. *British Medical Journal*

'I can recommend this book to all libraries and to those candidates who want to be able to converse on equal terms with even the most peverse of examiners'. *British Journal of Anaesthesia*

CONTENTS:
2,000 entries from Alveolar-arterial Oxygen Difference to Zidovudine

1995   480pp   150 line illustrations   270 x 202 mm
Paperback   0 7506 2285 7   £40.00

FRCA Survival Guide

S. Yentis BSc MB BS MD FRCA
Consultant Anaesthetist, Chelsea and Westminster Hospital, London, UK

This book is aimed at all trainees preparing for the Primary or Final FRCA professional examination.

Written in a light hearted style, this useful guide will put the examination candidate at ease, and help them to make the best use of their time in preparation and revision for the FRCA examinations. The scope of this book includes all aspects of the examination - what it is, what it consists of, how to revise and sit each part and how it is marked.

*   A guide to examination preparation for the FRCA candidate
*   Written in a conversational, user friendly style
*   Will help the busy trainee cope with the added pressure of revision and exam practice
*   Covers all aspects of preparation for both the primary and final examinations
*   Concentrates on revision technique rather than specific question content

CONTENTS:
Introduction; Revision; Multiple Choice Questions (MCQs); Essays; Short Answer Questions (SAQs); Vivas; Objective Structure Clinical Examinations (OSCEs); Sitting the Exams; After it's All Over; Appendix, Index.

1998   128pp   14 line illustrations   216 x 138 mm
Paperback   0 7506 3718 8   £14.99

FRCA: Passing the Primary Examination

H. Williams MBBS
Registrar in Anaesthesia, Department of Anaesthesia, North Hampshire Hospital, Basingstoke, Hants, UK

M. Hasan MBChB FRCA
Consultant Anaesthetist, Northwick Park Hospital, Harrow, Middx, UK.

M. Brunner MBBS FRCA
Consultant Aneasthetist, Northwick Park Hospital, Harrow, Middx, UK

P.N. Robinson MBChB FRCA
Consultant Anaesthetist, Northwick Park Hospital, Harrow, Middx, UK.

This book is a concise companion text for candidates preparing to sit the primary FRCA examination, combining the syllabus of the examination with over 200 examples of examination standard MCQs, vivas and OSCEs.

- Syllabus explained and discussed in an accessible manner
- Precise guidance on OSCEs and vivas
- Examples of MCQs with answers set at examination standard
- Complements information found in standard textbooks

CONTENTS:
Introduction; The exam; The syllabus; The MCQs; The viva section; The OSCE's.

1996   192pp   11 line illustrations   216 x 138 mm
Paperback   0 7506 3108 2   £15.99

MCQs and OSCEs for the Primary FRCA

E. I. Doyle FRCA
Consultant Anaesthetist, Royal Hospital For Sick Children, Edinburgh, UK

P. Goggin MB BS FANZCA
Consultant Anaesthetist, Royal Infirmary of Edinburgh, Edinburgh, UK.

This book is a concise companion text for candidates preparing to sit the primary FRCA examination and is made up of over 300 examples of standard MCQs and OSCEs. .

- Comprehensive mix of questions reflects those of the actual MCQ paper
- Questions cover pharmacology, physiology, biochemistry, clinical anaesthesia, physics, clinical measurement and statistics
- Offers guidance in identifying gaps in the candidates knowledge on major topics
- Ilustrations included in section on OSCEs

These questions have been designed to test the candidate's knowledge on a wide range of topics and to act as a prompt for further reading. The multiple choice papers offer considerable guidance for candidates using the MCQs as part of a study plan. The answers section gives brief explanations and, where appropriate, references for the topic.

CONTENTS: Introduction; How to sit a Multiple Choice Question Examination; Exam No 1: Questions and Answers; Exam No 2: Questions and Answers; Exam No 3: Questions and Answers; Exam No 4: Questions and Answers; Exam No 5: Questions and Answers; OSCEs: Questions and Answers, Index.

1997   155pp   3 black & white photographs   216 x 138 mm
Paperback   0 7506 2338 1   £15.99

Books can be ordered from your usual bookseller, or direct from the publisher using one of these four easy services:

BY PHONE: Please call Heinemann Customer Services on 01865 314627, please have your credit card details ready

BY E-MAIL: Send orders to bhuk.orders@repp.co.uk

BY FAX: Heinemann Customer Services on 01865 314091

BY MAIL: Heinemann Customer Services, Halley Court, Jordan Hill, Oxford OX2 8DP

All details correct at time of going to press, but may alter without prior notice.

Butterworth-Heinemann, A division of Reed Educational and Professional Publishing Ltd, Linacre House, Jordan Hill, Oxford, OX2 8DP, UK.